Women's Hats of the Twentieth Century

for Designers and Collectors

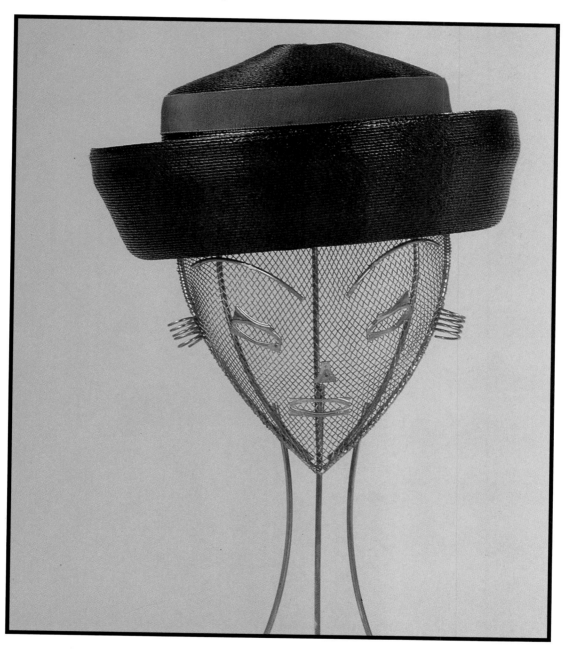

Maureen E. Lynn Reilly
and Mary Beth Detrich

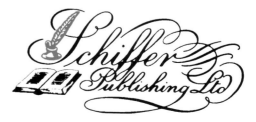

4880 Lower Valley Road
Atglen, PA 19310 USA

Dedicated to the Memory of my Mother, Evelyn Lynn Reilly,
a Former Model and Perennial Flower of Fashion.
Maureen E. Lynn Reilly

Thank you to my parents, Deane and Phyllis Kennedy,
for your abiding love and support.
Mary Beth Detrich

Printed in Hong Kong

ISBN: 0-7643-0204-3

Cover design and book layout by Michael William Potts
Photography by John Klycinski
Photo Styling by Mary Beth Detrich
    and Maureen Reilly

Cover Photograph:
Silver bugle beads waterfall from a white felt cap. Label: Jack McConnell. *Courtesy of: Banbury Cross Antiques.* Value: $200-300.

Library of Congress Cataloging-in-Publication Data

Reilly, Maureen.
    Woman's hats of the twentieth century: for designers and collectors/ Maureen Reilly and Mary Beth Detrich.
        p.   cm.
    Includes bibliographical references and index.
    ISBN 0-7643-0204-3 (hardcover)
    1. Hats- -History- -20th century. 2. Hats- -Collectors and collecting. I. Detrich, Mary Beth. II. Title.
GT2110.R43   1997
391.4'3- -dc21   96-37119
                                                                 CIP

Published by Schiffer Publishing, Ltd.
4880 Lower Valley Road
Atglen, PA 19310
Phone: (610) 593-1777   Fax: (610) 593-2002
E-mail: Schifferbk@aol.com

Please write for a free catalog.
This book may be purchased from the publisher.
Please include $2.95 for shipping.
Try your bookstore first.

We are interested in hearing from authors
with book ideas on related subjects.

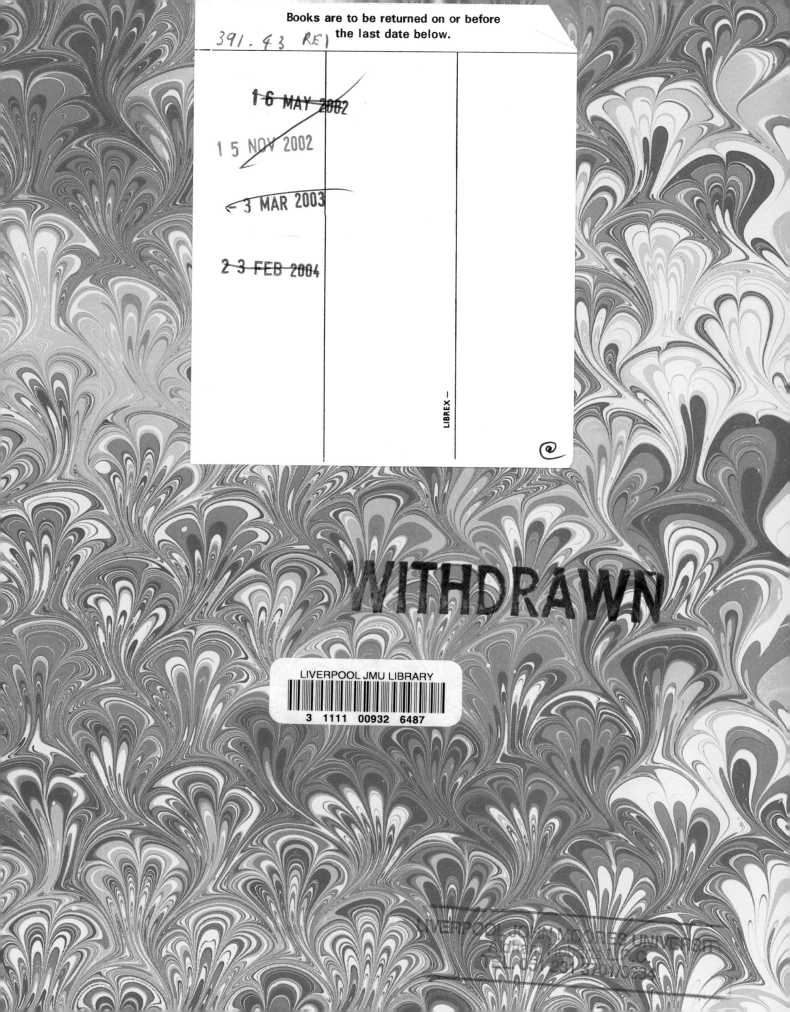

Table Of Contents

Preface

We began this project as a team just a little over a year ago, based on a chance conversation about our mutual love of hats. What woman does not feel a certain thrill when she primps before a mirror in a fabulous hat? For each of us, having had access to a wide variety of wonderful designs, we agreed that the experience is almost like assuming a new persona. One minute, you can play the demure country lass. The next, you are the ultimate sophisticate prepared for a round of socializing. With but another "tip of the hat," you can be transported back in time to the days of the covered wagon or the Civil War.

With encouragement from Nancy Schiffer, we began researching the lore and lure of hats through books on costume history, vintage fashion magazines, and conversations with like-minded enthusiasts. At the same time, we assembled favorites from our own hat inventories, and borrowed from others.

All told, this book has been a joy to assemble, but the photography was particularly satisfying. Working with a team of professional photographers, we catalogued and styled these fabulous hats. Each hat seemed to tell its own story, and we tried to capture its mood in both image and caption. And so we begin...

Acknowledgments

We gratefully acknowledge the assistance of the many vintage clothing experts who loaned their valuable collections and gave advice on dating. Particular thanks go to Barbara Griggs, Lafayette; Sharon Hagerty, San Francisco; and Doris Raymond, San Francisco.

Special mention must be made of the Mary Aaron Museum in Marysville, California. Under the guidance of curator Karen Burrows, this little gem of a museum has contributed greatly to the vintage clothing experience in Northern California. Also, the Art Deco Society of California and its director

Paula Forselles, sponsor of the delightful Millinery Tea and other vintage clothing events.

Our book would not be the same without having the professional photography of John Klycinski and Walter Kennedy. They worked many long hours with us in a studio setting, and we think their skill is obvious in the fine quality of the photos throughout our book.

On a personal level, Maureen Reilly wishes to thank her husband, Royce Saunders; and her children, John and Jamie Saunders, for their patience and perseverance.

How to Read the Captions

Each caption gives a value range for the hats and accessories pictured, based largely on West Coast prices. Assume that all merchandise is in mint condition, unless otherwise noted. Presume they are sold through an antique store or vintage clothing venue (shop or show). If no label is indicated, then the hat had none. For more information on labels, and a special chance to Meet the Models, see Chapter III. For more information on pricing, see Chapter XIV.

I. Introduction

These days, it would seem, we live in a virtually hatless society. Fortunately for collectors, it wasn't always so. Hats, whether worn or enjoyed as a form of functional sculpture, are a joy to own and display.

Headgear, perhaps more than any other clothing accessory, has played an important role in defining cultural values and social status throughout history. In this book, we will trace the evolution of hat design from the mid-Victorian era in 1865 to its near-demise due to the "cultural revolution," circa 1965. We will also focus on the influence of international couture on hats in the 20th century, for readers who wish to develop this aspect of their collections.

What styles can you expect to find in this book? We have included some marvelous examples of bonnets from the days of Queen Victoria, although they are becoming extremely high-priced and hard to locate. For this reason, a major portion of the illustrations are devoted to hats worn by women during the middle decades of the 20th century, of a type that are still affordable and plentiful today. Apart from the couture, you should be able to start a collection of hats from those periods for a modest outlay of money.

In the following chapters, we discuss principles of hatmaking to assist you in dating various styles. Also, we offer tips on dating hats in selected photo captions throughout the book, and address the perennial problem of storage, providing suggestions for displaying and refurbishing. In conclusion, we give advice on how to "start up" or give your existing collection the "finish" of a specialty focus.

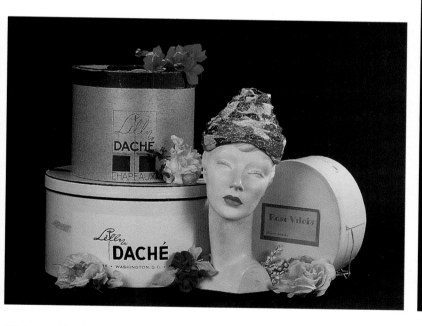

While searching for hats, keep your eyes open for vintage hatboxes. Label (hat): Miss Sally Victor. *Courtesy of (all): Banbury Cross Antiques.* Value (hat): $45-65. Value (box, each): $35-45.

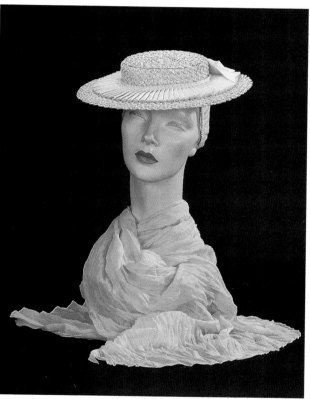

This straw boater from the 1940s has the crisp, clean lines of sculpture. *Courtesy of: Banbury Cross Antiques.* Value: $25-45.

This is an emerging area of collectibles, and prices are still unstable. As with any other fashion accessory, expect to pay more for earlier hats or those that bear a designer label. Condition, quality, and even whimsy may all factor into the sales tag. In any event, given the wide variation that we have seen in every market, we can only offer a price range for each era. Bear in mind that prices will be at the top end of the range in metropolitan areas.

Perhaps R. Turner Wilcox put it best, in his definitive survey of hats in history:

> *"No part of costume is so universally important as the headdress, which is worn even when body garments are dispensed with..."*

We may have dispensed with wearing hats for the present era, but it remains that no costume is complete without one. For those who love fashion, drama and dress-up:

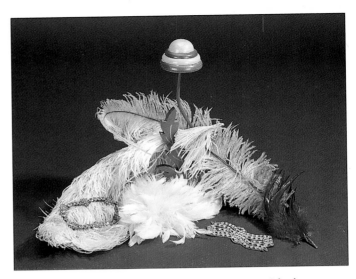

Any collector would covet this assortment of vintage ostrich plumes, beautifully curled and dyed. They can be used for restoration, or as part of a display. *Courtesy of (all): Banbury Cross Antiques.* Value (plumes, each): $35-55. Value (stand): $45-65.

Welcome to the world of hat collecting!

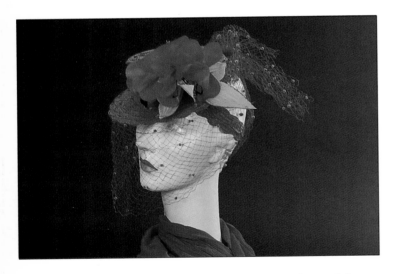

A froth of net and a swirl of straw in lipstick-red, irresistible in a tilt hat from the late 1930s. *Courtesy of: Lottie Ballou.* Value: $45-65.

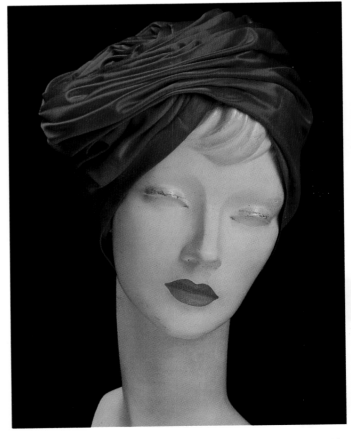

A fabulous red silk turban, with the detailed drape that only comes with custom design. *Courtesy of: Banbury Cross Antiques.* Value: $95-145.

II. The Evolution of Hat Design

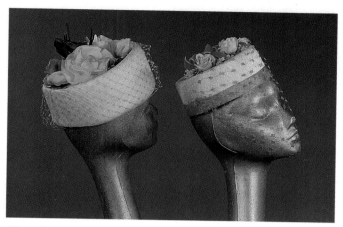

These flowered hats from the 1950s were probably purchased for Sunday services. Label (left): Noreen. Label (right): Sonni. *Courtesy of (both): Banbury Cross Antiques.* Value (each): $25-45.

The earliest hats were either straw or felt, designed to serve a purpose: protection from the heat or cold. Accordingly, form followed function. The peasant wore a straw sunshade in the fields. The merchant, who had no need for shelter from such exposure, wore a conical wool or felt cap.

Women's headgear followed men's styles, although the fair sex kept their hair covered throughout the day for the sake of modesty. Peasant women wore a large shawl, known as a couvre-chef or kerchief. Their noble sisters wore a broad veil or stole, draped over the head and held in place with a coronet.

The notion that a modest woman must cover her head persisted into the mid-20th century in church doctrine. For hat collectors, this is a fortunate circumstance, as it helped keep the art of millinery alive!

One of the earliest forms of headgear hearkens back to ancient Greece. This was a pointed hood of felt, worn by sailors and dubbed the Phrygian Bonnet. This same shape of hat marked a freed slave in Greece. In the color red, it became an emblem of liberty during the French Revolution.

The art of felting was re-discovered in about 1200 and contributed greatly to the range of available styles. Men began to wear the Liripipe, a stocking-like affair worn draped to one side or arranged about the neck like a scarf. The peasant class was denied such status, and continued to wear rudimentary caps and shawls.

A true classic, the beret made its first appearance on the heads of Etruscan huntsmen, circa 400 B.C. Peasant men wore a floppy straw or cloth cap in the manner of a beret. By the mid-1500s, this style was worn by tinkers and artisans throughout Europe, and is still associated with the Bohemian life.

The style must have spread to Scotland at some point in time, given the striking similarity between the beret and the clansman's tam o'shanter. Both beret and tam were adopted by women over the past few hundred years, and became a millinery staple during the 20th century.

For everyday dress in the feudal era, ladies wore a linen or lace cap indoors. Peasant women wore a coarse linen or linsey Wimple draped in folds under the chin. Either style could be worn under a larger headdress or cloak, upon venturing into the street.

In the late feudal period, women of noble birth wore elaborate and cumbersome headgear such as the circular Escoffian and conical Hennin. The latter is Oriental in origin, its steeple profile derived from the Etruscan tower or "tutulu." It is a shape favored by the Italian papacy, as much as by the ladies.

As depicted in manuscripts and tapestries, the Hennin reached a staggering height, and the Escoffian an enormous weight. Indeed, some historians wonder if the scale was exaggerated for artistic effect. Both were further embellished with a gauzy Wimple, a sheer length of linen or silk that was worn underneath or draped on top like a scarf.

The latter arrangement should be readily recognized as the headdress of a fairy-tale princess! Perhaps unwittingly, the Wimple was revived by modern-day princess Grace Kelly, when she swathed her head in her signature Hermés scarf.

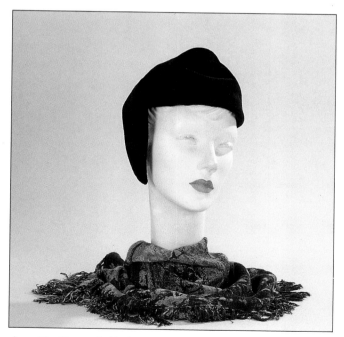

A starkly chic cap, in black velvet but strongly reminiscent of "le bonnet rouge" worn by peasants during the French Revolution. Label: Suzy. *Courtesy of: Maureen Reilly.* Value: $75-125.

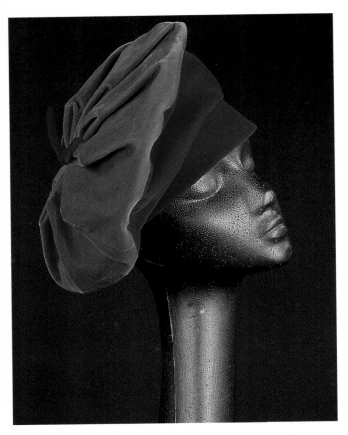

The tam o'shanter fresh from Carnaby Street circa 1960, a vibrant duotone of pink and red velveteen. Label: Archie Eason. *Courtesy of: Banbury Cross Antiques.* Value: $65-95.

The turban, another classic, has often been revived for women. It evolved, with few changes, from the Mesopotamian Valley some 5000 years ago when women first wrapped their heads in intricate folds of cloth.

This deceptively simple style may have spread to Europe with the Crusades. By the late 1700s, turbans were adopted by women of all classes in Europe, wrapped from lengths of linen or silk.

Circa 1800, the "desert turban" was in favor. This variation was left open in back, so that a mass of curls could tumble out in charming disarray. During the Empire period, turbans were especially popular for evening. Fashioned from brocade and velvet, they were often bound with ropes of pearls and graced by aigrettes. Some two centuries later, the turban topped exotic gowns during the tango craze of 1913.

Shifting back in time, the coptain was all the rage in the early 1600s. The crown of this hat was tall and slightly tapered with a moderate brim, and sat squarely on the head. The angular lines of the coptain were softened by its broad hatband and backswept plumes. It was fashioned from the full range of materials available to milliners at that time: felt, wool, straw, silk, and velvet.

This hat was to evolve into the Cavalier, a plumed and cocked affair of gallant proportions made famous by the exploits of Alexandre Dumas' *The Three Musketeers*. The Cavalier was worn by both sexes until the mid-1600s. A diminutive version of this hat was revived in the late 1700s, worn perched at the side of a pompadour.

In the mid-1600s, women's hats grew simpler due the emphasis in romantic hairstyles, especially the fad for ringlets. By the end of that century, following the English Restoration, hairstyles became so elaborate that hats fell out of favor entirely with upper-class women. The only new styles to emerge were for men: the trilby in felt with tricorne brim, and the classic fedora, in felt with creased crown.

With the passage of 100 years, hats were again in vogue. Perhaps the most enduring (and endearing) was the straw Pamela. Named after the heroine in a romantic novel by Richardsen, it charms with a low crown and a slightly curved brim that slopes down in front and back. This style has been re-cast in the fashion follies many times since then, with a few new lines and always a romantic role: the garden hat, cartwheel, and picture hat.

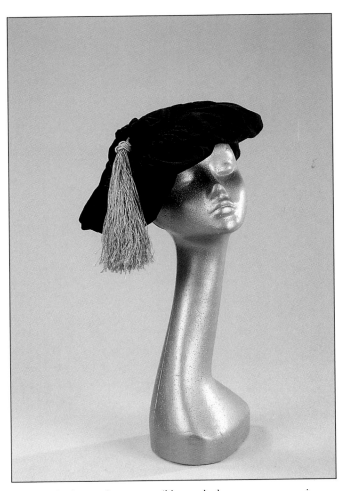

A midnight dream of a tam, possibly matched to an opera cape circa 1920. It is hand-stitched from black silk velvet, with smocking detail around the soft brim. The tassel was originally emerald, now a celadon "fade." *Courtesy of: Maureen Reilly.* Value: $75-125.

The romantic Gainsborough was named after the artist for hats featured in his paintings such as "The Morning Walk," which exhibited in 1785. It is a type of plumed and ribboned picture hat, with a steep crown and upswept brim.

From the Renaissance to the French Revolution, wigs were worn at court by both men and women. They were dusted with powder, typically white, although violet tints were used by brunettes and iris by blondes—an elaborate and messy procedure! So much so, that the nobility often built a "chambre de poudre " for the daily ritual and wig cabinets were a necessary adjunct to the dressing room.

Wigs grew to elaborate heights at the French court, following the style of pace-setting courtesan Madame Pompadour. Then came the predictable reversal, when hair reduced in size and hats rode high on the head. This change of millinery pace is attributed to another star in the Versailles firmament, the Duchesse de Fontanges.

Having lost her riding hat during a royal hunt, the duchess tied up her blond curls with a ribbon garter. She was so

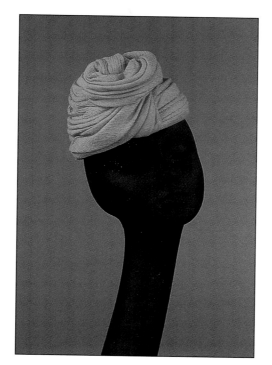

Très chic, this turban with a twist. It can be readily dated circa 1960 by its stretch knit fabric and I. Magnin department store label. Label: Emme. *Courtesy of: Banbury Cross Antiques.* Value: $45-75.

complimented on the look by Louis XIV that her makeshift hairdo became a fashion craze. This was to be the forerunner of a high-crowned bonnet, aptly named the Fontange, that dominated millinery in the 1880s.

Wigs worn by the fair sex often reached a towering height at the court of the Sun King. Poufed and powdered, they were embellished for evening with jeweled ornaments, and in the afternoon they were graced by follies, such as a lacy butterfly poised mid-flight.

The craft of millinery made great strides in the 1770s at the over-styled court of Louis XVI and his frivolous queen, Marie Antoinette. She was not content to merely order custom styles, but invited her own milliner to join the court. Thus, peasant-born Rose Bertin became one of the first "superstar" designers in history.

Rose Bertin's chapeaux were witty, charming and original. She is attributed with this sage observation, as apt to the fashion world of 1770 as it is today:

"The only new thing is that which has been forgotten."

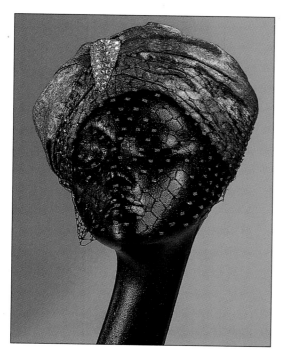

Can you just picture Gloria Swanson in this stunner—playing no doubt an exotic femme fatale. This evening turban glitters in lamé, sparkles with a strass clip. *Courtesy of: Anna's.* Value: $75-125.

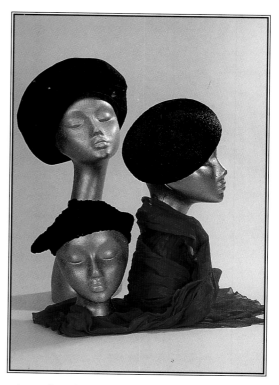

Three berets from the 1940s and 1950s, showing the range of this classic shape, even though all are basic black. Label (top): Jack McConnell. Label (center): Dayne. *Courtesy of (all): Maureen Reilly.* Value (top): $65-95. Value (others): $25-45.

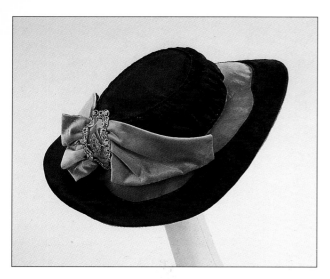

A Pamela in ruched black silk. The soft glow of its pink hatband is reflected in the polished facets of a large enamel buckle. This shallow-crowned and sweep-brimmed style is a perennial favorite. *Courtesy of: The Way We Wore.* Value: $200-300.

The shepherdess mode of dress was adopted by Marie Antoinette and her ladies as a relief from the tedium of court. This begat the bergere, a straw hat with shallow crown and broad brim. Trimmed in the naive manner with simple flowers and ribbons, it remains one of the most charming styles of all time.

Flat straw hats, a variation of the bergere, might top a wig pancake-style. A less formal look was available in the dormeuse, an oversized mobcap layered with lace and ruching.

The dormeuse was wildly popular from the mid-1700s through the mid-1800s. Earlier mobcaps were even larger, so that a new bonnet was designed in 1765 to be worn over them for traveling. This was the calash, made of silk or other fabric that was shirred over whalebone or reed hoops. It could be raised or lowered by a string, like a carriage top!

For a brief hiatus after the French Revolution, women of the upper class went hatless. Parisiennes wore their hair close-cropped, but for tendrils at the nape and temple. The social upheaval of the times was nowhere more manifest than in the lack of fashionable attire for the former ruling class, during the brief Directoire period.

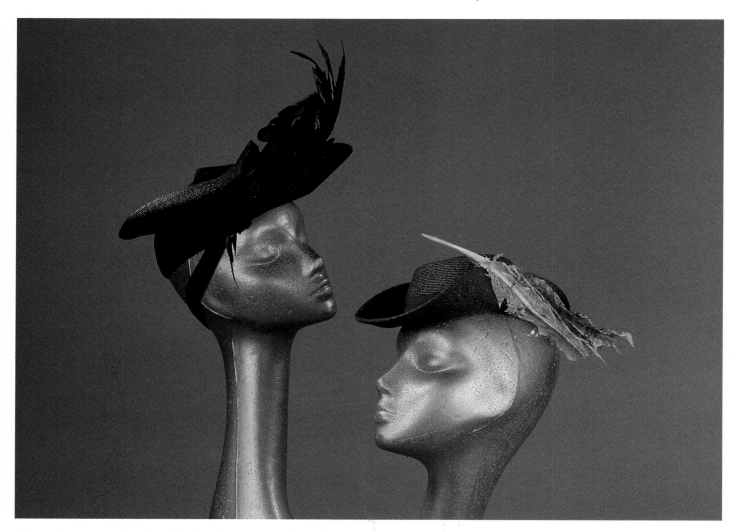

The cavalier was revived in the 1930s, à la the taupe straw with cocked brim and jaunty feather trim. Its companion, in lilac straw, is a variation on the theme of romantic plumed hats worn at the court of Louis XIV. Label (left): The White House. Label (right): Judkins, New York. *Courtesy of (both): Maureen Reilly.* Value (left): $55-85. Value (right): $75-115.

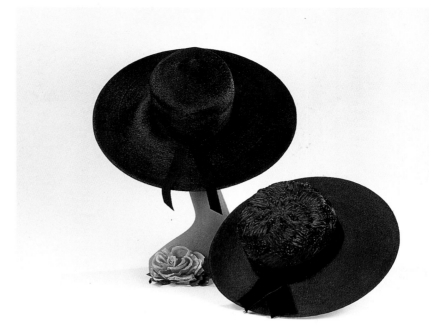

The ever-popular picture hat, shown here as summer straws in sophisticated black, circa 1950. *Courtesy of (both): Rich Man, Poor Man.* Value (each): $45-75.

Napoleon assumed power in 1799. It was only then, during the Empire period, that fashion regained its rightful place as a force in French history. The *dernier cri* was ardently pursued by the nobility, with full panoply and folly.

Following the dictate of Empress Josephine, ladies of the court adopted a Grecian mode of dress, a style that was emulated throughout Europe and America. Then she staged the *bal à la victime*, launching a bizarre trend whereby Parisiennes eschewed jewelry for a red ribbon at the throat, in sympathy for their peers who had met Mr. Guillotine.

The ladies soon returned to wearing jewels, albeit simpler and more classical, such as diamonds twinkling from diadems in the evening. During the day, the ladies donned small-brimmed bonnets, bright with flowers. It was an effect both gay and sophisticated, a perfect foil to the elegant lines of an empire-waisted gown.

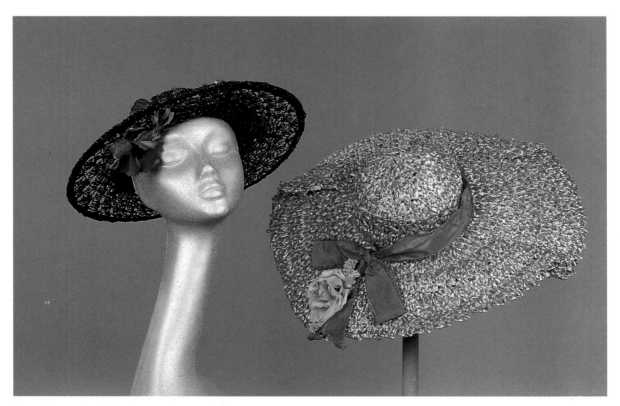

Paired here, a black horsehair with coy flowers under the brim, and a violet raffia with side pleating, circa 1930s. *Courtesy of (both): Banbury Cross Antiques.* Value (each): $75-125.

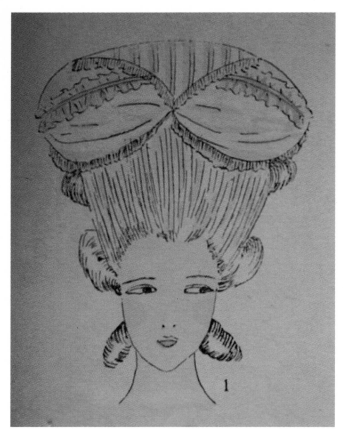

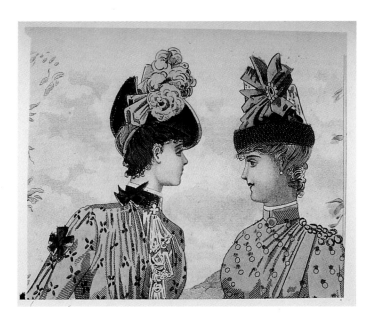

From *Peterson's Magazine* in 1889—the Fontange, a royal profile born of a windy day at the court of Louis XIV.

For the fair sex, hats were secondary to their highly-styled wigs. This powdered confection is capped with a lace doily. From *L'Histoire du Costume Feminin Francais,* a hand-colored folio published in the early 1900s.

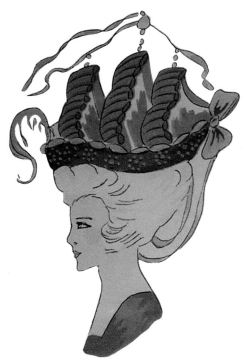

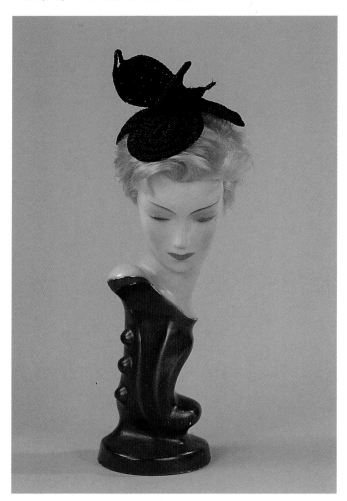

A fine hand-colored illustration from *L'Histoire du Costume Feminin Francais.* This ship in full sail rides the billowing waves of a powdered pompadour. Smaller follies, in the shape of butterflies and flowers, were also popular for balls and masquerades circa 1600-1770.

The gaily sophisticated folly was revived in the 1930s, when women wore their hair in a modified pompadour. This pretty blue butterfly was crocheted by the author's grandmother. *Courtesy of: Maureen Reilly.* Value: Special.

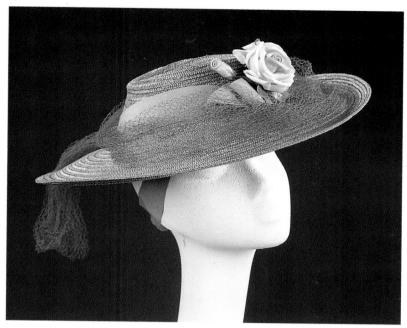

We show the bergere's winning ways in this sewn-straw revival, circa 1940. *Courtesy of: Banbury Cross Antiques.* Value: $45-75.

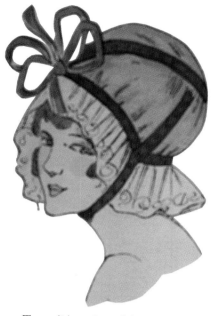

Two stylish versions of the dormeuse, from *L'Histoire du Costume Feminin Francais.*

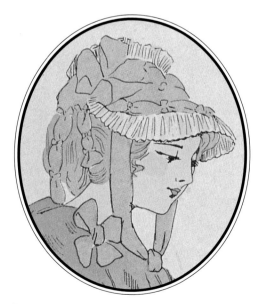

Boudoir caps such as this were routinely worn during the morning toilet, from the early 1700s through the early 1900s. Although much more charming, they may be seen as the forerunner of the ubiquitous curler caps circa 1950! From *L'Histoire du Costume Feminin Francais.*

Rather radical fashions appeared in the waning days of the Empire, circa 1790-1810. Even women played the dandy, preening in the manner of a "marveilleuse." This called for sheer and flowing gowns with shawls and ruffs, topped off with a fantastic array of hats. Some ladies chose plumed helmets inspired by Napoleon's campaigns. Others wore oversized Gainsboroughs, with elongated brims that preceded them by a good two feet!

Throughout the 1800s, women kept their hair covered at all times. Hearkening back to medieval custom, it was considered indecent for a woman's crowning glory to shine unrestricted by a headdress.

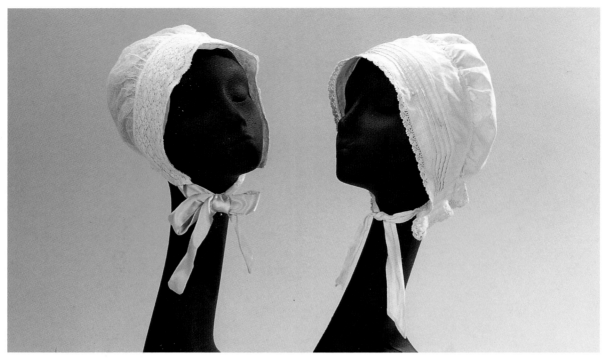

Two simple caps, one for morning and the other for daily chores, circa 1880. To the left, a delicate band of hand-made lace that originally had narrow ribbons of lilac silk. The original ribbons were damaged; those shown were hand-sewn from a length of pastel vintage silk. *Courtesy of (both): Maureen Reilly.* Value (each): $65-95.

Little lace caps would be worn upon rising—the breakfast or boudoir cap, which continued to be worn until the mid-1920s. A simple cloth bonnet or scarf would be worn for midday chores, even something as routine as pinning up laundry on an outdoor line.

Nightcaps were worn by men and women from the Renaissance through the late 1800s. These caps were not meant for bed, but for warmth in the evening at home. This was espe-cially important for men, who sometimes shaved their heads to accommodate a wig!

By the late Victorian era, the nightcap was deemed old-fashioned, and was replaced by the smoking cap for men. This style served a dual purpose, both for warmth and to shield hair from the pervasive odor of pipes and cigars. Nightcaps, and other stiff brimless caps, hearken back to the fez that was imported from Arabia, possibly during the Crusades.

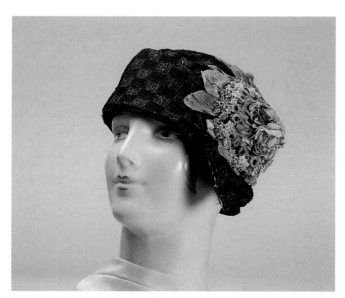

A brimless hat circa 1900, either a latter-day fez or an early pillbox. Regardless, it is a beauty in basketweave wood straw dyed navy, with silk hatband to match and velvet flowers to contrast. *Courtesy of: The Way We Wore.* Value: $150-200.

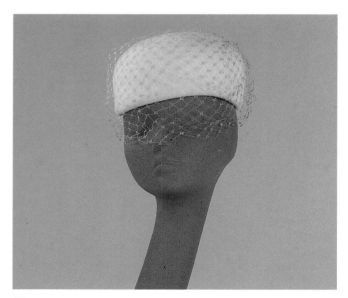

This smart 1960s pillbox in ecru felt is devoid of trim, providing a structured balance for daytime dress. Label: Emme. *Courtesy of: Maureen Reilly.* Value: $45-75.

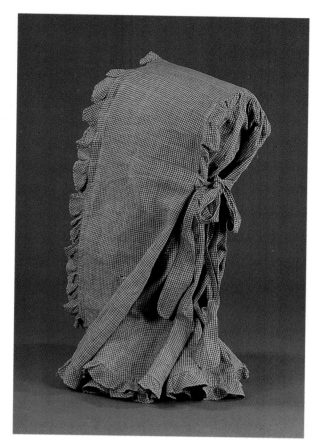

A green-and-white calico poke bonnet with a long bavolet, to afford extra protection from the cruel prairie sun. The deep poke is stiffened with thin wooden slats, a complex form of construction that indicates it may have been factory-made. *Courtesy of: Mary Aaron Museum.* Value: Special.

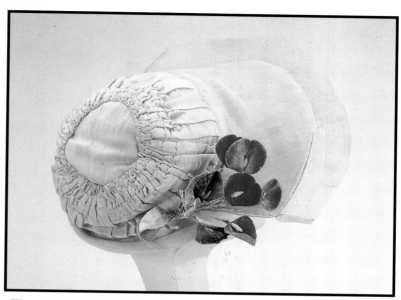

The poke of this light-pink bonnet is stiffened with a brim of horsehair. Based on the condition of its fabric and method of its construction, the authors are confident this is a revival. *Courtesy of: Banbury Cross Antiques.* Value: $75-125.

This black tulle bonnet would have been a wardrobe staple, circa 1890. It is simply trimmed with feathers and wired beading. *Courtesy of: Mary Aaron Museum.* Value: Special.

Despite the fez's exotic origins from the sands of Arabia, this style was a favorite of middle-class women in England and America once translated into the porkpie hat of the mid-1800s and the pillbox of the mid-1900s.

The bonnet was headgear of choice for most women from the Directoire period of the early 1800s through the waning influence of Queen Victoria one hundred years later. It was worn at all angles, and stitched (usually on a wire rim) into all shapes.

Common to all bonnets, the brim is emphasized over the crown, and ribbons serve as security. Many varieties of bonnets have been in favor, with their crowns and brims being scaled up or down according to the current taste.

Ribbons served double duty as a form of trim for bonnets, along with lace, feathers, flowers, fruit, and the same broad array of stuff used to decorate hats. Crowns were wreathed in flowers or swathed in veiling. Some featured the bavolet, a drape of soft fabric at the lower crown that covered the back of the neck. Brims were broad enough to encircle the face, or deep enough to block the entire face from view (like a poke)!

Fashioned from fine straw, tulle, or velvet, the bonnet appeared with all manner of day and evening ensembles. Formed of rough straw, felt, or fabric, it was suitable for the country, and was even adaptable to the American Frontier.

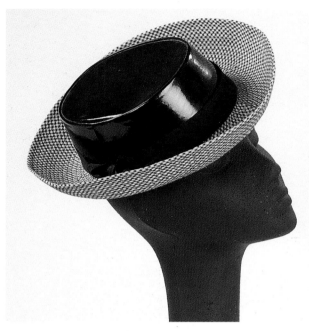

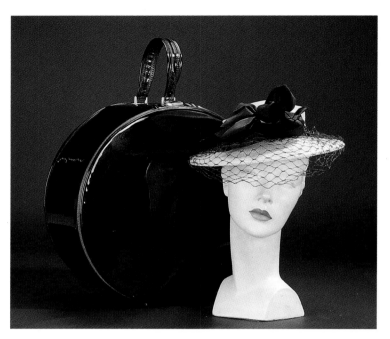

An unusual boater from the Edwardian era, snappy in black patent leather and checkered fabric. In the inside crown there is a drawstring linen bag, ready to help hold the high-styled hairdos of that era. Label (inside crown): R.E. Hat Co. *Courtesy of: Banbury Cross Antiques.* Value: $95-145.

The boater was revived in the mid-1900s, as in this black and white version shown with a patent-leather hatbox by Lark. *Courtesy of: Banbury Cross Antiques.* Value (hat): $45-65. Value (box): $35-50.

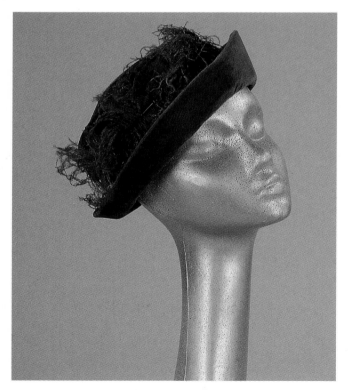

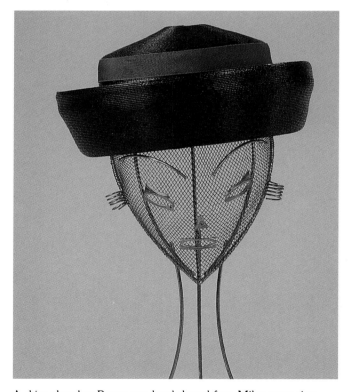

A dove grey velvet Breton with dyed-to-match ostrich plumage as an elegant hatband. This hat shows the simpler lines of the late teens. *Courtesy of: Sharon Hagerty.* Value: $125-175.

A shiny chocolate Breton was hand-shaped from Milan straw circa 1965, an example of millinery mastery from Leslie James. *Courtesy of: Maureen Reilly.* Value: $65-95.

The 1800s was the century of westward expansion in America. Women crossed the plains wearing dresses stitched from calico and broad-brimmed sunbonnets to match. They brought churches and schools to towns like Dry Gulch and Last Hope, along with social events like the bazaar and barn dance. In their wake came the trappings of fashion via catalogs or dry goods stores.

The classic bonnet is beloved for its grace and charm, and it has been through many revivals. Like its predecessor, it is secured by long ribbon streamers and offers the shade of a deep brim. Its repeat popularity makes the bonnet particularly difficult to date, and care must be taken to "feel" the fabric and trim for signs of age.

In the 1840s, women could wear a hairnet or snood, a revival of the caul worn in ancient Greece. Whether worn alone or under a bonnet, the snood was ideal for informal or indoor activities. It kept the hair neat and could be made inexpensively at home. For these same reasons, the snood enjoyed a resurgence in popularity during the Depression and the war years.

Certain styles endure by reason of their chic, charm, and versatility. These classics cross all barriers of time and culture. Some we have already discussed such as the beret and turban, but several others deserve special mention.

Both the boater and Breton are derived from the headgear of French sailors. Admiral Horatio Nelson actually made the ribbon-banded boater part of his crew's regulation dress in 1805.

The boater can be worn schoolgirl-straight, or cocked at a rakish angle. With its cousin, the Breton, it is forever evocative of summer afternoons, the one with flattened brim and level crown; the other with rolled brim and round crown. Both were perfect for country outings, circa 1870-1970.

The toque has been fashioned in every fabrication known to the millinery trade. In straw or felt, it has a curiously homey quality, much like a round loaf. In fur, it becomes exotic, perhaps due to its distinct Tartar origins. Place a toque in Persian lamb on your head, and be transported to the wild Russian Steppes!

The cloche is relatively new, but deserves mention as an enduring style. It was created by milliner Caroline Reboux in the early 1920s. Her celebrated technique was to drape a hood of chiffon-soft felt over the head of each client, then fold and tuck it in such a way as to assure a perfect fit.

The beret, tam, turban, toque, boater, Breton, and cloche all appear in one version or another in each decade of the 20th century. These are the styles that have passed fashion's test of time. Each one, in its own right, is a true millinery classic.

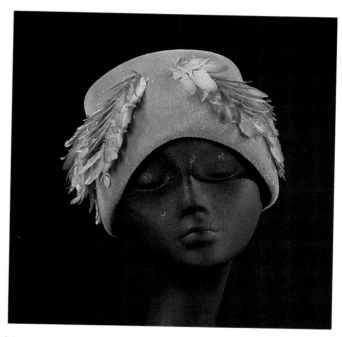

Mauve felt in a wire-rimmed structured fez, with the surprise of orange and green feather wings, circa 1947. Such wild colors may have coordinated with a special suit. Label: Replica de Parisienne. *Courtesy of: Maureen Reilly.* Value: $35-55.

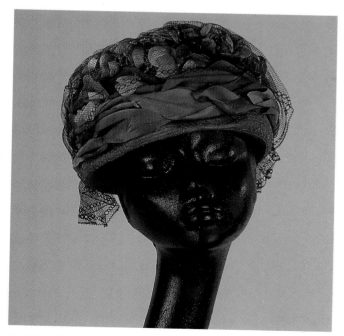

An Edwardian toque of honey-colored felt swirls with feathers caught in net, all in the colors of Autumn leaves. *Courtesy of: Maureen Reilly.* Value: $95-125.

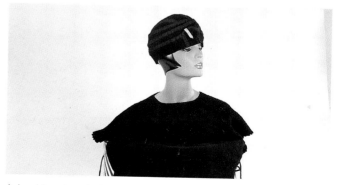

A head-hugging cloche circa 1929, in a geometric mix of black and blue knit. *Courtesy of: Sheryl Birkner.* Value: $75-125.

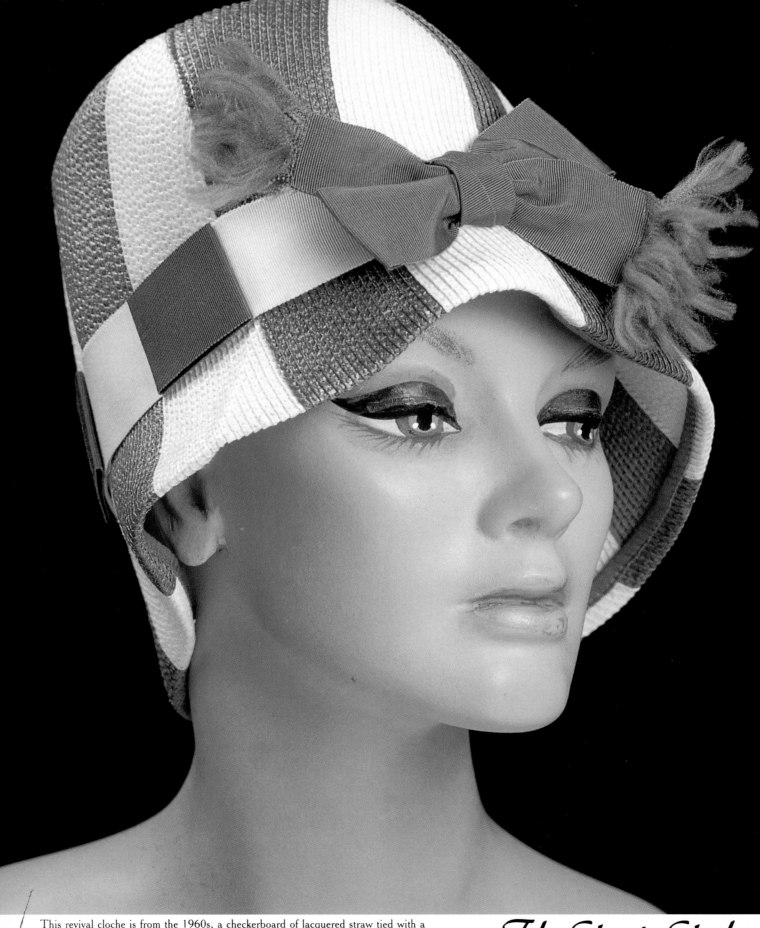

This revival cloche is from the 1960s, a checkerboard of lacquered straw tied with a grosgrain bow. Label: Lilly Daché Debs. *Courtesy of: Maureen Reilly.* Value: $45-75.

The Classic Cloche

Price

III. The Effect of International Couture

A basic knowledge of clothing styles is critical for accurately dating hats. Women chose their hats carefully to balance their silhouette and enhance the mood of an ensemble. Hats were an extension of the dress or suit, and often incorporated the same colors and trimmings. Proportion was critical—the hat that topped an exaggerated S-shaped silhouette bears no resemblance to that worn with the simple H-shape of a chemise.

In the mid-1800s, hooped skirts defined the female figure, in a range of softly billowed or belled shapes. By the century's close, the exaggeration of form shifted to the rear, with the much-ridiculed bustle. For a brief period in 1915, women endured hobble skirts, with their ankles literally tied by loops of fabric in order to trim their stride. These and other cumbersome styles spawned a series of dress reforms as early as the 1870s.

Milan Style

Milan made important contributions to "hat couture" dating back to the Renaissance, when that city was a center for the fledgling millinery trade. Indeed, the word milliner stems from Milan, as first recorded in 1529.

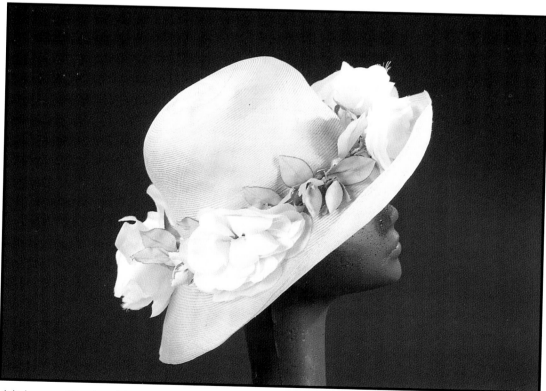

A high-crowned Pamela with floppy brim, exhibiting the fine weave of Milan straw. The soft silk flowers add to the languid lines of this timeless summer hat, circa 1930. *Courtesy of: Maureen Reilly.* Value: $75-125.

The Victorians turned to Paris for the *dernier cri* in style. The luscious gowns created by Charles Frederick Worth, whose salon opened in 1856, were widely copied from the French originals. These and other couture creations received worldwide attention, thanks to detailed coverage in the new ladies' magazines (e.g., *Godey's* and *Peterson's*). Embroidery, beadwork, hand-made lace, smocking, and other dressmaker details were employed to create an impression of luxury and wealth, even for daytime dress.

Edwardian women followed the lead of elegant Queen Alexandra, wife to King Edward of England—even though historians assure us that her wardrobe was imported from across the Channel! Based on her sure sense of style, and that of fashion contemporary Empress Eugenie of France, women completely changed their wardrobes in palette and silhouette.

In 1909, Fortuny patented a process for pleating silk, which he used to good effect in light and elegant evening fashions. That same year, the Ballets Russe shocked Paris with dramatic costumes designed by the pre-cubist Leon Bakst. This performance was the inspiration for Paul Poirot's harem pants and other exotic designs.

Pants would not be accepted for wear by the average woman, however, until Chanel introduced her wide-legged variety a decade hence. Then, with the advent of World War I and the emergence of a female work force, dress reformists finally had their day.

Simpler lines and shorter skirts prevailed in the trying years of World War I. As would occur again in the 1940s, the governments of Britain and America rationed wool and other fabrics deemed necessary for the war effort.

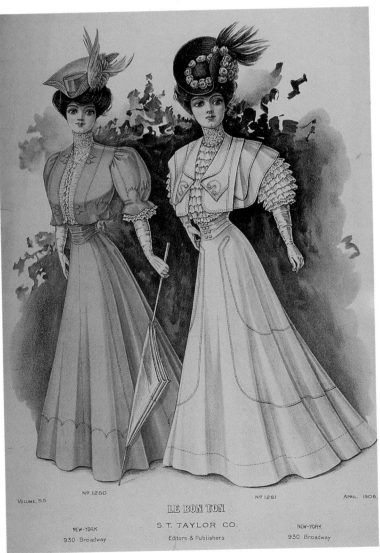

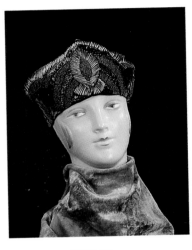

This unusual transitional style is a rare find, in celluloid "straw" dyed blue, yellow and brown, with an ethnic influence, possibly inspired by Poirot. Label: Lileth, Paris & New York. *Courtesy of: The Way We Wore.* Value: $200-250.

Two fashion lithographs show the new spring styles. From April 1906, *Le Bon Ton* styled a pink frock in the new slim line inspired by Queen Alexandra, along with a self-fabric bonnet. From the very next year, two suit ensembles with complementary chapeaux in natural and black straw.

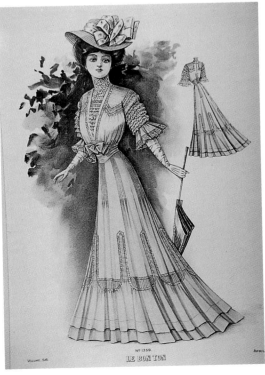

Women began to wear the same basic suit or dress throughout the day. This seems unremarkable now, but at the time it was a marked contrast to the fussy etiquette that required a change of clothing for every social activity, as often as five times in a single day. World War I triggered a demand for tailor-made suits and shirtwaist dresses in Europe. These were less restrictive, practical styles, of a type that active American women had been wearing for years.

According to fashion historian Caroline Rennolds Milbank, the simplicity of American style had been long developing, in deliberate contrast to our British forbearers:

> *"It had its genesis in the patriotic determination, after the Revolutionary War, to wear homegrown, homespun, and home-sewn clothes…"*

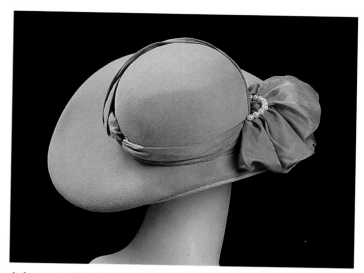

A fawn velvet Pamela with scoop brim. Banded in a chiffon scarf, clipped with pearls. This elegantly simple style was popular in the 1920s and again in the 1960s, when this hat was made. *Courtesy of: Banbury Cross Antiques.* Value: $25-45.

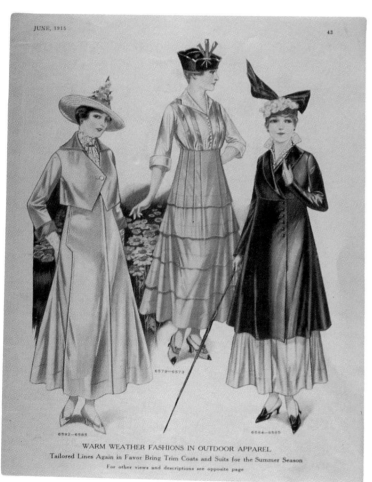

JUNE, 1915   43

WARM WEATHER FASHIONS IN OUTDOOR APPAREL
Tailored Lines Again in Favor Bring Trim Coats and Suits for the Summer Season
For other views and descriptions see opposite page

Two charming illustrations from *McCall's*, June 1915. The small and neater silhouette was admirably suited to the functional dress of World War I. These hats are far from drab, however, thanks to their trim.

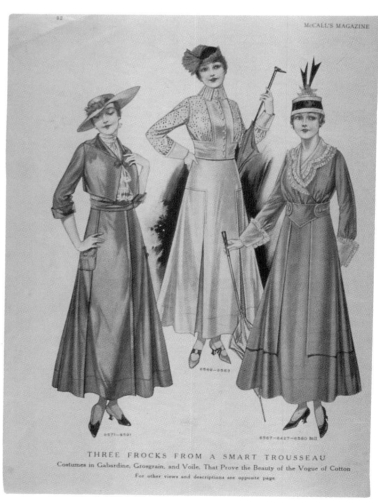

82   McCALL'S MAGAZINE

THREE FROCKS FROM A SMART TROUSSEAU
Costumes in Gabardine, Grosgrain, and Voile, That Prove the Beauty of the Vogue of Cotton
For other views and descriptions see opposite page

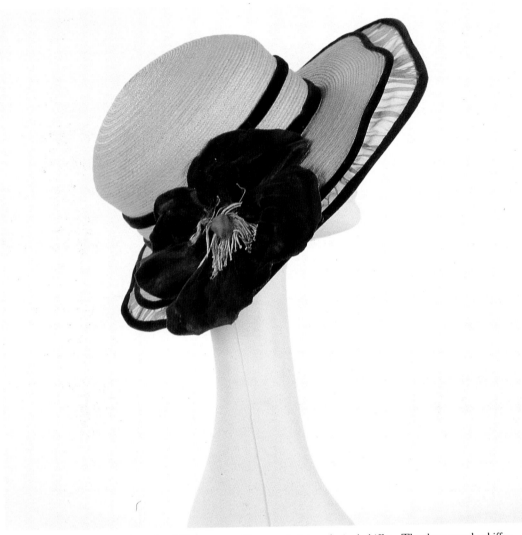

A Pamela meticulously fashioned in Milan straw, with an underbrim of wired chiffon. The deep purple chiffon and velvet is a pleasing contrast against the cream straw. The label proclaims its market niche: Debutante Salon. *Courtesy of: Barbara Griggs Vintage Fashion.* Value: $150-200.

Nevertheless, French fashion plates were the inspiration for American dress throughout the formative years of this country, and well into the 20th century. Paris brought about the major design changes, which were then copied by women the world over—or, rather, interpreted by women who often had no more direction than the illustrations in a fashion plate. This was, literally, a "sketchy" basis for creating a new dress or hat.

The American retailer Madame Demorest, actually a husband-and-wife design team, began marketing paper dress patterns in the late 1850s. This revolutionary concept was of no use to women who wanted the latest Parisian chapeaux, however. They were still guided only by illustrations, and sometimes a text that described the types of fabric or manner of trim that the latest bonnet might be worked in.

In the early teens, Madame Paquin of Paris introduced floating dresses which blended comfort with femininity, the per-

fect foil to a pared-down daytime look. Similarly, Jeanne Lanvin designed romantic "robes de style," a full-skirted and wide-collared style that remained popular throughout the early 1930s, especially for young women and debutantes.

Madame Vionnet began experimenting with her elegant bias-cut couture in 1912. This would eventually become her signature style, strongly associated with the Jean Harlow look of the 1930s. But the the most important fashion influence of this decade came from Hollywood.

Women the world over clamored for knock-offs of the glamorous styles created by Adrian for Greta Garbo and Joan Crawford. Many hats of this era were based on the Hollywood wardrobe room, and their marketing was timed to the release date of the movie.

We know that Hollywood's effect on fashion was international, and can only assume that European women demanded hats with studio labels, the same as their American sisters. This was a reversal of the usual order, whereby French couture held the fashion world in thrall. Ironically, some Hollywood designs still boasted of French origins.

The German invasion of Paris put a temporary end to fashion as an industry in that country, despite the best efforts of the French government to keep it alive. An American design idiom had long been developing—headquartered in the garment district and publishing citadels of New York City. However, there was little public recognition of the individual American designers, until the stars of Paris dimmed in 1939.

Many of the large New York City department stores took this wartime opportunity to promote their designers, giving credit in window displays and newspaper ads. As an outgrowth of this shift in marketing, many stores opened their own millinery salons. Some devoted an entire floor to this segment of their market.

Salon hats almost always bore a store label, and sometimes the designer's label as well. Collectors should be on the lookout for these hats, which were of the highest quality.

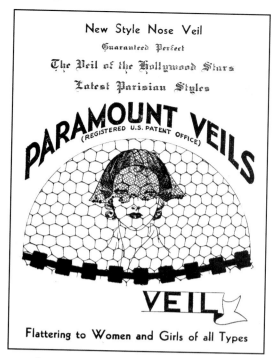

New Style Nose Veil
Guaranteed Perfect
The Veil of the Hollywood Stars
Latest Parisian Styles

PARAMOUNT VEILS
(REGISTERED U.S. PATENT OFFICE)

VEIL

Flattering to Women and Girls of all Types

A Paramount Studio veil, promoted as "The Veil of the Hollywood Stars." As if that wasn't endorsement enough, customers were also assured it was from the "Latest Parisian Styles."

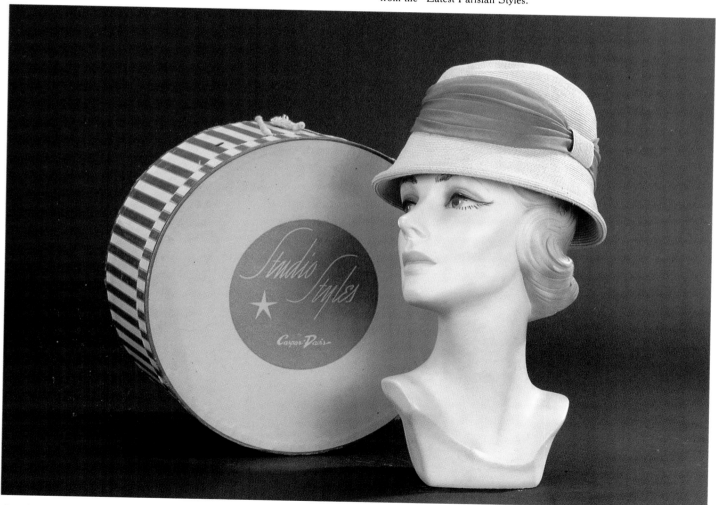

An olive green toque, circa 1955. The twin labels show it was created for Hollywood's successful Studio Styles, but was "modeled after" French couturier Jacques Fath. Shown with original hatbox. *Courtesy of (both): Banbury Cross Antiques.* Value (hat): $45-75. Value (box): $25-45.

The American design talent was considerable, from the East to the West Coast. In New York City, there was Lilly Daché, Hattie Carnegie, Peggy Hoyt, Lucile, Pauline, Suzy, Bernice Charles, Nettie Rosenstein, Irene of New York, Sally Victor, and Sally Milgrim. True, some of them had emigrated from Paris, but their designs were inspired by the American cultural idiom.

Among their male counterparts were John P. John, John Frederics, and Adolfo, in New York City. On the West Coast there was Leslie James, Frank Olive, Jack McConnell, and the legendary Adrian of Hollywood.

The corps of American milliners did not emulate Europe, but built upon it. They acquired the finest felts from Borsalino, Italy; the most delicate laces from Belgium; and silk flowers crafted in the ateliers of France. The forms were hand-steamed and blocked by professional felters, and the trim was hand-sewn by midinettes. By blending American design with old-world craftsmanship, they acquired a devoted clientele that continued into the post-war years.

After the war, American designers were still fighting—this time, to retain their hard-won recognition in spite of the New Look missile launched by Christian Dior from Paris. Rather than compete with French haute couture, the American designers perfected a breed of "casual couture." These clothes were clean of line and relatively easy of care, ideal for the emerging ready-to-wear industry.

A cocktail hat with the good breeding of Lilly Daché couture. Prancing from the tiny cap, a thick mane of horsehair is bound up for show, in bows. *Courtesy of: Maureen Reilly.* Value: $95-125.

Salon Style

As described by fashion researchers at the Fine Arts Museums of San Francisco, the process of buying a custom-made dress at I. Magnin was "remarkably similar to that of purchasing a dress directly from a couture house." This involved consultations and several fittings, culminating in a custom design. From the caliber of hats we have seen bearing the I. Magnin Salon label, we can only assume there was a similar procedure for millinery.

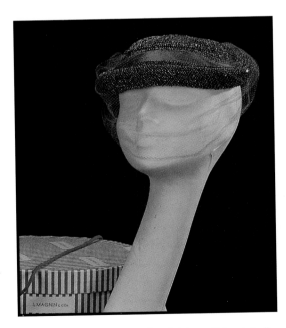

A bronze-beaded cocktail cap from I. Magnin Salon. It is all hand-worked with exquisite detail. The eyebrow veil is an intricate silk "spiderweb." Shown with its original bandbox of sturdy lacquered cardboard. *Courtesy of (both): Maureen Reilly.* Value (hat): $55-75. Value (box): $25-45.

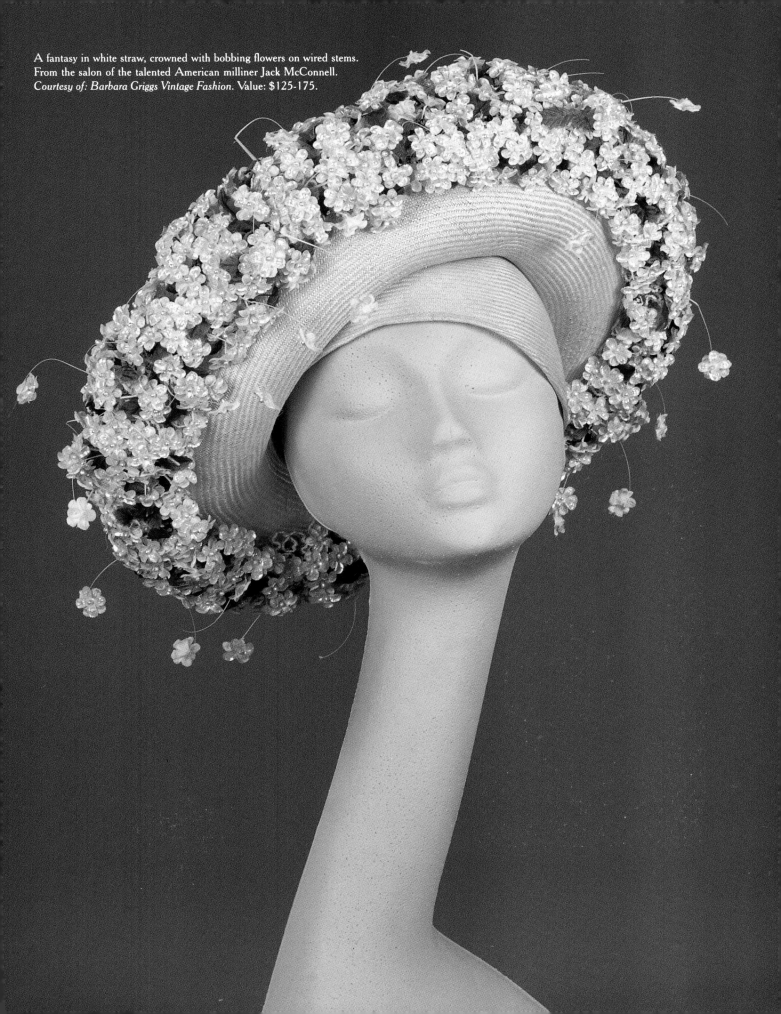

A fantasy in white straw, crowned with bobbing flowers on wired stems.
From the salon of the talented American milliner Jack McConnell.
Courtesy of: Barbara Griggs Vintage Fashion. Value: $125-175.

Anecdotally, French couturier Jacques Fath is credited with having pioneered the concept of ready-to-wear, in 1949. But he fitted the line to the longer torso and leggier gait of American models—from his atelier in Paris. Then he shipped the collection to New York City, where it debuted to rave reviews!

In the 1950s, hats were already beginning to diminish in importance, in favor of structured hairstyles. But the perpetual female penchant for glamour ensured a strong market for cocktail and "special occasion" hats.

In the 1960s, the cultural trend toward freedom of expression had a devastating effect on the influence of Paris. Ironically, women had greater access to fashion news than ever before in *Vogue, Harper's Bazaar,* and other glossies.

These magazines gave detailed photo coverage to the collections of Blass, Cardin, Courregès, Galanos, Gernreich, Gucci, Norell, Pucci, Scaasi, Yves St. Laurent, and Trigère. We highly recommend vintage fashion magazine coverage, for a real sense of how and where hats were worn.

Worldwide, the millinery trade tried to capture the youth market with styles built upon the glitzy "go go" theme of the new couture. They also introduced bridge lines, aimed at a younger and less affluent market niche. These efforts were valiant, but doomed to failure. By the end of the decade, it was clear that casual chic was here to stay, and the days of couture were numbered.

Three Metropolitan Tales

Paris and La Fête de Catherine

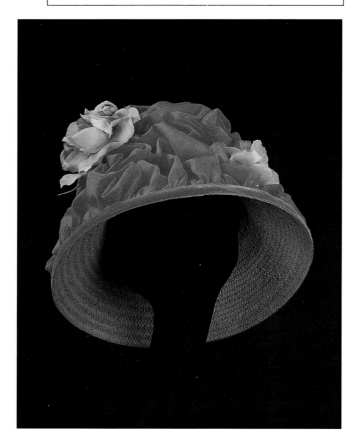

Each November 25, French milliners pay homage to St. Catherine of Alexandria, patron saint of maidens. In the 19th century, so many young Frenchwomen were earning their living as milliners that she was acknowledged as patron saint for the entire profession.

The festival originated in the Middle Ages, when brides-to-be would dance around a statue of the good saint, and decorate her head with flower circlets and veils. This custom of so many years ago continues today. Unmarried women, in particular those in the millinery trade, still don fanciful hats of their own creation on November 25, in the hopes of attracting a suitor. Indeed, a series of parades are held throughout France for "la fête des Catherinettes," in which behatted ladies are the main participants.

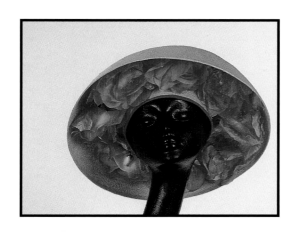

Is it an inverted dish, or hat? Is it an upside-down flowerpot, or what? Both of these fanciful hats exemplify the styles that are still created by Catherinettes, the name for unmarried women over the age of twenty-five who work for the millinery trade. *Courtesy of (right): Barbara Griggs Vintage Fashion. Courtesy of (left): Banbury Cross Antiques.* Value (each): $100-125.

London and the Races

Royal Ascot is not just a thoroughbred horse race, but a showcase for sartorial splendor by the gentry-bred. The annual fashion fever reaches its peak on Ladies Day, when it has long been the custom for women to sport their most elegant chapeaux. Today this tradition has become an exaggerated publicity stunt.

Hats are selected not for style, but for show, in the hope of attracting the photographer's eye. Even royalty gets into the act, and some of the most outlandish designs rest on crowned heads.

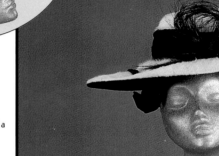

King Edward ruled but briefly, from his mother's death in 1901 until his own, in 1910. As a tribute to Edward—and a reflection of his emphasis on style—London society wore black hats and armbands to Ascot that year. This was the inspiration for the black-and-white hat designed by Cecil Beaton for the Ascot Opening Day scene in the 1960 hit movie "My Fair Lady."

Similar to the hat designed by Beaton for Audrey Hepburn to wear at Ascot: a dyed white beaver fur, trimmed with black velvet banding and bows. The enormous size of this hat would have balanced on top of a pompadour, secured by many hatpins. Label: Hale's. *Courtesy of: Rich Man, Poor Man.* Value: $200-300.

New York and the Easter Parade

Shortly after the Civil War, the New York garment manufacturers focused attention on the chic postwar hat styles in one of the greatest publicity stunts of all time: the Easter Parade. They sealed off Fifth Avenue, that mecca of stylish shops, for the upper crust who could parade the latest designs in bonnets for women and hats for men.

The idea caught on quickly across America, and by the 1880s an Easter Parade was held in most large cities. By the 1930s, the parade had become over-publicized, and it died out entirely over the next few decades.

The nostalgic movie "Easter Parade" starred Judy Garland and Fred Astaire. Dressed to the nines, they promenaded on Fifth Avenue and sang the title song: "In your Easter bonnet, with all the frills upon it, you'll be the prettiest lady in the Easter Parade."

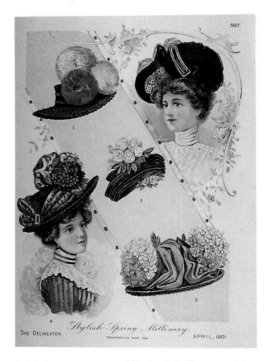

Judy's bonnet was inspired by the Belle Epoque, of the type shown in this color lithograph from *The Delineator* in Spring 1901.

IV. Meet The Designers

For the most part, the hats that are still affordable today by the average collector are those from the mid-20th century. These are the years when the individual milliners began to be promoted by the retailers, and their names came to be recognized by the buying public.

In pricing these hats, the label will often indicate value, as much as intricacy of design and quality of construction. We offer here a brief profile of key designers and millinery houses. Both in America and abroad, these are the "labels to look for."

We also list the names of better American department stores, culled from the advertisements in vintage fashion magazines. These stores often had millinery salons, with their own in-house designers and labels. If you enjoy a treasure hunt, you will find it rewarding to seek out these labeled hats.

The Americans

American style, sporty and simpler than its European counterpart, had been developing for almost a century before the Occupation of Paris. But that event triggered the formation of a distinct cadre of American designers. We profile here some of the great names behind the grand millinery salons of New York and Hollywood.

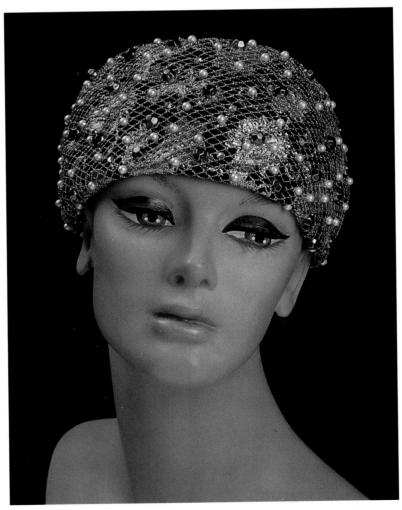

The Emme label designed by Adolfo in the 1950s. Brocade on a buckram form, with rhinestones and pearls. This pillbox is beautifully lined in printed satin.
Courtesy of: Maureen Reilly. Value: $65-95.

ADOLFO

Born in Havana, Cuba, in 1933, Adolfo was involved in fashion at an early age. A wealthy and fashionable aunt took him to Paris to see couture showings and introduced him to such luminaries as Balenciaga and Chanel. He apprenticed to Balenciaga and later moved to New York, where he worked as a designer for Emme. Some two decades later, his label read: Adolfo of Emme.

By 1962, Adolfo was heading his own firm, and was a favorite designer of Nancy Reagan. He was known for such styles as the shaggy Cossack hat in 1967, and the romantic big straw in 1968. Adolfo hats from this era are fairly plentiful in today's vintage marketplace, and are beautifully made.

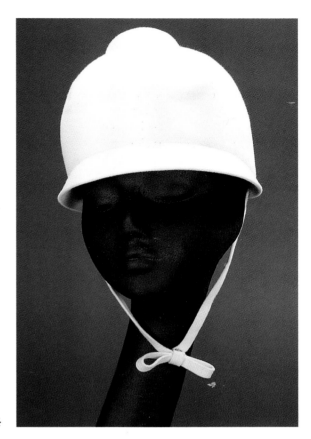

Perhaps inspired by Courregès, this felt helmet would have been just the thing to wear with a vinyl miniskirt, circa 1965. Label: Adolfo II. *Courtesy of: Banbury Cross Antiques.* Value: $75-125.

ADRIAN

Although he gained fame as a top Hollywood designer, Adrian studied art in Paris in the early 1920s, where he became friendly with Irving Berlin and began designing costumes for the stage.

Adrian's first break in Hollywood was designing costumes for Valentino, and he went on to become MGM's leading designer from 1925-1939. He designed for such stars as Joan Crawford and Greta Garbo, who had great influence on a fashion-conscious public.

In 1930, Adrian launched a national fad when he designed the plumed Eugenie hat, for Greta Garbo's role in a movie of the same name. In 1933, he decreed:

"Motion Pictures are becoming the Paris of America."

He operated Adrian, Ltd. in Beverly Hills from 1941 to 1948, selling top quality ready-to-wear items. He was married for many years to the actress Janet Gaynor, and died while working on a stage production of Camelot.

Collectors fortunate enough to find an Adrian hat can expect it to steadily increase in value and desirability. For a fabulous look at Adrian hats, check out the videotape of "The Women." This is a new release of the 1939 movie, and it features a colorized insert of an Adrian fashion show. On labels, look for his name alone or in tandem with a movie studio.

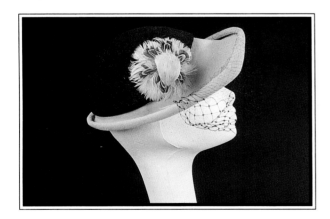

Watch the birdie, on this novel duotone felt with forward-thrusting brim. The label is Paramount, one of the major studios that promoted a line of movie star styles. *Courtesy of: Graf's Glitz.* Value: $75-125.

The Kanengeisir family from Austria joined the flood of immigrants pouring into New York City at the turn of the century. Hattie began working at age fifteen as a cashier, model, and trimmer in the millinery department at Macy's. She made extra income designing hats for neighborhood women.

By all accounts a petite, charming, and feminine woman who loved design and fashion, she also possessed a sharp business sense. By age twenty she was partnering in a shop on East 10th Street. She had changed her name to Carnegie after Andrew Carnegie, who was the richest man in the world at that time. Her shop, "Carnegie—Ladies' Hatter," was an immediate success.

By 1940 Hattie Carnegie, Inc., employed 1,000 people in the sales and production of hats, clothing, accessories, jewelry, and perfume. Carnegie made frequent trips to Paris for inspiration, but her creations were essentially her own. Her look was not extreme, but overall it was spirited and sophisticated.

Her business was a training ground for such designers as Galanos, Norell, Trigère, and McCardell, but it was very much her own, and when Carnegie died in 1956 it soon disbanded.

Look for the early label Hatnegie, which sold in better department stores during in the 1920s and 1930s. Hats with a Carnegie label are particularly desirable for the collector.

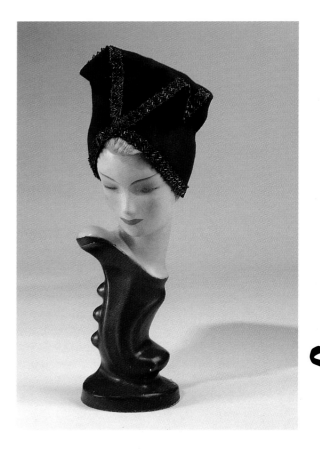

Fine wool felt from the Hattie Carnegie label, circa 1945. First flapped, then beaded in bronze, a statuesque toque with Medieval references. *Courtesy of: Cheap Thrills.* Value: $95-145.

Hattie Carnegie

Oleg Cassini

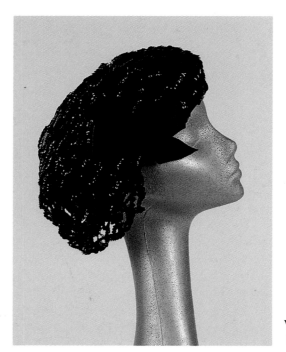

Oleg Cassini is perhaps best known for his line of accessible couture clothing in the American design idiom, dating back to the 1950s when he launched his line of ready-to-wear in New York City.

As the son of a Russian count, Cassini had traveled across Europe before his family settled in Florence. There, his mother established a successful couture house while her son studied fine art. He began his own career as a sketch artist for Patou in Paris, and emigrated to New York in 1936.

He eventually moved to California, where Paramount Pictures hired him as one of Edith Head's design assistants. After a decade in Hollywood, it was back to New York, where he was well-positioned to become one of Jackie Kennedy's favorite designers after she became First Lady. Cassini will forever be associated with Jackie and her signature pillbox, although many of his millinery designs had much greater flair than this simple design would suggest.

What a spectacular hat! A designer original by Oleg Cassini circa 1960, with a unique combination of black satin hatband and sequin-sprinkled snood. *Courtesy of: Banbury Cross Antiques.* Value: $125-175.

Lilly Daché

The daughter of a French farmer, Lilly Daché apprenticed in Paris for the famous milliners Caroline Reboux and Suzanne Talbot before striking off for America on her own. Arriving in New York City with $15.00 to her name, she tried selling hats at Macy's, but was fired for her poor English!

Through creative talent and fortuitous event, by 1938 she owned a nine-story building at 18 East 56th Street, just down the street from Hattie Carnegie. Her staff of 150 catered to a pampered clientele, who paid as much as $165 for a single hat. Equipped with gold fitting rooms for brunettes and silver for blondes, her spacious salons were famous.

Daché created hats in the 1930s and 1940s that were seen in movies, which certainly increased her fame. She capitalized on this with a "model" collection for that season. Better department stores around the country also carried her hats. A vital and charming woman, Daché was friends with society ladies and a personal milliner to many movie stars.

One of Daché's most notable contributions was the "half hat," which profiled the face from one side. For this, she won the American Designer Award in 1941. Other innovations included a visored cap for women workers during World War II and a "stand up" beret. Her floral creations involved the use of unusual varieties of flowers and little insect accents.

Lilly Daché died in 1968, and her business closed the year after. Her hats are still fairly plentiful, and a wide time span and variety of styles are available to collectors.

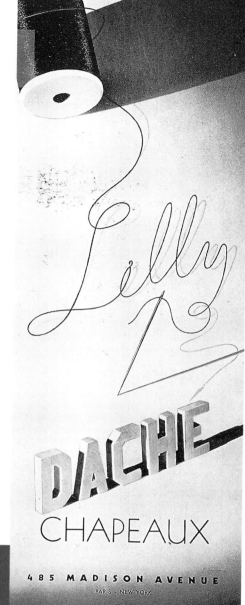

Lilly Daché advertised in *Vogue* (March 1936).

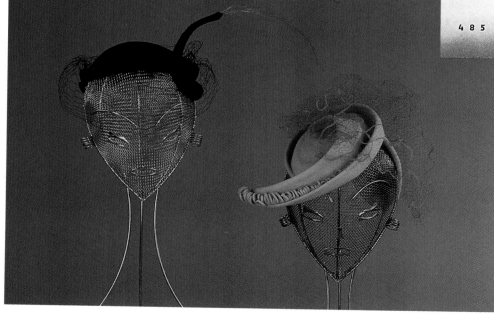

Two of Daché's original salon heads, modishly modern. They are shown wearing bandeaux which span two decades, but exhibit remarkably similar lines. Black silk twill on a buckram frame, circa 1955. Dusty pink felt on a wire rim, circa 1935. *Courtesy of (left): Maureen Reilly. Courtesy of (right): Sharon Hagerty.* Value (each): $75-125.

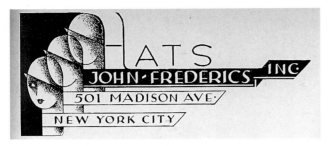

John-Frederics as seen in *Vogue* (March 1936).

John-Frederics

This millinery house operated from 1929 through 1947, formed by two partners, John Piocelle (a.k.a. Mr. John) and Frederic Hirst.

During this time, John-Frederics created hats for the studios, notably the leghorn straw cartwheel with deep velvet ribbons and the darling green bonnet that Rhett Butler brings Scarlett O'Hara from Paris in "Gone with the Wind." The team also designed the slouch hat worn by Greta Garbo, on and off the screen.

Although very successful, the partnership broke up in 1948 and Mr. John, Inc. began. Look for the John-Frederics label for a top quality addition to your collection.

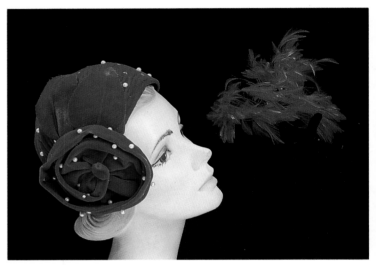

Red velvet bandeau dotted with pearls and rhinestones, from John-Frederics, Custom Made. *Courtesy of: K. Dean.* Value: $95-145.

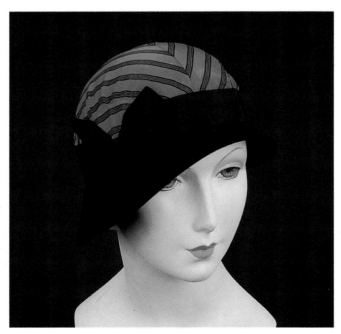

From Halston, a 1965 revival of the cloche in deep pink and black. *Courtesy of: Banbury Cross Antiques.* Value: $65-95.

Halston

Roy Halston Frowick was born in Iowa in 1932. He trained at the Chicago Art Institute, all the while designing and selling hats. Halston moved to New York City in 1957, where he worked for Lilly Daché, who allowed him to feature his own collection after only one year of apprenticeship.

Halston followed Adolfo as a leading designer at Bergdorf Goodman, renowned in the 1950s for its millinery department. In the 1960s, *Vogue* often featured hats that were "made to order by Halston at Bergdorf Goodman."

At the same time, Halston was also designing under his own label. One of his greatest advocates was Jackie Kennedy, who wore a Halston pillbox to her husband's presidential inauguration. Unfortunately, later business failures caused Halston to close his doors in 1984.

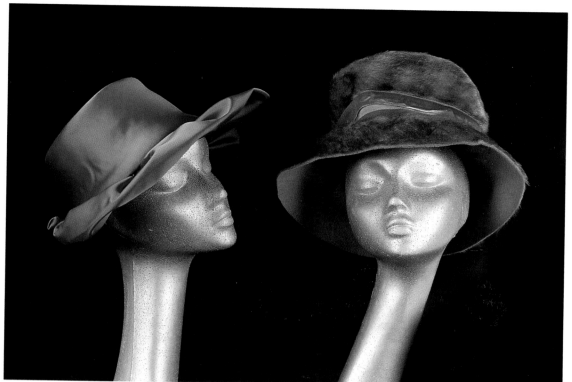

A dynamic duo, in a shako of blended turquoise and olive from Mr. John, Jr., and a satin turquoise from Mr. John Classics. These variations on the Homburg would have been worn with suits circa 1965. *Courtesy of (both): Maureen Reilly.* Value (each): $55-75.

MR. JOHN

At his peak, Mr. John produced 16,000 hats each year; however, he did not accept the decline of millinery with grace. On his retirement in 1970, Mr. John was quoted as saying: *"Women no longer have character or chic."*

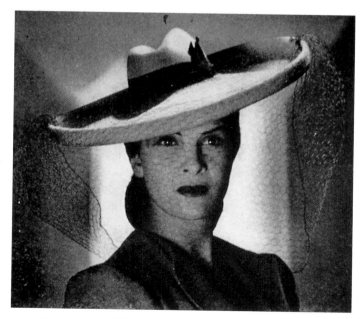

From *Harpers Bazaar* (February 1943), a Mr. John salon hat.

John Piocelle was born in 1906 in Munich, Germany. His mother was a designer of millinery, and encouraged John's natural talent. He studied fine art at the exclusive Sorbonne and Ecole des Beaux Arts in Paris.

At some point he styled himself as John P. John. He helped form the John-Frederics salon with Frederic Hirst in 1929, and also worked for many years with Adrian of Hollywood.

After the partnership with Hirst broke up in 1948, he began the Mr. John label. He became known for his outrageous and extravagant behavior, and had many celebrity clients. During the 1950s, his shop on West 57th Street was decorated in Louis XVI gilt grandeur, and he paraded in Napoleonic costume proclaiming himself a "fashion dictator."

His hats reflected this flair, but without being crude. Witty, exuberant, and sophisticated, his designs were wildly popular. In his early years with Hirst, he helped pioneer the doll hat and the feminized Stetson. As Mr. John, he specialized in huge floral creations and fur "chechias."

FRANK OLIVE

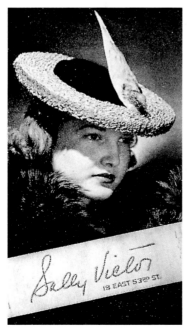

Following training in art and fashion in Milwaukee and Chicago, Frank Olive went on to design stage costumes in San Francisco. He later worked as a custom hat designer at Tatiana, Saks Fifth Avenue, and Emme.

He opened his own boutique in Greenwich Village and became particularly well known for his millinery designs. Olive's talent ensured the financial survival of his business, at a time when other hatmakers were floundering.

Olive died just a year ago, and his hats are a particularly good investment for the collector. Look for three labels: Frank Olive Original (salon); Frank's Girl (bridge); and Counterfits (mass-market).

A pair of red felt cloches from Frank Olive Original, left, and Frank's Girl, right. The quality of fabric and trim differs, but the style is almost identical! *Courtesy of (both): Banbury Cross Antiques.* Value (left): $75-125. Value (right): $45-75.

Sally Victor

There is a real Sally behind this label—joining her first name with that of her husband, Victor. She was born in Scranton, Pennsylvania, and in the mid-1920s she worked as a buyer of millinery for R.H. Macy's. She married the owner of a wholesale millinery house, Victor Serges, and designed hats for him until 1934 when she began using the Sally Victor label.

She found a niche market by producing fine quality, stylish hats for the vast middle class at affordable prices. It was a very successful formula through the 1960s. Look for Sally Victor, along with her bridge lines, Miss Sally Victor, Sally V, and Sally Victor Headlines.

Sally Victor in *Vogue* (April 1937).

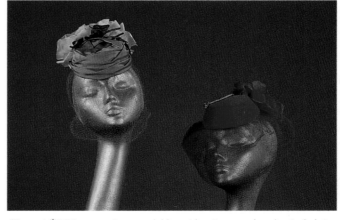

Two satin doll hats, one in peacock blue with twin roses, the other in fuchsia with cabbage rose. Both feature sprightly demi-veils, from Miss Sally Victor. *Courtesy of (both): Banbury Cross Antiques.* Value (each): $75-125.

No book on hats would be complete without a tribute to the French designers, who provided so much inspiration to the world of fashion.

Agnés

A famous French millinery designer of the 1920s and 1930s, Agnés was a friend of artists, and was herself a sculptress and fancier of the avant garde. She was one of the first to show turbans, work with zig-zag and abstract patterns, and use the new material, cellophane. Agnés hats were often featured in *Vogue* and *Harper's Bazaar* in the 1930s and 1940s.

The Agnés (pronounced Ahn-yeah) label can be found with diligent searching, as her line was imported in America and sold in better department stores.

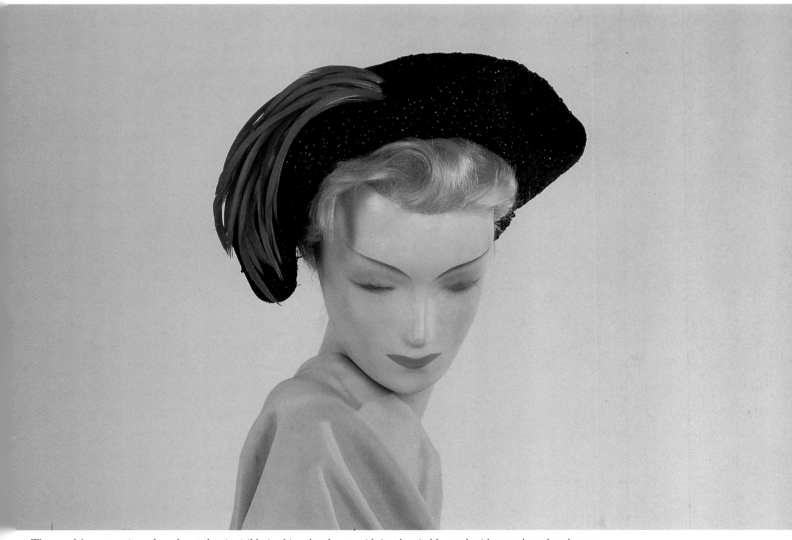

The careful construction of an Agnés hat is visible in this velvet beret, with its electric blue embroidery and scarlet plumage. *Courtesy of: Maureen Reilly.* Value: $150-225.

Cristobal Balenciaga

A Spaniard by birth, Cristobal Balenciaga was sponsored by a marquesa, who sent him to Paris at age thirteen to study design. Some twenty years later, in 1937, he had a salon on Rue George V. and had become one of the greatest couturiers of all time.

Balenciaga was known to have personally designed all the hats that appeared in his collections. A master of innovation and a perfectionist of style, he would use extremes of scale in his millinery. Hats were either head-hugging or gigantic, but always designed to compliment the proportions of dress. Balenciaga retired in 1968.

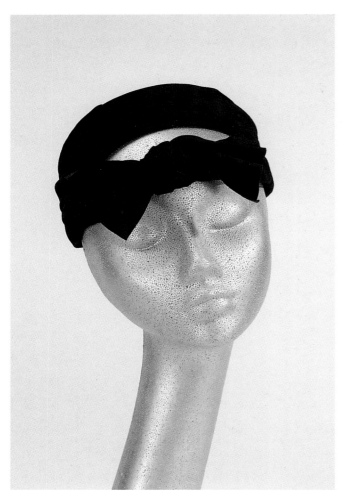

A head-hugging cap with peek-a-boo bow, this elegant slice of black suede is from the couture salon of Cristobal Balenciaga, circa 1950. *Courtesy of: The Way We Wore.* Value: $200-300.

Coco Chanel

The great Coco Chanel began in Paris as a milliner before moving into couture. She was born into the peasant class as Gabrielle, but her talent and spunk are perhaps better stated in her nickname "Coco."

Coco opened Chanel Modes at 21 Rue Cambon in 1920, financially sponsored by her lover of the time. Her hats, such as the straw boater, caused a sensation. They were pure in line and relatively unadorned as compared to the opulent millinery of the time.

Chanel made an early mark on couture by the use of simple, menswear-inspired styles and fabrics. Known for her wry humor, she once decreed:

> "A woman's education consists of two lessons: never to leave the house without stockings, never to go out without a hat."

After World War I, Chanel flourished in her re-opened shop and went on to lead a creative, adventuresome, and glamorous life. Coco enjoyed a large revival of popularity during the 1950s. The House of Chanel continues to thrive today under talented couturier Karl Lagerfeld.

The Chanel label is not easily found in this country. Count yourself fortunate should you own one of her hats.

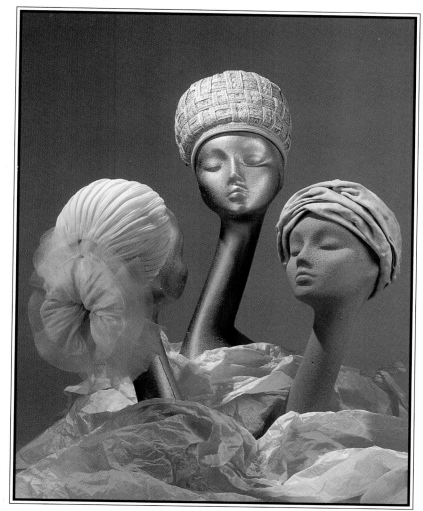

A trio of turbans from Dior, including a Miss Dior with sprightly chiffon chou, center. *Courtesy of (left): Sandra Lagario. Courtesy of (rest): Banbury Cross Antiques.* Value (each): $75-125.

Christian DIOR

The famous couturier Christian Dior was born into a privileged French family, but found himself destitute during the Depression of the 1930s. While recuperating from an illness during this time, he learned tapestry weaving, which fostered his yearning to create.

He sold hats for the milliner Agnés, and was later hired by Piquet as a designer. His most successful designs in these early years were his hats. Following military service during World War II, Dior worked for Lucien Lelong until 1946—when, with the aid of a wealthy sponsor, he opened his own couture house and became an immediate success.

Dior launched his New Look in 1947, a sensational change from the previous decade. Wasp-waisted skirts, full or pencil-slim, were paired with fabulous hats. These were either small and fitted, or graceful and wide-brimmed.

Dior made all final choices but his millinery was actually created by Maud Roser. This talented lady was famous for a series of small hats, called *Les Toits des Paris*. She also pioneered the showing of hat collections before clothing at the Paris showrooms, claiming equal importance.

Dior chapeaux were sold at all better department stores, and seem particularly plentiful in styles from the late 1950s and 1960s.

Nina Ricci

As a young child in France during the 1880s, Nina Ricci made hats and clothing for her dolls. At the age of thirteen, she was apprenticed to a couturier, and by the time she turned eighteen she was the head designer. Over the next few years, she had advanced to the position of premiere.

Ricci opened her own house in 1932. She was known for feminine, rather than trend-setting, styles. In 1945, her son took over the company's management, and continued producing hats and clothing throughout the 1960s.

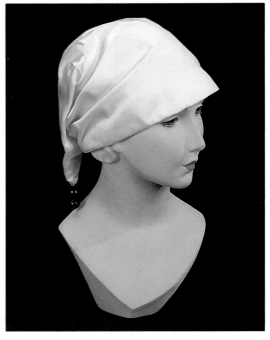

With a nod to the classical Liripipe, a Nina Ricci design in ivory peau de soie. The pointed hood ends in a pert bead. *Courtesy of: The Way We Wore.* Value: $150-225.

Paris of 1920 found Elsa Schiaparelli estranged from her husband, penniless, and with a young daughter to raise. During this time, she designed and wore a sweater which by chance was seen by a prominent Parisian clothing retailer.

He commissioned her design, and so she gained entrance into the fashion industry. Once she acquired experience, given her innate creativity and dramatic flair, she achieved huge success. When the actress Ina Claire wore her mad cap—a knit tube that could be twisted into any shape—it became an overnight sensation.

By 1930, Schiap employed 2,000 people in twenty-six showrooms. She became involved with the Parisian art world and collaborated with Salvador Dali to create surrealistic designs. Outlandish, witty, wonderful hats were the order of this day—including her famous shoe, lambchop, and inkpot hats. The shape of these hats showed to best advantage in black. As her style matured, her palette brightened. Soon, Schiaparelli's signature was boldly written in color, à la Shocking Pink.

Schiaparelli pioneered the use of synthetic fabrics, and used stretchy Lastex in hatmaking. She possessed a form of courage and self-confidence which was reflected in her designs. While maintaining a basic harmony of proportion and color, Schiap added that dash of the unexpected that caused heads to turn and people to talk. The madder the hat, the smarter it was!

She discontinued her business in 1954, but continued as a consultant to the many companies that were manufacturing and marketing perfumes, hosiery, and scarves using her name. Collectors should look for the Schiaparelli label, along with the Shocking Pink hatboxes that bear her signature.

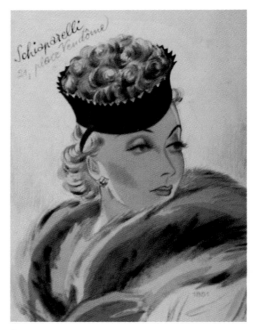

Schiap's witty tilt hat from the cover of *Chapeaux Modernes*, a fashion folio published in 1939. It resembles a crimp-edged porkpie, with a surprise filling of bright sugarplums.

Elsa Schiaparelli

YVES ST. LAURENT

Yves St. Laurent was born to a wealthy family in Algeria in 1936. He studied art in Paris until, at the age of nineteen, he was hired by Dior. St. Laurent was hailed as a "boy wonder" when he succeeded the great man as head designer for the House of Dior in 1957. His first success was the "trapeze" dress from the 1958 collection.

Known for simple, elegant, and wearable styles, he went on to open his own house in 1962. Not one to rest on his laurels, St. Laurent achieved great success. The costume institute of the Museum of Modern Art in New York did a retrospective of twenty-five years' of his work in 1983—a first for a living designer.

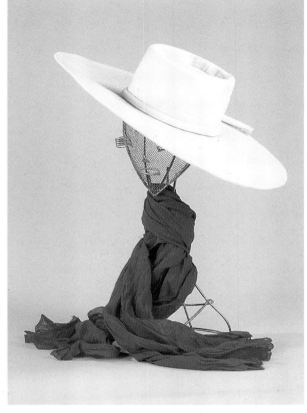

Simplicity in white felt, with trapunto stitching on the oversized brim. This cartwheel bears the Yves St. Laurent label, circa 1965. *Courtesy of: Maureen Reilly.* Value: $75-125.

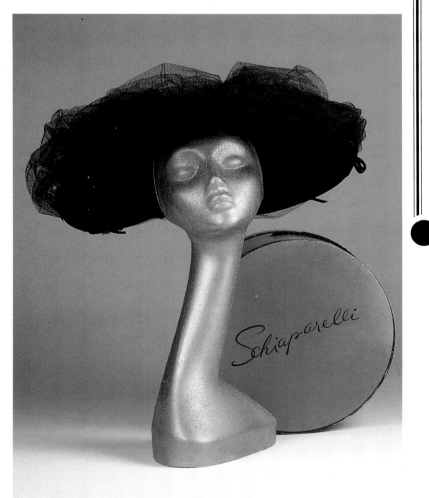

The Schiaparelli label is so highly prized that collectors must be wary of fakes. The crown of this hat bears the coveted label, but it was cut onto a different brim. However, little skill was employed in stitching the two forms, indicating this was not a fraud but just the prior owner's effort to remake a favorite hat. *Courtesy of (both): Lisa Carson.* Value (hat): $75-125. Value (box): $50-75.

Labels to Look For

We list here the labels of the milliners and hat companies that appear in many of the best hats featured in this book. These names are also prominent in advertisements and articles in vintage issues of *Vogue*, *Harper's Bazaar*, and other fashion magazines from about 1930 to 1970.

Some of these labels repeat those of the designers we profiled above, but they are included for ease of reference. We included some expatriates with their adopted country, both on the American and French sides. Here are the "labels to look for," listed in alphabetical order by first name or word:

American Designers & Millinery Cos.

Adolfo
Adrian
Alexander Hats
Alfreda
Alice May
Alma Original
American Modes, Ca.
Archie Eason
Bagatelle
Banner Millinery
Betty Co-Ed
Bernice Charles

Carmel Model
Casper Davis
Chalfonte
Chanda
Chanté
Clover Land
Coralie
Christine Original
Dachettes
Darby

Dayne
Dece Original
Delle Donne, N.Y.
Del Marie Models
Dobbs Hats
Don Anderson
Dorée

DuBarry-French Adaptations
Dunlap
Earl R. Lindberg, Co.
Elenora Barnett, S.F.
Elinor's, S.F.
Emme
Emme Boutique

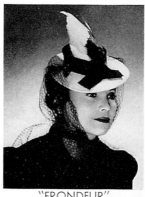

Bernice Charles charmer, as seen in *Vogue* (March 1939).

Bird-Speakman, Inc.
Boyer Originals
Brandt
Brewster
Carolyn Kelsey

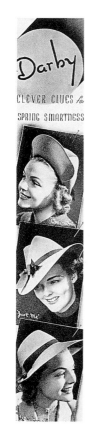

A Darby hat advertised in *Harper's Bazaar* (February 1939).

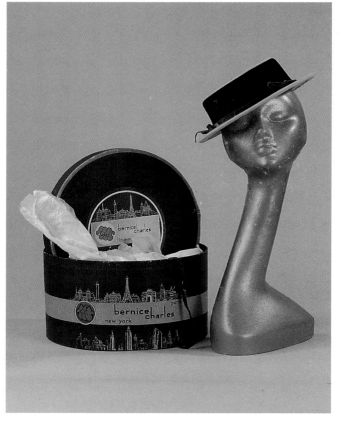

From the salon of Bernice Charles, a jaunty felt boater circa 1945, with its original hatbox. *Courtesy of (both): Maureen Reilly.* Value (hat): $55-75. Value (box): $25-45.

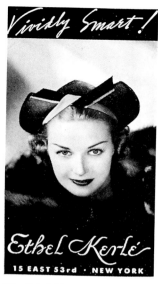

Vividly Smart!

Ethel Kerlé
15 EAST 53rd · NEW YORK

The Ethel Ker-lé label in a *Vogue* advertisement (April 1937).

Ethel Kerle
Eurora
Eva Mae
Eve Nouvelle, N.Y.
Evelyn Varon-Model
Fanny & Hilda

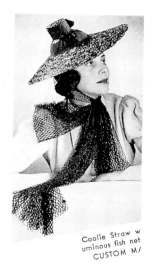

Coolie Straw w
uminous fish net
CUSTOM MA

Fanny and Hild
Madison Ave. at 52nd St.,

An ad for Fanny & Hilda in *Harper's Bazaar* (February 1939).

Fannye's
Felix-Autographed Original
Frank Olive

Frank's Girl
Florence Reichman

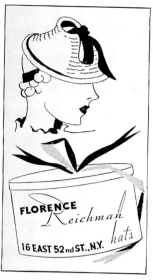

FLORENCE
Reichman hats
16 EAST 52nd ST., N.Y.

Flo Reichmann shows her latest look in *Vogue* (April 1936).

Gage
George Mander's Hats
G. Howard Hodge
Gertrude Menczer
Gladys & Belle

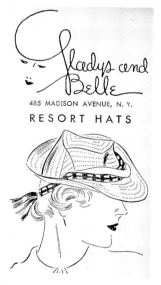

Gladys and Belle
485 MADISON AVENUE, N.Y.
RESORT HATS

Gladys & Belle as shown in *Harper's Bazaar* (January 1937).

Halston
Harry on Hats
Hats by Louis
Hattie Carnegie
Hatnegie

Heather
Henry G. Ross
Howitt
Hy-Class Hats, Ca.
Irene of New York
Jack McConnell
Janet

Jay Thorpe
Jean King
Jeanne Tête
J. Hudson Co.
John-Frederics
John Hogan
Knox

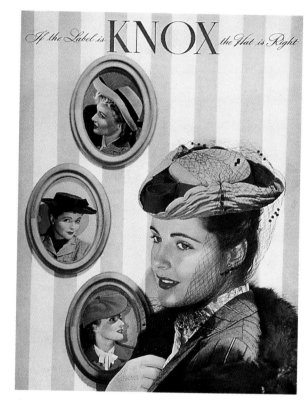

If the Label is KNOX the Hat is Right

A prominent Knox ad in *Harper's Bazaar* (February 1943).

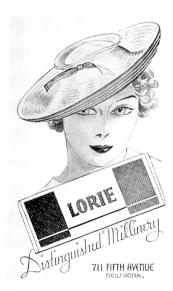

LORIE
Distinguished Millinery
711 FIFTH AVENUE
NEW YORK.

Lorie beckons in *Vogue* (April 1936).

La Mode Chez Tappé
Leighton
Lady Stetson
Lazarus
Leslie James
Lilli of Calif.
Lilith-Paris, N.Y.
Lilly Daché
Lilly Daché Debs
Lilly's Dillys
Lion, San Diego
Lori
Louis Miller
Lydia
Mack III
Madcap—Paris, N.Y.
Mademoiselle

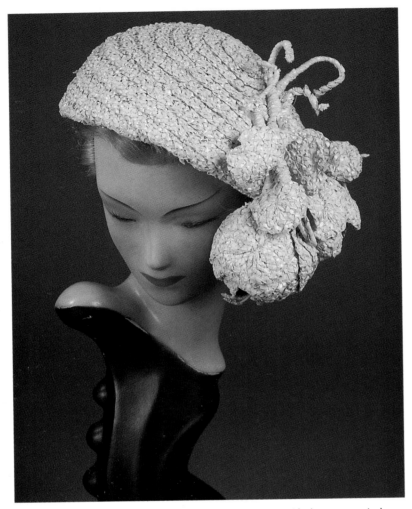

A fabulous hat from Lilly Daché, all in rough ivory straw, with the asymmetrical styling was her signature in the 1930s. *Courtesy of: Barbara Griggs Vintage Fashion.* Value: $95-145.

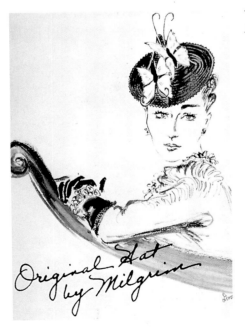

Original Hat by Milgrim

The Milgrim line, seen in *Harper's Bazaar* (February 1939).

Maisôn Mendesolle
Marion Vallé Original
Marché Hats
Martha Gene, N.Y.
Maurice L. Rothschild
Midfield
Midinette
Milgrim
Miramar Hats, Hollywood
Miss Sally Victor
Miss Dior
Miss Eileen

Mitzie's Hats, L.A.
Mme. Pauline
Monte Rey of Calif.
Molli
Mr. Almo
Mr. Arnold
Mr. D
Mr. Dave
Mr. John
Mr. John, Jr.
Mr. John Classics
Ms. Andree by Bellini
Nan Duskin
Nell, N.Y.
Nettie Rosenstein
New Era
New York Creation
Noreen
Oleg Cassini
Original by Sherman
Paramount Originals
Paris Maid
Patrice
Pauline
Rafield
Rickie Original
Rilla Marie
Robinaire
Rose Hagan
Rose Saphire
Rubin
Rumar Hats
Sally V
Sally Victor
Skol Nips
Sonni
Stetson
Studio Styles -Warner Bros.
Sunset Hats, L.A.
Suzanne
Suzi of Calif.
Thornton Hats
Trêt-Moulin
Trimble
Tulip Model, S.F.
Velda Original
Veola-Model
Vivian, Calif.
Vogue Company, L.A.
Woodmere, N.Y.
Wm. Silverman

French Designers & Millinery Cos.

Agnés

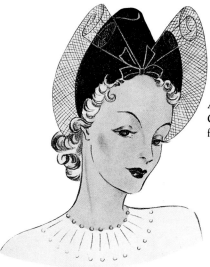

An Agnés beauty as sketched in *Chapeaux Modernes*, a French fashion folio published in 1936.

Gaby Mono
Hubert de Givenchy
Jacques Fath
Jane Blanchot
Janine Lacroix
Jean Barthet
Jean Patou
Jeanne Lanvin
Jeanne La Marechal
Lanvin Castillo
Laroche

Legroux Soeurs
Louise Bourbon
Lucien Lelong
Madeleine Vionnet
Maggy Rouff
Mainbocher
Marcel Rochas
Maria Guy

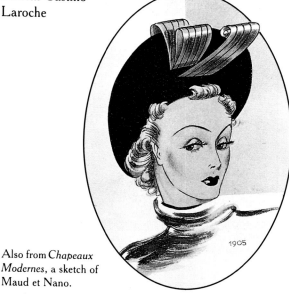

Also from *Chapeaux Modernes*, a sketch of Maud et Nano.

Albouy
Alix Grés.
Anne-Marie
Balenciaga
Balmain
Camille Andree
Camille Roger
Cardin
Caroline Reboux

Chanel
Courregès
Charlotte Bonneville
Claude Saint-Cyr
Denis
Eneley Soeurs
Gabrielle
Germaine Page
Gilbert Orcel

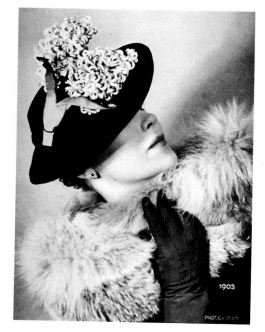

Gilbert Orcel as seen in *Chapeaux Modernes*.

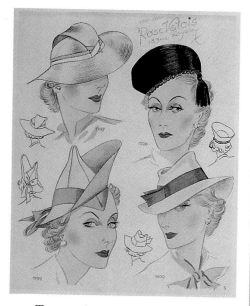

Two sets of original millinery sketches from the Parisian salons of Jean Patou and Rose Valois, from their 1930s showrooms.

Maud et Nano
Molyneux
Paulette
Paul Poirot
Rose Descat
Rose Valois

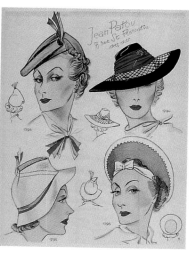

Schiaparelli

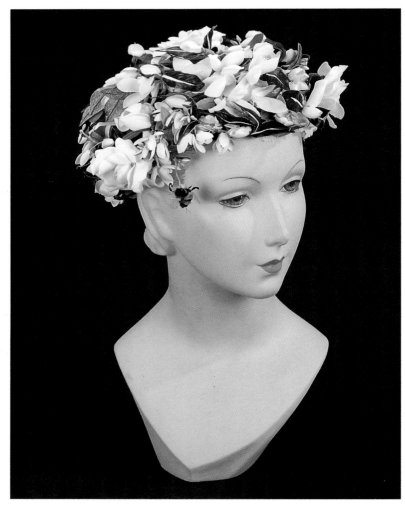

A cap of sweet magnolias attract attention, and a bumblebee, too. By Schiaparelli, circa 1950. *Courtesy of: The Way We Wore.* Value: $150-225.

Suzanne Farnier
Suzanne Moulin

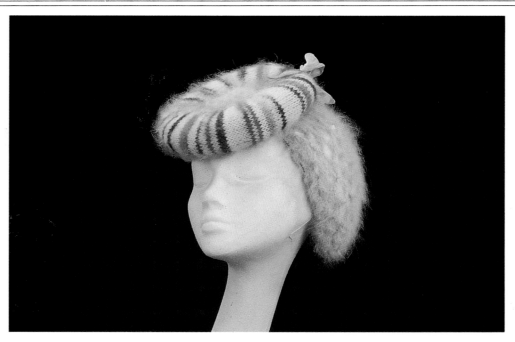

Powder-puff angora in eyeshadow colors. This snood is just right to snuggle a pageboy hairdo. Label: Suzanne Moulin, Paris. *Courtesy of: The Way We Wore.* Value: $175-250.

Suzanne Talbot
Suzy
Svend
Victoria Crosnier
Worth

Paris asks...

"Have you seen the hats made by 'Victoria Crosnier'? Paris asks, too. She did the hats for the French production of 'Cyrano de Bergerac,'—so successfully, many women in the audience wanted them copied." Vogue, March 1939.

Bridge Lines

In the 1950s, presaging a practice that is common today in the couture, some American milliners created lower-priced "bridge lines," geared to a youthful market. This is a bit confusing at first, especially since the difference in quality and design is sometimes barely discernible between bridge line and salon label. The prolific Lilly Daché marketed three bridge lines: Dachéttes, Lilly Daché Debs, and Lilly's Dillys. Other bridge lines include: Miss Sally Victor and Sally V (by Sally Victor); Frank's Girl (by Frank Olive); Adolfo II (by Adolfo); Emme Boutique (from Emme).

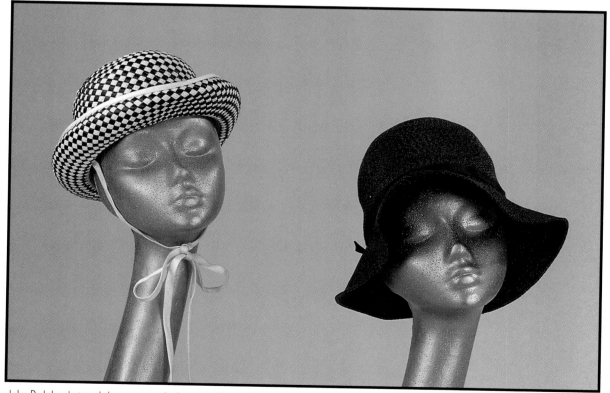

John P. John designed these navy and white straw hats in the 1960s. The Breton with chin strap is from his bridge line, Mr. John, Jr. (Another bridge line was Mr. John Classics.) The floppy-brimed Pamela is from his salon label, Mr. John. *Courtesy of (both): Maureen Reilly.* Value (each): $55-75.

The Department Stores

Not all collectible labels are from the couture. Many department stores had their own millinery salons, as shown in a custom silk label. The designer's name may also be featured. Such "twin labels" indicate that a hat was well-made, and costly in its day.

Some department stores specialized in custom millinery. For example, Milgrim's offered hats by Sally Milgrim in the 1920s, and for many years thereafter. Adolfo designed for Bergdorf Goodman, as did Halston. In the mid-1960s, *Vogue* often featured hats "made to order by Halston at Bergdorf Goodman."

Most of the stores listed below are headquartered in New York City. We do not know if they all had millinery salons, but if you find one of their names in a hat label, you can be assured of quality.

Arnold Constable
B. Altman
Barney's
Bergdorf Goodman
Best & Co.
Bloomingdale's
Bonwit Teller
Burdine's
Carson Prairie Scott
City of Paris
Dayton's
Fortnum & Mason
Franklin Simon
Frederick & Nelson
Frost Bros.

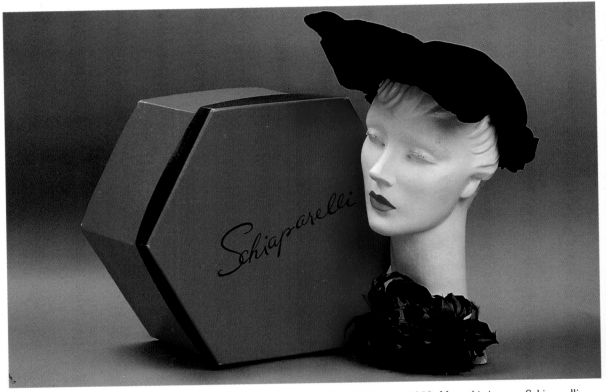

Black silk velvet crushes onto a wired "duckbill" brim. From Barney's-New York, circa 1939. Note, this is not a Schiaparelli; the hatbox is separate. *Courtesy of (both): Banbury Cross Antiques.* Value (hat): $75-125. Value (box): $45-65.

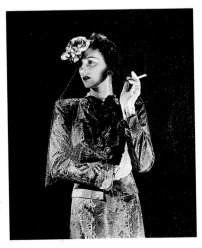

An advertisement for Bergdorf's in *Vogue* (March 1939).

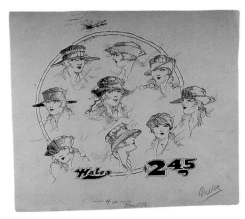

Hale's department store ad for hats circa 1920.

46

Gump's
Hale's
Harzfeld's
Henri Bendel
Hudson's
I. Magnin
J. Magnin
Jay-Thorpe
Julius Garfinkle
Kaufmann's
Livingston Bros.
Lord & Taylor
Macy's
Marshall Field & Co.
Montaldo's
Neiman Marcus
Peck & Peck
Ransohoff's
Regina & Rudolph
Robinson's of Calif.
Roos Atkins
Roos Bros.
Rich's
Russek's
Saks Fifth Ave.
W&J Sloane
Wanamaker
White House

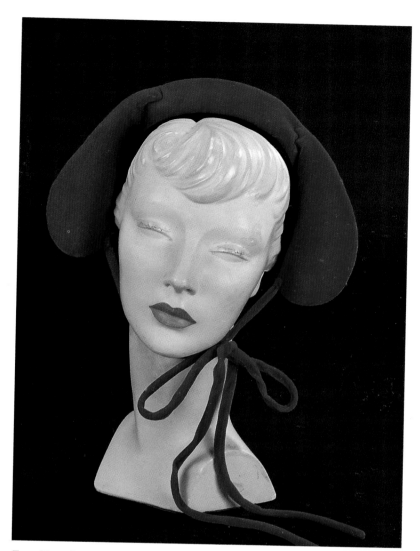

From Henri Bendel, a 1930s Dutchgirl in velvet tied under the chin, charmingly true to its ingenue origins. *Courtesy of: Banbury Cross Antiques.* Value: $75-125.

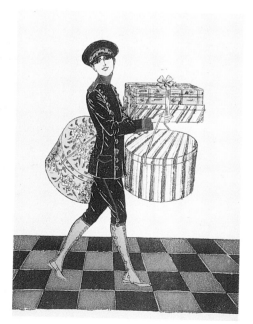

A jaunty bellhop invites the ladies to an exhibition of "French Model Hats" at Livingston Brothers department store in 1924.

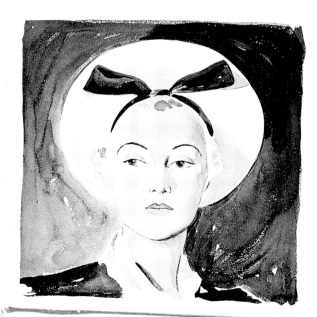

Wanamaker ran this ad in *Vogue* (March 1936).

Meet the Models

We hope you enjoy looking at our wonderful mannequin heads as much as we did photographing them! These beautiful young ladies each seemed to have a distinct personality, which we tried to show to its best advantage. You are seeing a lot of them throughout the book, and we'd like you to meet them now.

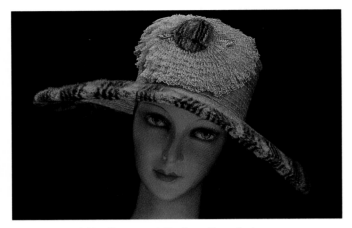

Paulette, c. 1930s. *Courtesy of: Banbury Cross Antiques.*

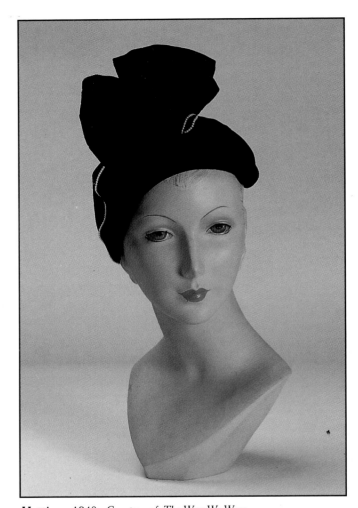

Hattie, c. 1940s. *Courtesy of: The Way We Wore.*

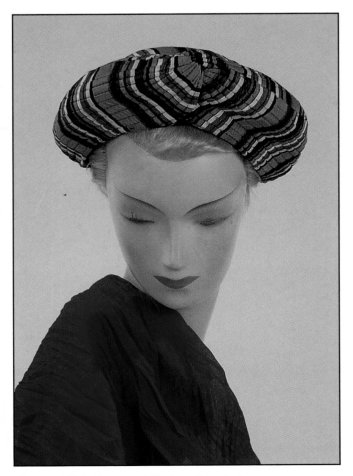

Coco, c. 1930s. *Courtesy of: Banbury Cross Antiques.*

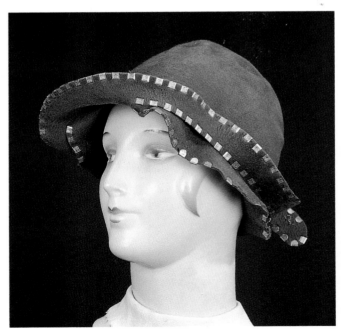

Agnés, c. 1930s. *Courtesy of: The Way We Wore.*

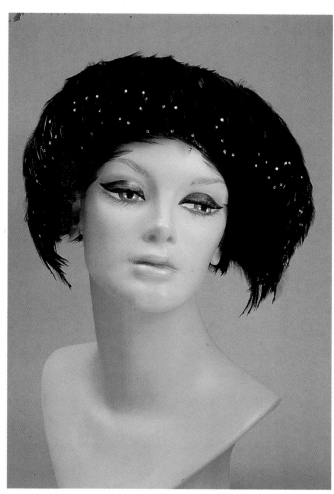

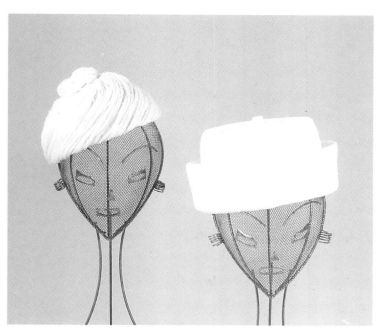

Lilly & Dilly, c. 1940s. *Courtesy of: Sharon Hagerty.*

Sally, c. 1960s. *Courtesy of: Banbury Cross Antiques.*

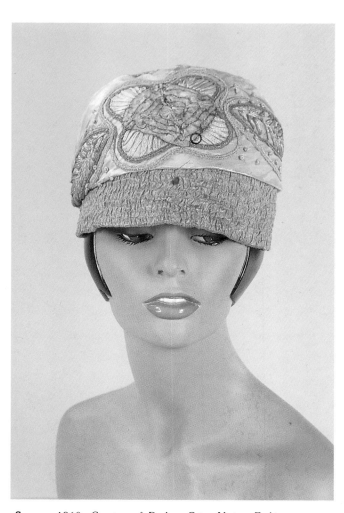

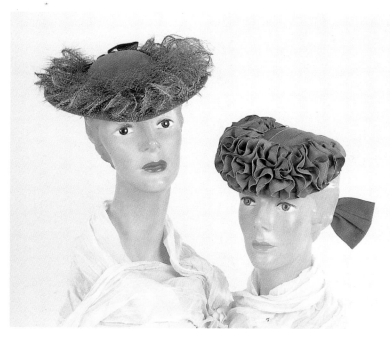

Fanny & Hilda, c. 1940s. *Courtesy of: Rich Man, Poor Man.*

Suzy, c. 1960s. *Courtesy of: Barbara Griggs Vintage Fashion.*

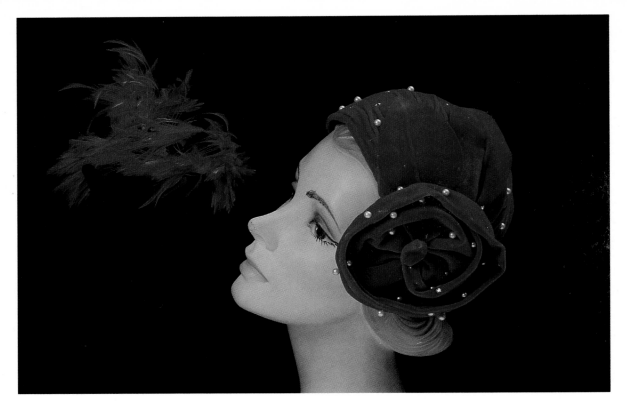

Elsa, c. 1940s. *Courtesy of: Banbury Cross Antiques.*

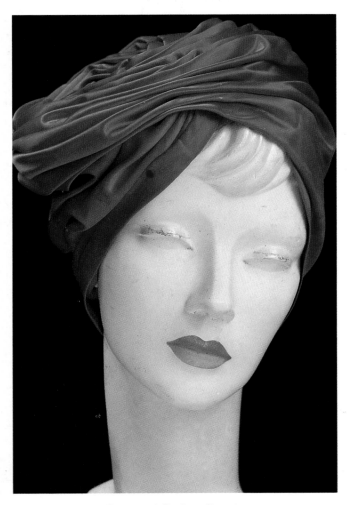

Caroline, c. 1950. *Courtesy of: Banbury Cross Antiques.*

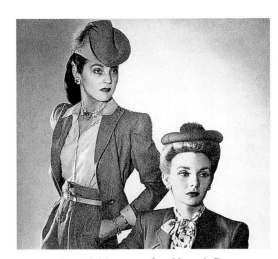

A sporty duo at I. Magnin & Co., *Harper's Bazaar* (February 1943).

Mannequin heads such as these are difficult to find, and must be valued accordingly. If the heads have a prestigious provenance, such as Lilly & Dilly which are from Daché's New York salon, then values will escalate. Some heads are so lifelike—each with a different look or expression—that their valuation must also depend on "beauty in the eye of the beholder." Given these variables, we have assigned a fairly broad price range of $150 to $500 per mannequin.

V. Victorian Innovations

The long reign of Queen Victoria, from her coronation in 1838 to her death in 1901, was a time of great growth and development in the western world. Prosperity followed, giving disposable income and leisure time to an emerging middle class.

Leisure time or not, the Victorians were not predisposed to folly. Even when pursuing a sport or hobby, their society decreed strict rules of decorum and dress. As a result, the collector will find all manner of millinery, classifiable by social status and function.

During the mid-1800s, the bonnet was relieved only by the Pamela and porkpie, with an occasional capote. The latter two styles were especially versatile for daytime wear. They were both petite and brimless, although the porkpie had a boxier crown. Both could be trimmed with feathers, flowers, and ribbons.

The bonnet continued to dominate women's headgear throughout Victoria's reign. The crowns were routinely shallow, but the brims scaled up or down, as necessary to balance the width of hooped skirts and bustles.

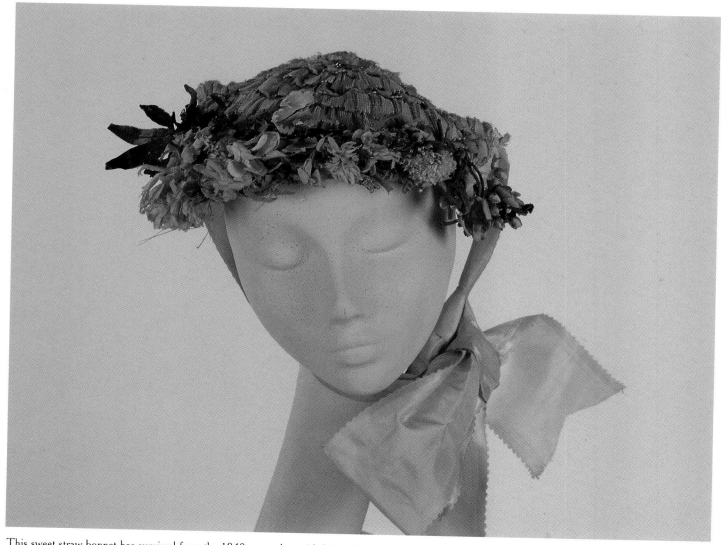

This sweet straw bonnet has survived from the 1840s, complete with fabric flowers and silk bow. Charming and simple, it is a style that would have been favored by a young, perhaps flirtatious, woman. *Courtesy of: Banbury Cross Antiques.* Value: $200-300.

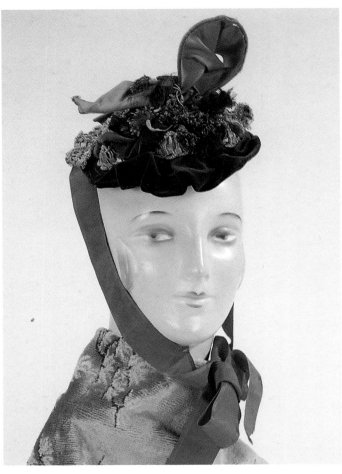

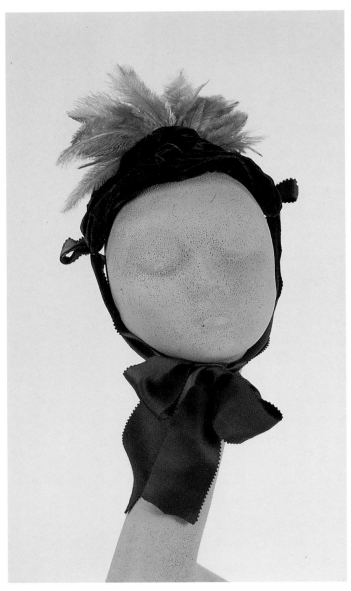

This little brown bonnet boasts a deep-peach bow of wired ribbon, perched atop Autumn foliage. *Courtesy of: Mary Aaron Museum.* Value: Special.

A velvet bonnet circa 1865, with a softly-shaded spray of feathers. It is untrimmed in back, and most likely was designed to perch atop a large chignon. *Courtesy of: Maureen Reilly.* Value: $125-175.

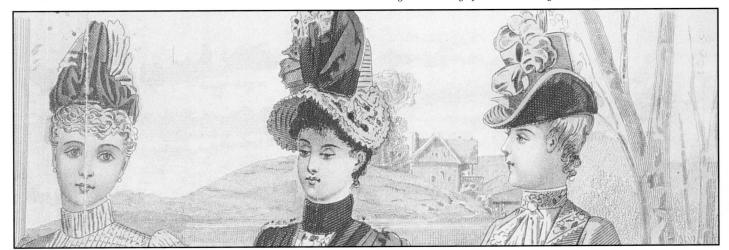

Three city hats from 1888, as pictured in *Peterson's Magazine.* The style on the far left is a petite, cocked-brim cavalier, gay with plumage. The other two are bonnets, featuring upswept crowns à la Fontanges.

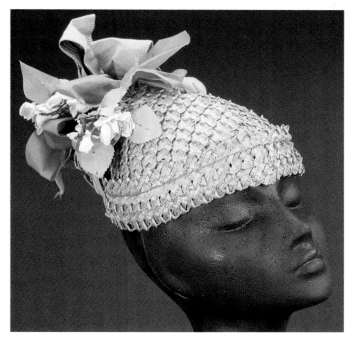

A capote in sunshine-yellow straw, with a ruche of velvet flowers at the back, circa 1870. It would have been tilted forward, to show off a large chignon. *Courtesy of: The Way We Wore.* Value: $200-300.

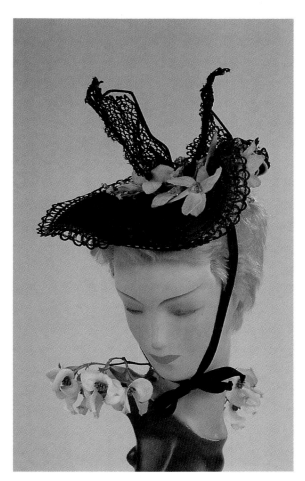

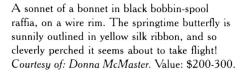

A sonnet of a bonnet in black bobbin-spool raffia, on a wire rim. The springtime butterfly is sunnily outlined in yellow silk ribbon, and so cleverly perched it seems about to take flight! *Courtesy of: Donna McMaster.* Value: $200-300.

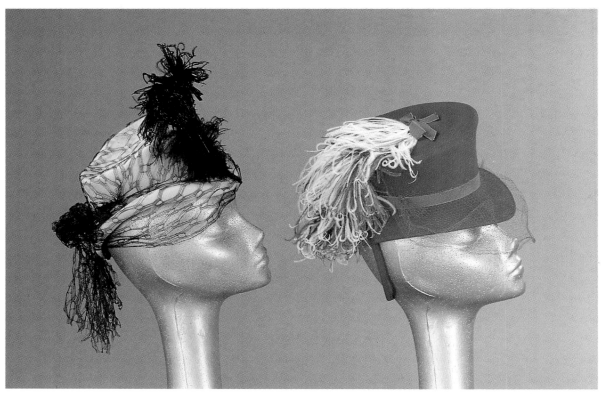

Women's hats have been inspired by the glamour of riding kit for centuries. These are revivals from the 1940s, as shown by the rear "hoops" that tilt them forward. *Courtesy of (both): 57th Street Antiques.* Value (each): $45-65.

Then as now, fashion magazines showed an exaggerated ideal of sartorial elegance, the better to promote clothing and accessories. They could promote silk and satin all they liked, however, the average woman would most likely have chosen a simple straw boater for country outings. Especially in America, women adapted the newest look of each season to suit their everyday needs.

In the 1890s, society women adapted the derby from riding kit for their afternoon carriage calls. It was generally styled in felt, and worn with a veil that extended around the hatband and trailed in back. By anecdote, the derby was all the more desirable for having been worn by the courtesan "Skittles" during her afternoon carriage rides in London's Rotten Row.

Victorian bonnets, and the later broad-brimmed Edwardian hats, were pinned securely to a lady's bouffant hairdo with hatpins. The hatpins were so elaborate, they must be considered as another form of jewelry. Indeed, the finest were later dismantled so the stones could be remounted in pendants and brooches.

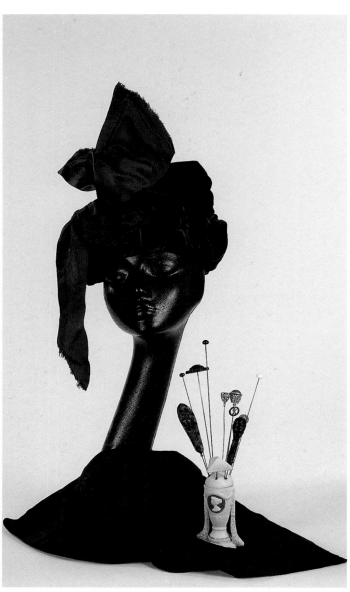

Jewel-like hatpins would undoubtedly have secured this velvet bonnet. The large self-ribbons are wired in the manner of French ribbon, and may have extended like plumage at one time. *Courtesy of: Banbury Cross Antiques.* Value: $150-200.

Good Housekeeping promised "tips on recreation" in June 1910. Featured on the cover, a traveling hat of straw with a spray of malines and peacock feathers. The large veil would have secured it from the stiff breezes caused by motorized travel. Although this hat is Edwardian, similar broad-brimmed styles were worn for traveling in the late Victorian era.

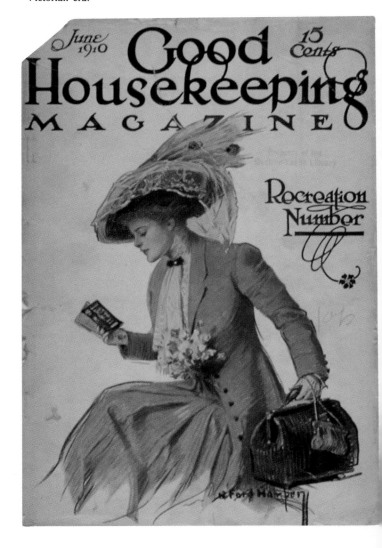

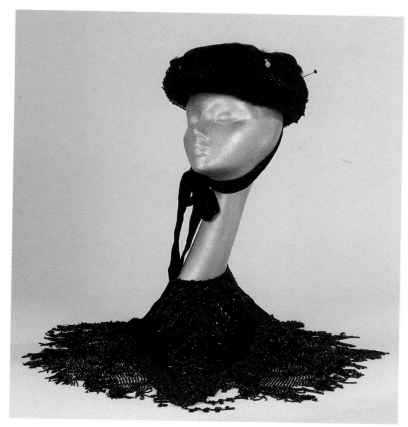

A black bonnet trimmed with tulle and dripping with jet. This wire-framed style would have perched squarely on the head, with the ribbons drawn forward under the chin. *Courtesy of: Lisa Carson.* Value: $150-200.

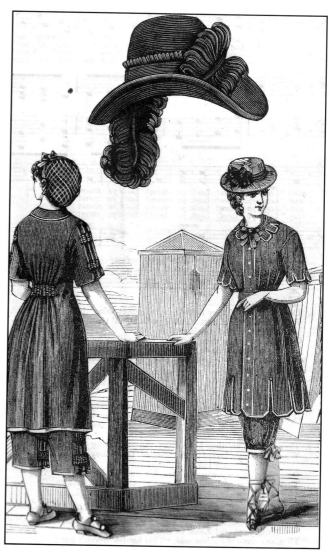

Women wore hats as part of any public outing, even at the shore. This 1883 fashion illustration from *Peterson's Magazine* shows bathing costumes worn with a snood and a boater.

Less elaborate hatpins, of the type women saved their "pin money" to purchase, have survived in greater numbers. Hatpins were worn two or three at a time, and were kept handy on the dressing table in special holders.

The average Victorian woman did not have a profession, although she might have worked outside the home in a shop, factory, or school, as dictated by financial circumstance. Of course, the working woman could not afford custom hats, and so resorted to home millinery.

Hat shapes in straw, buckram, or esparta were produced in factories and sold in special emporiums or by mail-order. They also sold all the trimmings in the form of ribbons, feathers, wax, and glass fruit, silk, and velvet flowers. The factory-made forms were considered a great time-saver. Before they were readily available, the wire frame had to be fashioned from scratch, or the straw form hand-sewn into the desired shape.

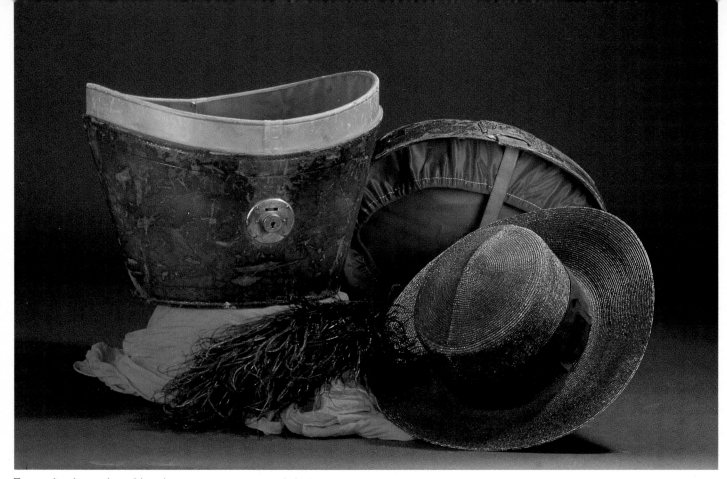

For traveling by coach, and later by motorcar, a custom-made leather bandbox. The circa 1880 box is shown with a country straw Pamela from the 1890s. *Courtesy of: (hat) Sandra Headly, (box) Banbury Cross Antiques.* Value (box): $95-145. Value (hat): $75-125.

Women were encouraged to exercise their artistic talents in their millinery projects. A magazine article in *Ehlrich's Fashion Quarterly* for Spring 1879 advised its readers "to devote some time to practice (as in) pinning the trimmings instead of sewing them, and noting the effect." Trim was often salvaged from one year's hat and used for the next. From the same article on "How to Trim a Hat": "A bit of lace, or a few ribbons,...and may be made to do service repeatedly for successive trimmings."

For the first time in history, the populace had leisure time to pursue sports and other outdoor pleasures. This caused a demand for casual hat styles, resourcefully satisfied by both men and women via a trip to the haberdasher. A man's straw boater was adapted by the ladies for bathing and boating; the jaunty tam o'shanter, for bicycling and golfing. For motorcar enthusiasts, hats were tightly swathed in veils, or replaced altogether by close-fitting hoods.

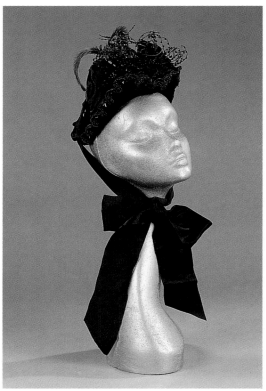

This simple bonnet may have been the product of a home milliner. It is fashioned on a wire frame, patterns for which were printed in women's magazines of the 1800s. *Courtesy of: Mary Aaron Museum.* Value: Special.

In the winter, the Victorian mother might snug a knit cap under her toddler's chin, and put a velvet tam o'shanter on the heads of older siblings. In warm weather, children wore merry straw sunbonnets and boaters.

The Victorians romanticized childhood, and the nurseries of the well-to-do were stocked with marvelous toys. However, children were expected to behave with decorum in public. On outings, they were dressed rather stiffly, like miniature adults. Girls wore smaller versions of their mother's bonnets, complete to the last ruffle and ribbon. Their brothers were outfitted as sailors or soldiers, with caps to match.

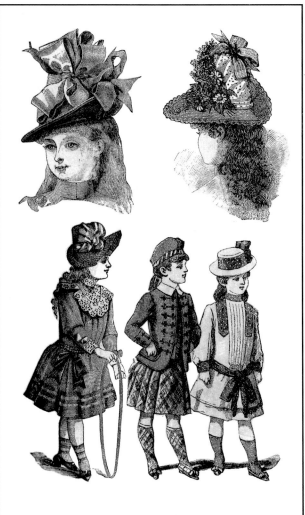

It is often difficult to tell if a Victorian hat was meant to be worn by a child or adult. This sketch from *Peterson's Magazine* in 1888 shows that grown-up styles were deemed suitable for little girls. Note the Scottish Highlander cap, of the costume variety regularly worn by little boys of that era.

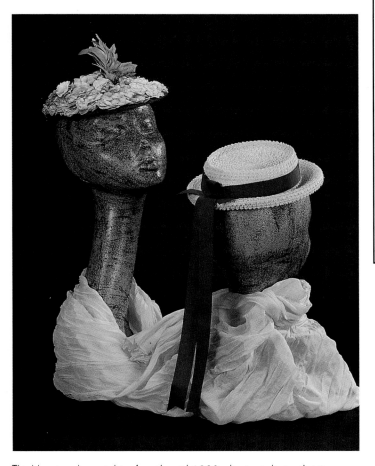

This blue straw bonnet dates from the mid-1800s. Its size indicates that it may have been a child's. It was in a state of disrepair when acquired, and is shown "spruced up." By its provenance, the white straw boater was worn by a little girl circa 1890. It would have been secured under her chin with a thin elastic band. *Courtesy of (both): Maureen Reilly.* Value (each): $55-75.

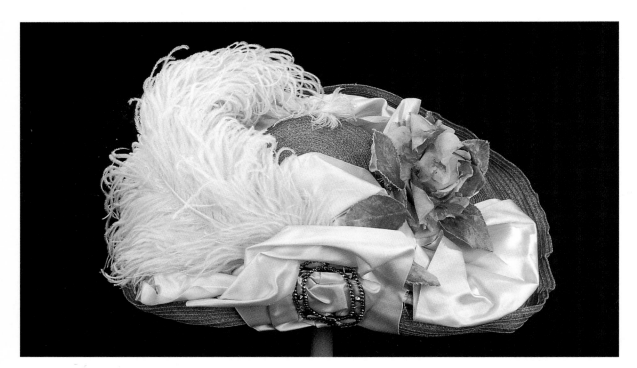

A dusty-rose straw, its graceful ostrich plume secured by a cut-steel buckle. Just right for afternoon outings. *Courtesy of: The Way We Wore.* Value: $300-400.

The court of Edward VII and Alexandra was the most fashionable in Europe, a welcome change from the strict decorum of Queen Victoria. It was the Belle Epoque, a time of gaity and prosperity. But even in the midst of a relaxed moral credo, the rules of dress remained rigid.

Proper headgear was required for men, women, and children for each occasion, according to their social standing. It would not be unusual for ladies of the *ton* to completely change their ensembles, three or four times a day!

Edwardian hats were made of every material imaginable—and trimmed with some that weren't. As milliners developed new skills in taxidermy, whole birds were used, nestled in an improbable garden of silk flowers and artificial fruit. These were lavish concoctions of feathers and flowers, ribbons and fruit, and whatever else seemed suitable to a given milliner.

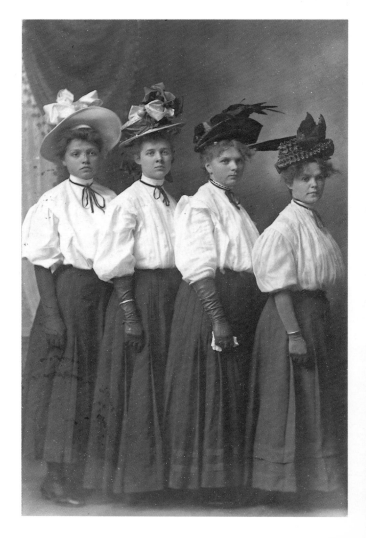

Pictured here, a quintet of ladies in identical dress but wildly individual hats! This photo was taken circa 1905.

The truly chic insisted on hats trimmed with the plumes of exotic birds, and even the entire bird stuffed whole. The results were equal parts magnificent and ludicrous.

In its day, this high-flung type of taxidermy was the subject of much broad humor. It inspired a poem, later turned dance-hall song, by Arthur Lamb:

"He don't know Nellie like I do…said the saucy little bird on Nellie's hat."

Domestic plumage and ostrich feathers remained popular throughout the Edwardian era. It was reputed that these feathers could be farmed from the living bird, in response to pressure from the Audubon Society, a group established in America and England in the 1880s to stem the slaughter of wild and exotic birds. The reformists were ultimately successful. In 1906, Queen Alexandra announced that she would no longer wear feathered hats. In 1911, she was joined by Queen Mary, who publicly discarded hers.

In the teens, responding to mounting pressure from the Audubon Society, milliners began to replace exotic plumes with the feathers of domestic birds such as the robin, raven and lowly guinea hen. Milliners also became well-versed in the art of "made" plumage, as a means of using expensive feathers to best advantage.

Often, the feather trim on those hats which had not sold during one season were restyled for the next. For home milliners, magazines offered tips on how to "recycle" costly plumage.

Hats grew quite large to accommodate the mass of feathers and floral trim during the Belle Epoque. Hatpins were essential, stabbed into elaborate coiffures made possible by the use of cotton batting or rats. The hat crowns were often interlined with a cloth bag, that could be stuffed with tissue to ensure a custom fit.

The size of chapeaux scaled down when Europe entered World War I in 1914. As had occurred before during the Civil War, and would again in World War II, women were obliged *perforce* to enter the work force.

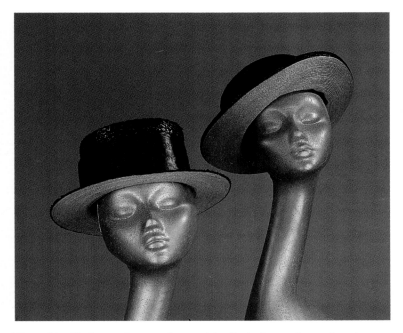

These shiny black straw hats are almost minimalist in form, a far cry from the excesses of the Belle Epoque. Both borrow from the boys: one is a variation on the stovepipe and the other is a modified boater. *Courtesy of (both): Sharon Hagerty.* Value (each): $125-175.

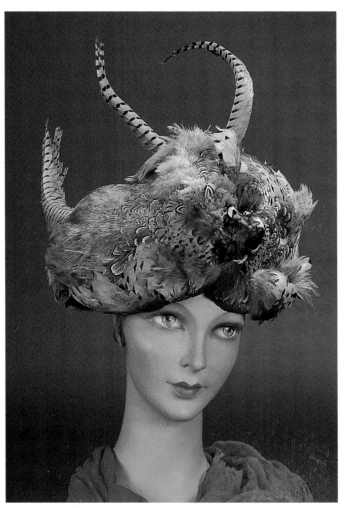

This is a "made" bird, the product of a milliner's skill with batting and muselage. Two pheasants are mated to a felt form to create this outrageous hat. As dramatic as it may seem to the modern eye, the natural coloration of the plumage suggests that this hat was worn with a daytime ensemble. *Courtesy of: Lottie Ballou.* Value: $200-300.

Due to the great war, England was in financial turmoil, and fashion took a back seat to factory production. In France, the government recognized couture as a cornerstone of the economy, and encouraged continued production. But the shortages of raw materials and the military recruitment of designers and their staffs closed French salons for the duration.

The thwarted dress reform movements of the previous century now made great strides, both literally and figuratively. Skirts were unhobbled and shortened, in response to women's more active role on the home front during World War I.

Some couturiers turned to an overseas market, at least until America entered the war in 1917. Poirot even conducted a whistle-stop train tour of major American cities in the mid-teens, hoping to generate a new market for his designs. It was wildly successful, and helped enshrine Paris as a fashion inspiration for this country.

In contrast to the exoticism of the worldly Poirot and his followers, many Edwardian milliners designed feminine hats, relying on silk flowers for winsome appeal. Indeed, the art of hand-crafting all manner of silk blooms was considered the pinnacle of a milliner's achievement. Many were imported from Europe, where special petal and leaf molds had been carefully handed down from one generation to another.

Edwardian outings were often grand affairs. From the accounts in books and cartoons by contemporary authors and artists, it seems they were seen by the nouveau riche as an opportunity to announce their status, through the overt costliness of their attire.

Much care was given to the selection of suitable chapeaux. Hats were all custom made, whether bespoke or from the "little shop around the corner." Even when the size of hats scaled down during the teens, this did not mean economy of trim or hand-workmanship.

But the Age of Innocence—as chronicled by Edith Wharton in her richly detailed book of that name—was drawing to a close. Looking back, the span of time from 1901 through 1918 was an era of transformation, a precursor to the slick mores and sleek lines that demarcate the 1920s.

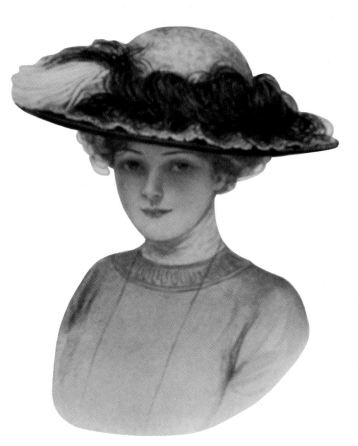

An Edwardian fashion quarterly recommended this hat: "On the left side is placed a black and white ostrich-feather tassel, the long flues reaching to the brim edge. This is a novel idea and an economical one, as these ostrich-feather tassels may be made from old feathers which are no longer of use."

Vintage Flowers

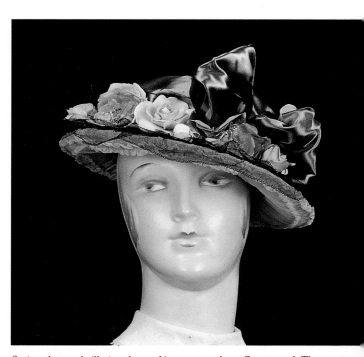

Satin velvet and silk, in a bevy of ice cream colors. *Courtesy of: The Way We Wore.* Value: $250-350.

The fashion folio that featured the hat shown at right, above, described it as "endowed with the free and easy grace of a sou-wester" and, "ideally fitting to wear with the tailored suit or for knock-about in the country." It was shown with the mocha brown pith helmet at left, below.

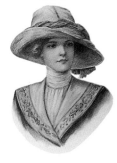

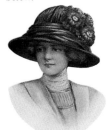

The authors believe this natural straw boater is relatively new although it features fine vintage trim, particularly the patterned French ribbons and dyed plumage. *Courtesy of: Antique Arcade.* Value: $150-200.

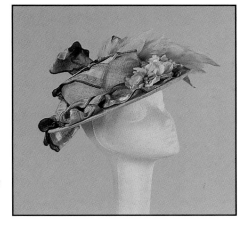

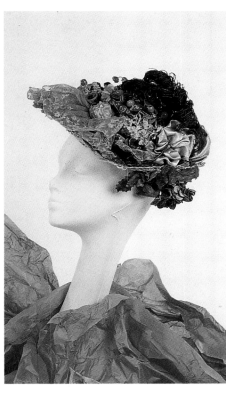

Rough natural straw, silky tea-stained lace, with the surprise of an underbrim posy. Label: G. Raverdy— Paris. *Courtesy of: Antique Arcade.* Value: $200-300.

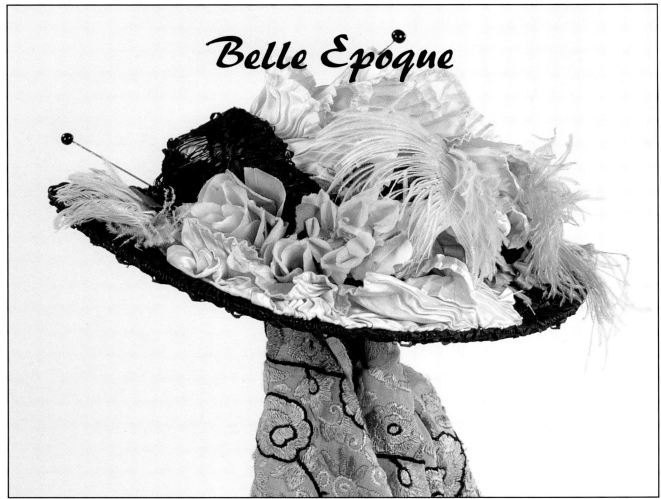

Belle Epoque

Black straw forms a base for horsehair lace and ivory pleated ribbon. The silk roses nestle in the fronds of dyed ostrich plumes. *Courtesy of: Past Perfect.* Value: $250-350.

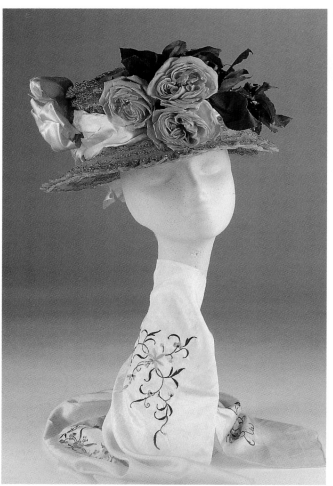

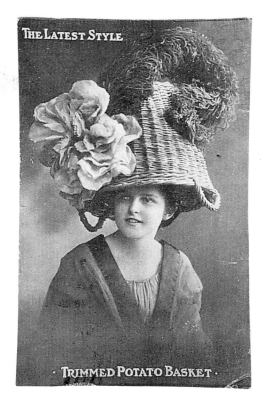

The enormous size of some basket hats inspired broad humor in the supposedly genteel Belle Epoque. This postcard pictures a trimmed potato basket as the latest style.

A basket hat shaped from bobbin-weave raffia on a wire rim, trimmed with large cabbage roses of creamy silk. *Courtesy of: Cheap Thrills.* Value: $200-300.

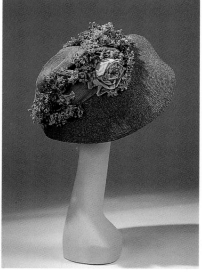

Trailing petals and a rose in pale pink on a floppy straw. The underbrim is a true lilac, indicating its fade with the passage of time. *Courtesy of: The Victorian Closet.* Value: $175-225.

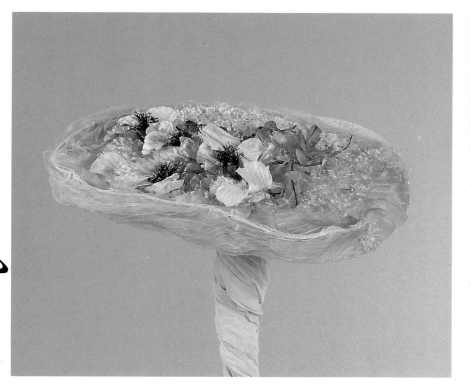

Ivory fabric fluffed on a wire rim, a platter to top the popular pompadour. *Courtesy of: Past Perfect.* Value: $200-300.

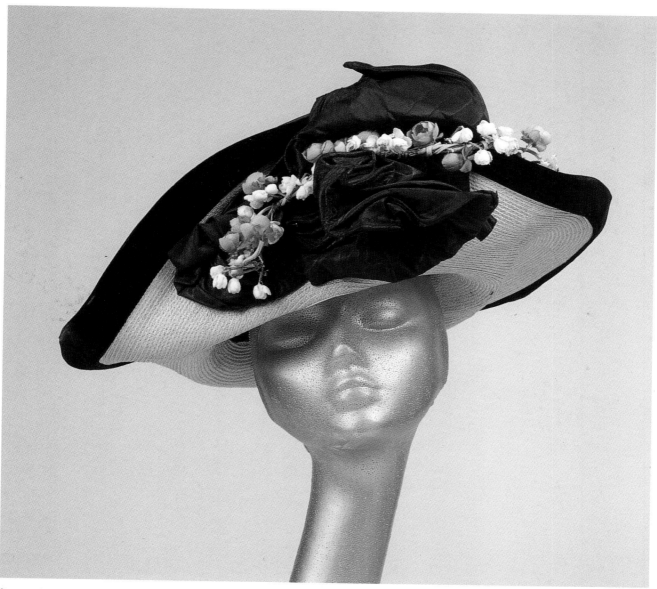

Spectacular in size, this natural straw hat features an upturned brim, trimmed with black velvet ribbon and pink silk flowers. *Courtesy of: Lisa Carson.* Value: $200-300.

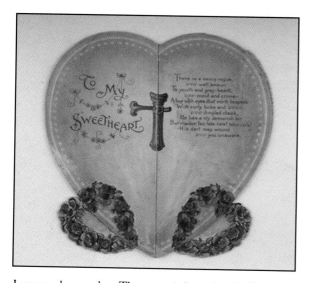

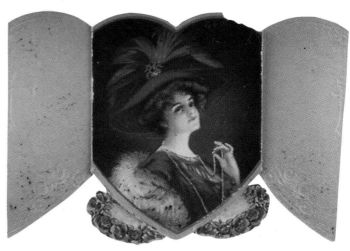

Love me, love my hat. The romantic hats of the Belle Epoque were often featured in ephemera, such as this early lithograph Valentine.

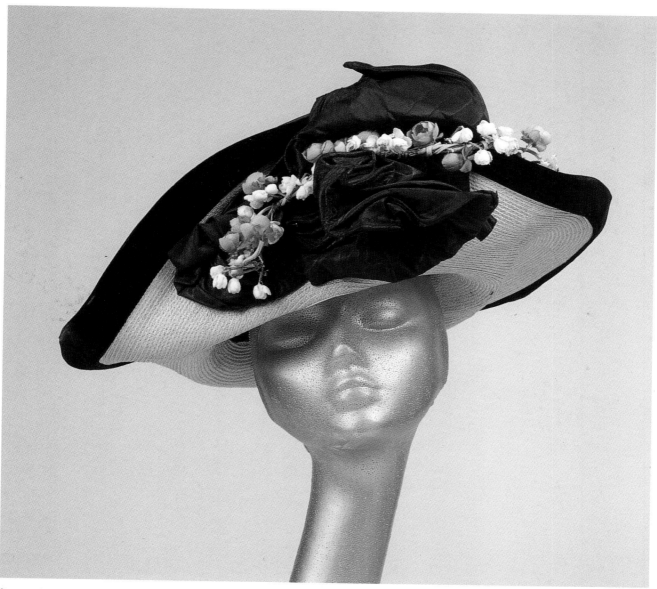 *Parisenne Belle*

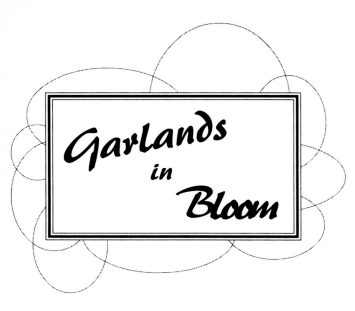

Garlands in Bloom

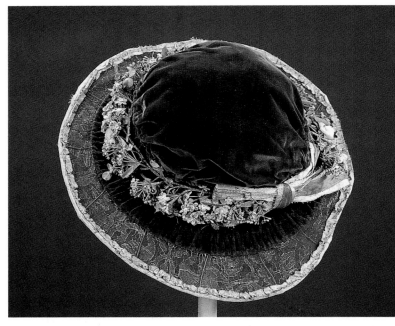

Purple velvet for the crown, matching horsehair for the brim. *Courtesy of: The Way We Wore.* Value: $200-300.

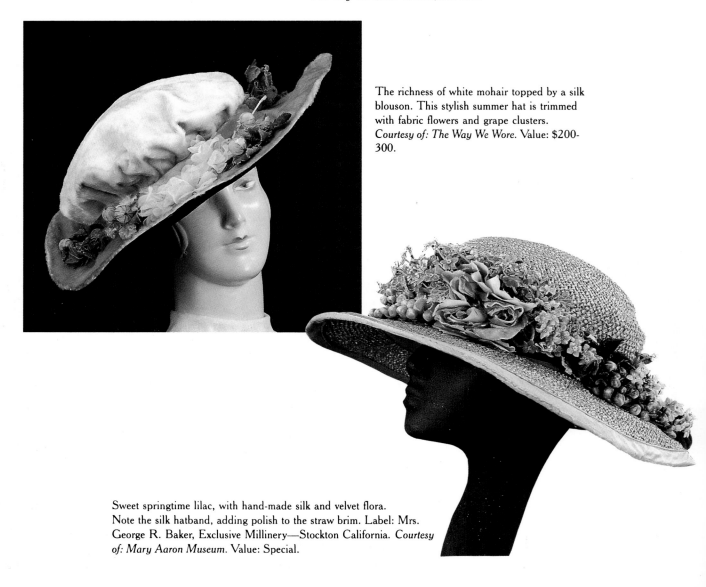

The richness of white mohair topped by a silk blouson. This stylish summer hat is trimmed with fabric flowers and grape clusters. *Courtesy of: The Way We Wore.* Value: $200-300.

Sweet springtime lilac, with hand-made silk and velvet flora. Note the silk hatband, adding polish to the straw brim. Label: Mrs. George R. Baker, Exclusive Millinery—Stockton California. *Courtesy of: Mary Aaron Museum.* Value: Special.

Feathered Fantasies

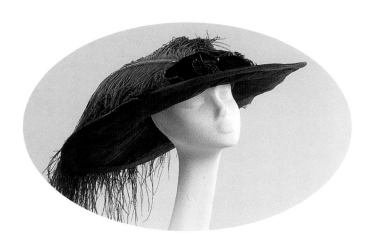

Two hats, graceful as willow trees. They owe their languid lines to the natural grace of ostrich plumes. Note the French-jet buttons on the hatband to the right. *Courtesy of (photo, left): Mary Aaron Museum. Courtesy of (photo, right): Rich Man, Poor Man.* Value (left): Special. Value (right): $250-350.

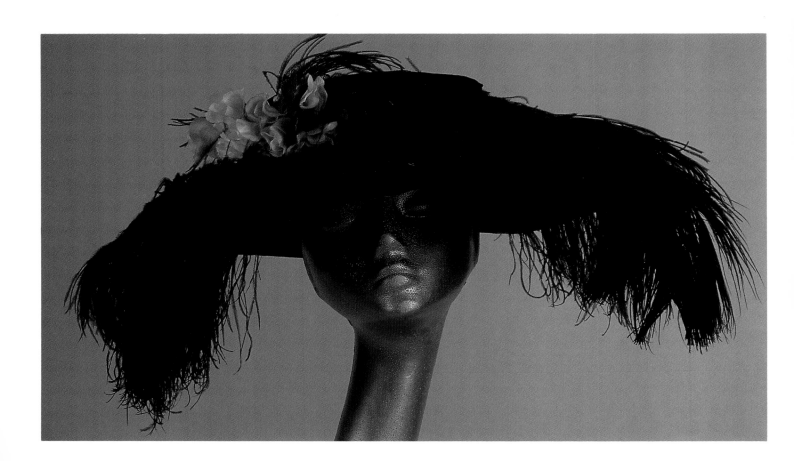

During the Directoire, Parisienne beauties took to wearing bicornes and helmets with a nod to the regimental finery of Napoleon's campaigns. In the waning days of the Belle Epoque, similarly inspired by the prospect of a call-to-arms in Europe, ladies again affected a military style.

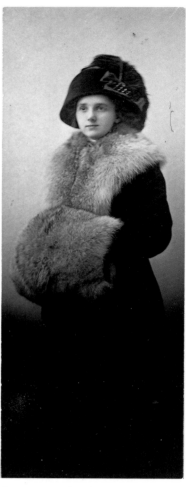

A circa 1910 daguerreotype of an unknown society lady, majestic in her helmet.

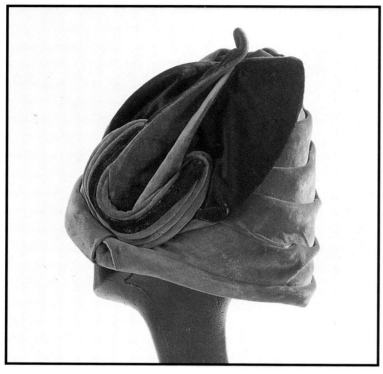

A helmet in tones of green velvet. This imposing hat is shaped, not on a wire rim, but a heavy form of tight-packed straw. *Courtesy of: The Victorian Closet.* Value: $300-350.

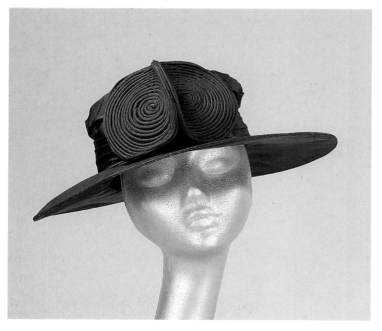

Simply
Elegant

Navy blue silk is worked on a wire frame to form this flattering boater, crowned by a double swirl of cording. *Courtesy of: Sharon Hagerty.* Value: $150-200.

Black Beauties

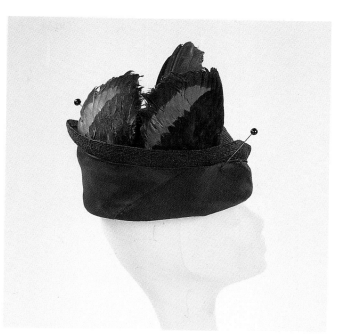

A beautiful black straw garnished with silk ribbon and ostrich plumes. *Courtesy of: Rich Man, Poor Man.* Value: $95-145.

A smart black straw serves as nest for the blue and black "made" wings of some imaginary bird. *Courtesy of: Donna McMaster.* Value: $95-145.

This broad-brim boater breathes Gigi charm, with the plaid taffeta ribbon of a schoolgirl and a big plume for dress-up. *Courtesy of: Maureen Reilly.* Value: $150-200.

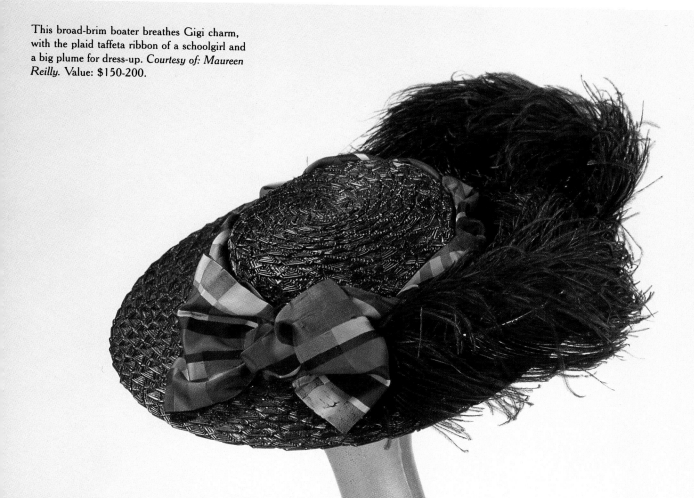

Winter Outing

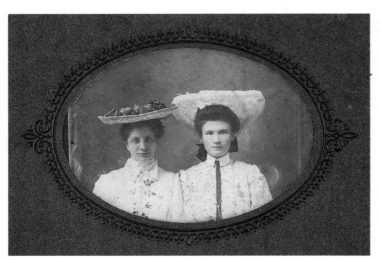

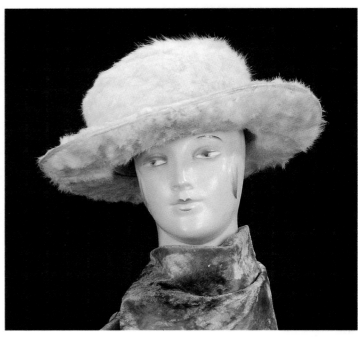

Pictured in this daguerreotype of two young women, a fine example of dyed-white beaver in a style that could be worn with an everyday shirtwaist and a bow-tied hairdo.

Plush beaver fur, skillfully dyed a bright white. This versatile boater could have been worn year-round. *Courtesy of: Rich Man, Poor Man.* Value: $125-175.

Bed of Roses

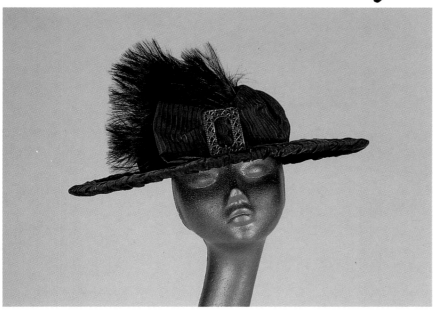

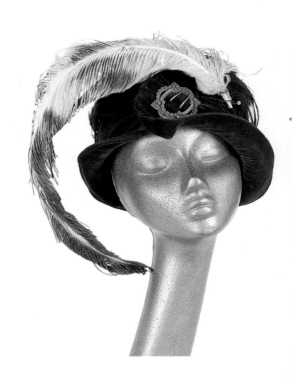

A mix of brown silk, velvet, and taffeta. Whipped into style with a center plume and ruched ribbon hatband. The buckle also plays a central role on the brown velvet toque with swooping ostrich plume. *Courtesy of (top): Maureen Reilly. Courtesy of (right): Banbury Cross Antiques.* Value (top): $200-300. Value (right): $150-200.

These three lovely hats were recently purchased from a San Francisco Estate. They had been stored in a large hatbox for eighty years, along with a carefully-penned note informing: "From Mother's Trousseau." All, courtesy of Banbury Cross Antiques.

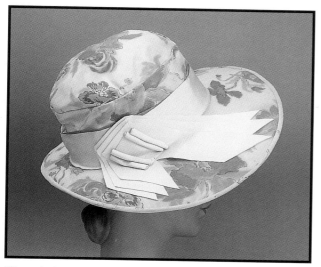

Watercolor blossoms painted by hand on pale silk. Label: Hyman's—Oakland, Berkeley. Value: $200-300.

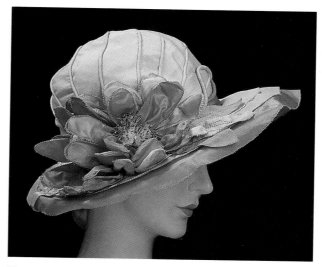

Pleated and layered silk, in tones of apricot and peach. Wired petals bloom on brim. Label: Wayman Sports Hats. Value: $200-300.

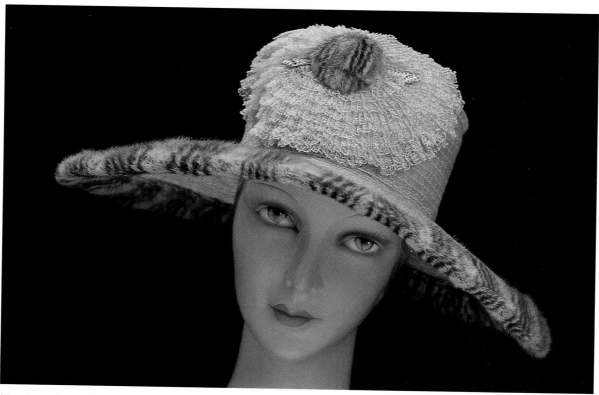

Horsehair with monkey fur accents the brim, and a lace fichu is pinned to the crown of this highly unusual Pamela. Value: $250-350.

Banded in Silk

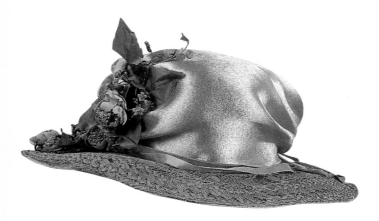

A fabulous fine straw, customized with a satin blouson for the crown. This hat is from a small-town shop, but has all the elan of a big city salon. Label: Bradley's, Inc.—Marysville, California. *Courtesy of: Mary Aaron Museum.* Value: Special.

Not-So-Basic Black

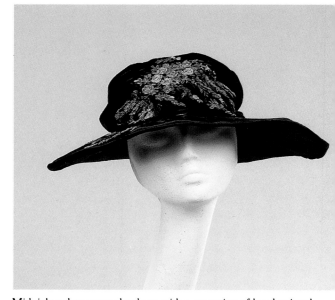

Midnight velvet greets the dawn with a scattering of hand-painted posies, on the crown of this floppy-brimmed Pamela. *Courtesy of: Donna McMaster.* Value: $125-175.

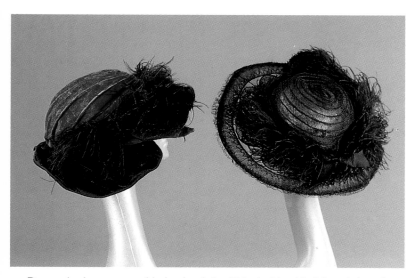

Deep red velvet crowns a black velvet brim. Paired with a black horsehair and tulle Pamela. *Courtesy of (both): Antique Arcade.* Value (each): $150-225.

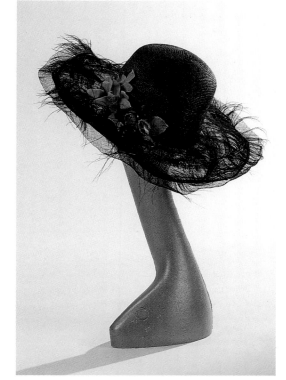

Black horsehair shaped on a wire rim, with golden floral highlights, a lovely style for summer nights circa 1918. *Courtesy of: Banbury Cross Antiques.* Value: $150-225.

Lovely to Look At

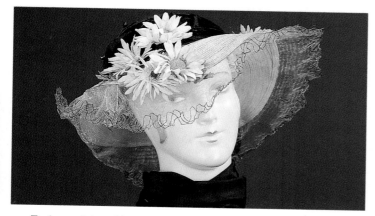

Fresh as a daisy, a blend of town and country in black velvet and natural straw. *Courtesy of: The Way We Wore.* Value: $200-300.

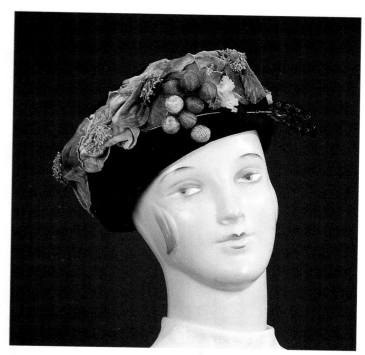

The classic toque, sprayed with oak leaves and flowers. *Courtesy of: The Way We Wore.* Value: $200-300.

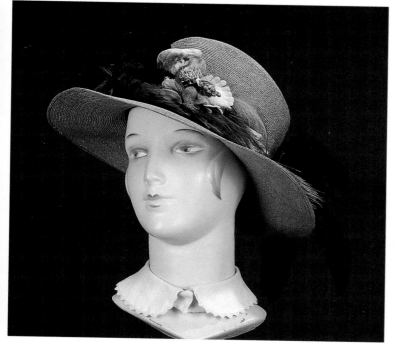

Natural Milan straw with exotic floral trim. *Courtesy of: The Way We Wore.* Value: $200-300.

Flight of Fancy

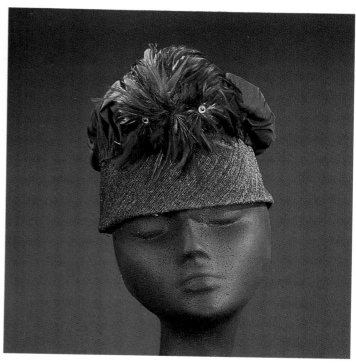

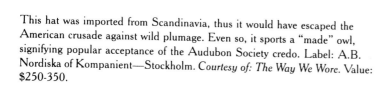

This hat was imported from Scandinavia, thus it would have escaped the American crusade against wild plumage. Even so, it sports a "made" owl, signifying popular acceptance of the Audubon Society credo. Label: A.B. Nordiska of Kompanient—Stockholm. *Courtesy of: The Way We Wore.* Value: $250-350.

The Edwardians were highly conscious of the roles associated with gender, marital status, and age. Toques were considered suitable for women "advancing into the frankly elderly years beyond sixty" according to a fashion quarterly of 1905. The article recommended hats in slate, brown, and plum to complement graying hair.

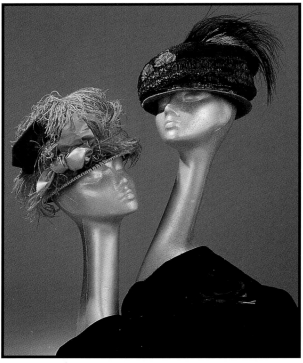

Sophistication was the desired effect for evening—as shown in this royal purple toque, discreetly sparkled with silver beading and sprigged with a maline. *Courtesy of: The Victorian Closet.* Value: $150-225.

The same hat in profile, plus its cousin in a lighter shade of purple. *Courtesy of: Lisa Carson.* Value: $150-225.

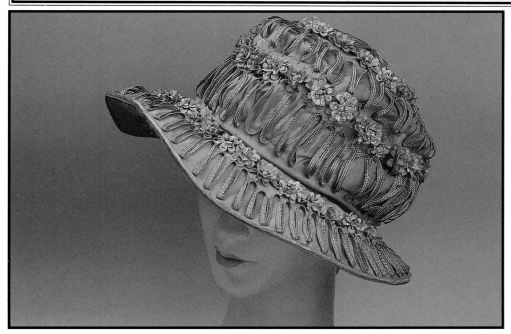

Bronzed Beauty

Dainty rosettes and loopy braid surround a soft-bronze shattered satin Pamela, shaped on a wire rim. Label: Naco—Paris, New York, San Francisco. *Courtesy of: Maureen Reilly.* Value: $200-300.

Spring into Fall

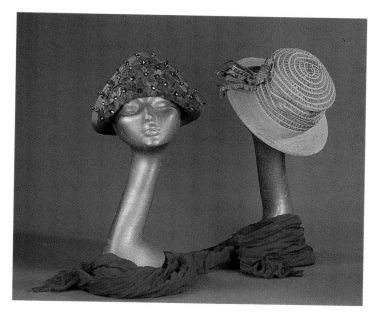

Two delicious hats circa 1918. To the left, a chevron hatband serves up deep-peach silk sprinkled with beads. To the right, a swirl of peach and cream on caramel straw. *Courtesy of (both): Sharon Hagerty.* Value (left): $175-250. Value (right): $125-175.

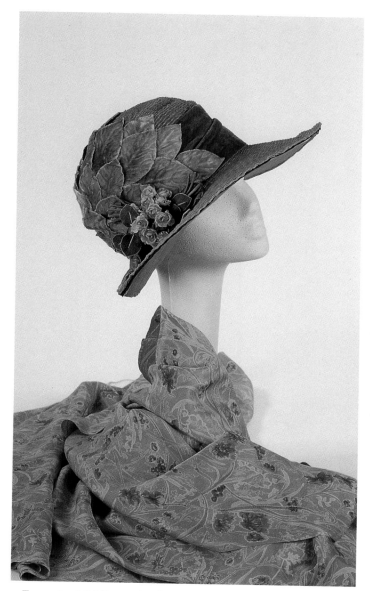

Forecasting fall foliage, velvet leaves grace a natural straw Pamela. *Courtesy of: Lisa Carson.* Value: $200-300.

An "out-of-Africa" straw Homburg, perfect for tramping around on late summer days. The vintage silk posy was added by the author. *Courtesy of: Maureen Reilly.* Value: $125-175.

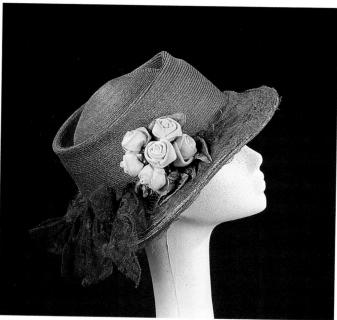

Simply Divine

This little evening hat is snugly formed by a drape of plum satin, with a spray of malines for side interest. *Courtesy of: Lisa Carson.* Value: $150-225.

Dark Sensations

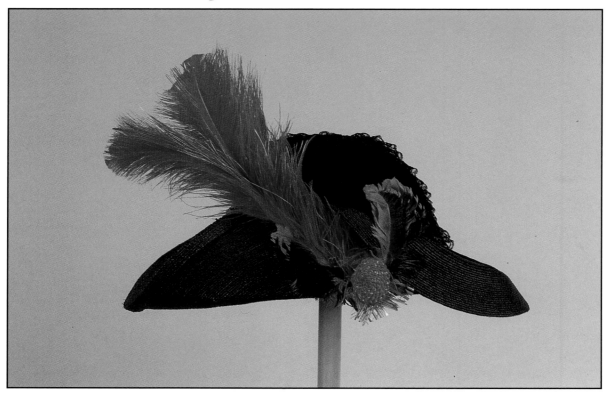

A fabulous conceit in black straw, its back brim pinned by a cockade of fuschia ribbons and malines. *Courtesy of: Donna McMaster.* Value: $200-300.

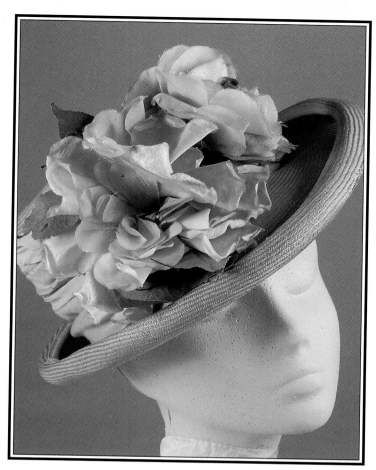

April in Paris

A Homburg's rolled-straw brim showcases hand-made cream and pink roses. *Courtesy of: Banbury Cross Antiques.* Value: $95-125.

Two hats, bicorne and tricorne, identically banded in ostrich plumes. *Courtesy of (both): Sharon Hagerty.* Value (each): $175-225.

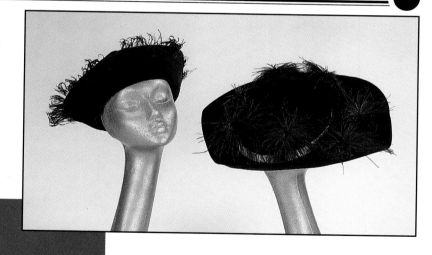

A modified Pamela in winter burgundy velvet, with a starburst of beading on the brim. *Courtesy of: Mary Aaron Museum.* Value: Special.

Edwardian hats are the epitome of romance, elegance, and old-world grandeur—which means they are highly collectible, but almost unwearable. If you are inclined to play "dress-up" with your hats, you may want to join a social group dedicated to vintage styles.

If you are already active in such an organization, consider sponsoring a milliner-themed event. A recent fund raiser for the Art Deco Society of California was a *millinery tea*, held in an historic Oakland hotel. Club members and other participants were asked to dress in vintage clothing—and, of course, hats!

The "coup de chapeaux" at the society's tea in 1996 was a display of Edwardian hats by Rodna Taylor. This personable lady turned her hobby into a business: The Mad Hatter. She entertains women's clubs with running commentary on fashion history and anecdotes. We show a sample of her Edwardian hats here; others from her collection are scattered throughout the book.

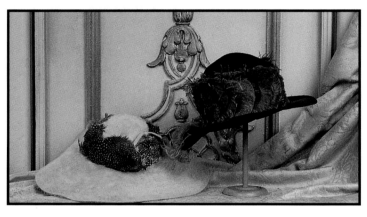

A cream shako bright with pheasant feathers curtsies to a rich brown Pamela banded in ostrich plumes. Value (left): $150-225. Value (right): $200-300.

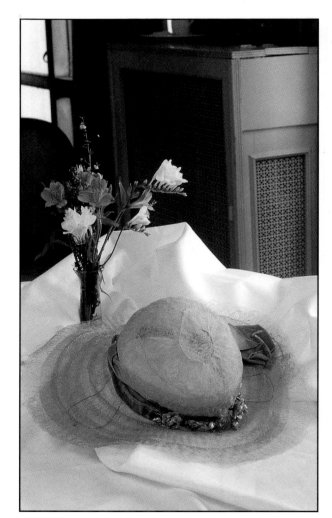

A stunning Pamela, its crown and brim heaped with roses formed by hand-ruched ribbons in dusty rose, cream, and blue. Value: $200-300.

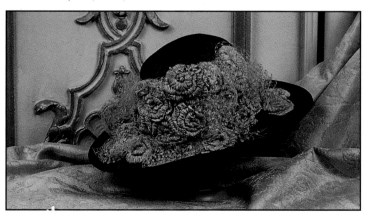

Horsehair lace with a crinoline-skirted brim, a perfect lady's tea picture hat. Value: $150-225.

The 1920s and early 1930s were shaped by social upheaval, from which emerged the tempo and temperament of modern life. These were times that changed the popular perception of women's role in society, and a fashion revolution was sure to follow.

The Roaring Twenties actually began on Armistice Day in 1919, a time of frivolity personified by the flapper. A gamine by day, she might observe a polo match or participate in a skeet shoot, at ease in a previously masculine province. A madcap by night, she might dance till dawn, then opt for a bootleg nightcap at the ubiquitous speakeasy. For all events, she would wear a carefully chosen hat.

Modern woman or not, hats were as indispensable an element of her wardrobe as they had ever been in the history of fashion. Their importance as an arbiter of social status was succinctly stated by a famous fashion illustrator of the era in a recent interview.

As a young woman living in Paris, the talented Catherine Morioton was retained on a regular basis by major fashion periodicals, such as the luminous *Art-Gout-Beauté*. In these days, before commercial photography was commonplace, she brought to life the work of Worth, Lanvin, Poirot, and Patou.

> ## C. Morioton
>
> *"You couldn't neglect any of the details...For example, if a woman had the misfortune to go out into the street without a hat, it would be assumed she was a servant."*
>
> -C. Morioton.

Helped by more than half a century of hindsight, it now seems clear that America experienced an artistic revolution in the 1920s. This was due, at least in part, to the arrival of artists and scholars who fled the privations of Europe in the aftermath of World War I. This infusion of talent and intellectual curiosity was reflected in the practical arts as well, such as clothing and millinery.

The chemise reigned throughout this period. It was a holdover from 1915, when this silhouette was first introduced by Poirot and Lanvin. But it was somewhat modified from the original by the use of dropped waistlines and flounced hemlines.

To complement these relaxed lines, even before her fame as inventor of the cloche, French milliner Caroline Reboux designed a simple and broad-brimmed hat. This modified Pamela was introduced by her atelier in 1923. She is credited with designing the cloche a few years later.

Reboux formed the cloche from a drape of felt, working directly on the head of each privileged client. The couture touch was evident in hats so custom-fitted they were finished by mere tuck and fold, snip or clip. But it is anecdotal that the cloche was popularized in Hollywood, when producers realized that their silent film stars could not be properly photographed in hats with brims!

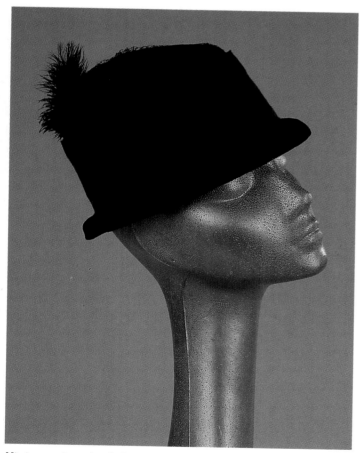

Kissing cousin to the cloche, a small-brimmed black velvet shaped on a wire rim. A similar style was described in a 1925 issue of *Vogue* as the "Directoire." *Courtesy of: Maureen Reilly.* Value: $65-95.

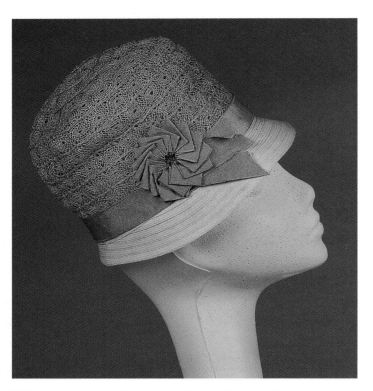

This straw cloche hugs the mannequin's head. It was sold by a vintage clothing dealer as a child's hat, but it could also have been worn by a worn by a petite Flapper. *Courtesy of: Banbury Cross.* Value: $95-145.

The cloche was worn so close to the head, it could only be worn over the somewhat scandalous bobbed haircut. The name cloche means "bell" in French, and it was a shape that could be cunningly coaxed from felt, straw or any stiff fabric. If trimmed, it was often to one side, for the modern look of asymmetry.

Large women must have found the clinging cloche difficult to wear. If from the social register, they could order custom sizes. If from the middle class, they could order "the larger head size" advertised in catalogs and magazines of the era.

Queen cloche was to reign for many years, but not without serious challenge. French couturier Jeanne Lanvin showed a city cousin of the Pamela, brimmed in silk and crowned with masses of velvet flowers, to complement her romantic "robes de style." Coco Chanel continued to satisfy with such classic and simple styles as the boater and beret.

Clearly, alternatives to the cloche were in demand by customers. We can easily envision those staid souls who were scandalized by flappery; the matronly types who were careful to eschew frivolity, and their daughters, who were expected to debut in organdy. All would have opted for the toque, turban, or Pamela.

Sportswear was an important addition to the female wardrobe, but it was certainly not pursued bareheaded. Instead, re-

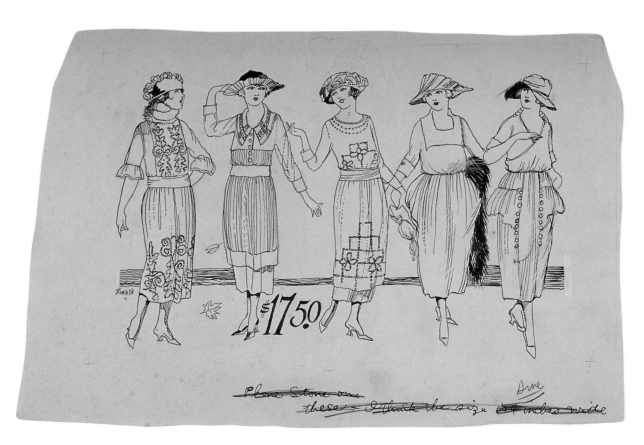

Ensembles with distinctive chapeaux were featured in department store ads. Shown, a selection for the Fall season, circa 1920.

tailers offered coordinating hats. A braided bandeau could shield the brow from glisten in a game of golf or tennis, while a terrycloth turban would protect Marcel waves from the watery variety. Perhaps most unique was the rubber bathing cap, reputed to first have been worn in 1927.

New developments in textile manufacturing directly influenced the milliner's craft. For the first time, a process was developed to rubberize fabric. These "elastics" were a precursor to the Lastex used by Schiaparelli in the early 1930s. They were bonded to jersey for daytime, lamé or satin for evening. Turbans were adaptable to the new textiles, as were bandeaux. For evening drama they might be trimmed with bijoux and aigrettes.

When Wall Street crashed in 1929, one shock wave was the shortage of capital necessary to bring new designs to the marketplace. The applied arts and fashion had been quick to absorb new trends during the 1920s, so that the spare geometry of Art Deco was translated into movie theatre facades and handbags alike. Now, the infusion would be slower and more restricted in scope. The haute couture might still play with Deco or Surrealism, for a select clientele that had escaped Black Friday; but these designs were not readily absorbed into the fashion vernacular.

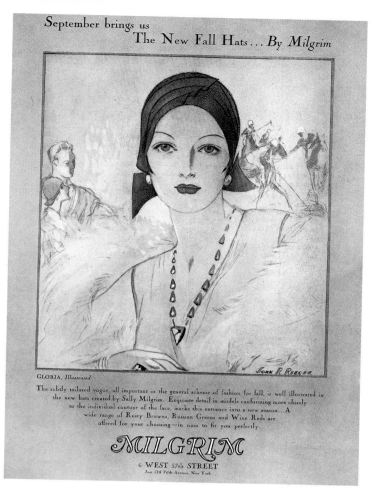

Sally Milgrim designed for her own store label for many decades. Shown here, a transitional style by Milgrim from an advertisement in 1929. The nape-hugging bow relieves the severe cloche lines of earlier years.

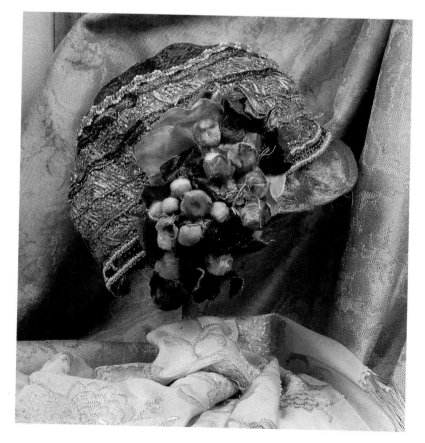

The hallmark of the cloche was its simplicity, but some women demanded a departure from starkly modern lines. Shown, a romantic cloche, blooming with ribbon tendrils and velvet grapes. *Courtesy of: The Mad Hatter.* Value: $200-300.

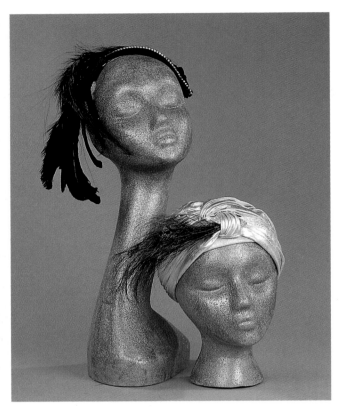

A turban of silver lamé bonded to elastic; a black velvet bandeau outlined with rhinestones. *Courtesy of (both): Maureen Reilly.* Value (bottom): $75-95. Value (top): $45-75.

During the Depression, hats and other fashion accessories were used to help revitalize an old wardrobe. Emphasizing their importance, matched sets were in vogue. It was not uncommon for women to pair shoes with belts, and hats with gloves, in variations of the same fabric and trim.

Ironically, the look we most often associate with the early 1930s is one of glamour, thanks to the influence of Hollywood. The populace turned to movies as an escape from economic privation. Talented designers such as Adrian were happy to style for the Silver Screen.

By mid-decade, a shift in the nation's financial outlook was beginning to occur, with a corresponding change in millinery. Perhaps it was the optimism of President Roosevelt's New Deal, or opportunities created by the rumblings of war in Europe. Whatever the reason, seemingly overnight women tossed aside their simple caps—and strapped on the fanciful tilt hats that were to mark a new era.

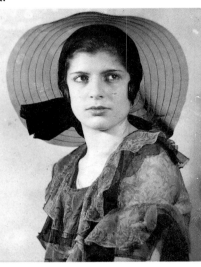

The author's mother, Evelyn Reilly (née Lynn) at sweet 16, in a horsehair picture hat. The "halo" effect is a hallmark of the early 1930s, when this photo was taken.

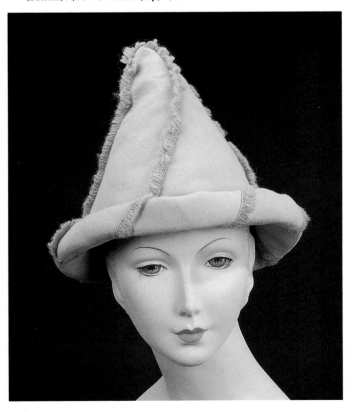

High style in the early 1930s, a felt sugarloaf twisted with fringe, from John-Frederics. Gone was the glitz of the Roaring Twenties, although Deco was still a strong influence for the couture. *Courtesy of: The Way We Wore.* Value: $125-175.

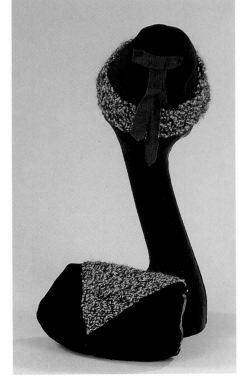

A simple felt cap and muff reflect the Depression in their dull grey and maroon palette. The fabrication is also poor: cotton velvet and rayon-pile fur. Still, the design is clean and the stitching is careful, so as to convey a spartan chic. *Courtesy of: Maureen Reilly.* Value (set): $45-65.

Romantic Ideas

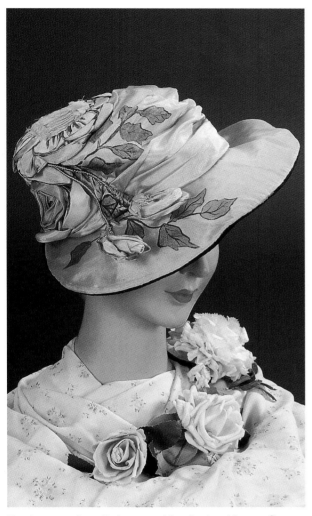

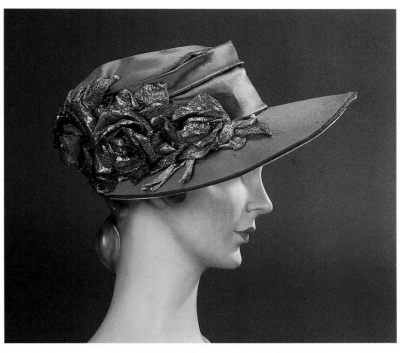

Nape-hugging copper satin with gilt lamé blossoms. Label: Zobel's. *Courtesy of: Sandra Headley.* Value: $150-225.

Peach satin with applied roses and hand-painted leaves. *Courtesy of: Sandra Headley.* Value: $200-300.

A Little Night Music

An early floppy cloche in black velvet. The night sky of its crown is star-studded with rhinestones. Label: Gracian. *Courtesy of: The Way We Wore.* Value: $200-300.

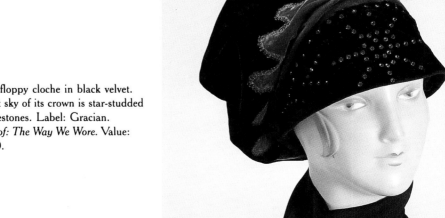

Stepping Out
in Style

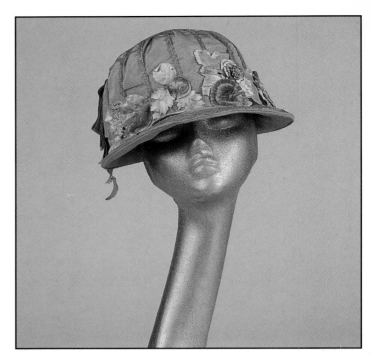

Attention to detail in a rose satin helmet. *Courtesy of: Lisa Carson*. Value: $150-225.

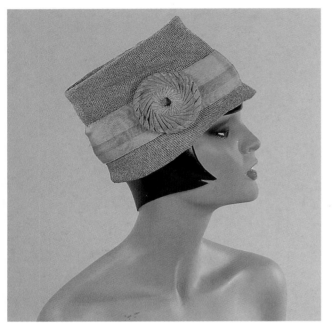

The squared crown popular in the early 1920s; this version in fine natural straw with grosgrain band and medallion. *Courtesy of: Past Perfect*. Value: $150-225.

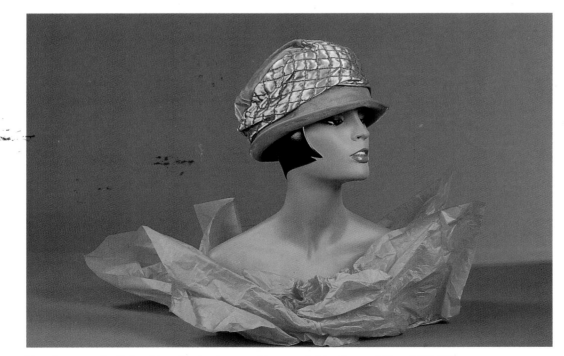

Netted cream satin distinguishes this simple toque. *Courtesy of: Lisa Carson*. Value: $150-225.

Bowl of Cherries

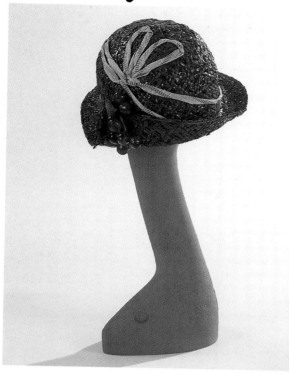

Woven cherry-pink straw with applied straw ribbon and early plastic cherries. *Courtesy of: Lisa Carson.* Value: $150-225.

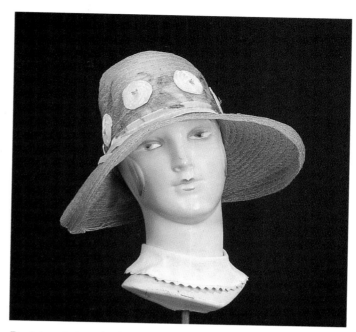

Peach horsehair garden hat with white medallions. *Courtesy of: The Way We Wore.* Value: $150-225.

Casual Living

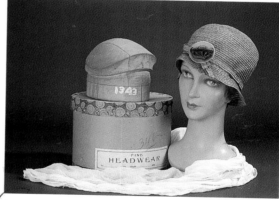

A taupe straw cloche ornamented with a large Bakelite disk. Pictured with wooden hatblocks, as used for generations in blocking felt and straw. Label (hat): Wyle. *Courtesy of (hat): Sandra Headley. Courtesy of (blocks): Banbury Cross Antiques.* Value (hat): $125-175. Value (each block): $95-145.

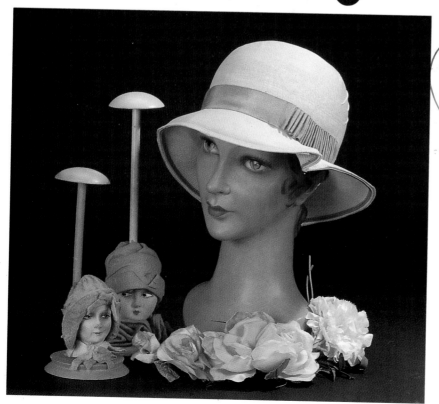

In mint condition, a silky straw with pleated ribbon band. Alongside are two hatstands with composition bases, in a flapper motif. Label (hat): Lee Nora. *Courtesy of (hat): Sandra Headley.* Value (hat): $125-175. *Courtesy of (stands): Lottie Ballou.* Value (each stand): $175-250.

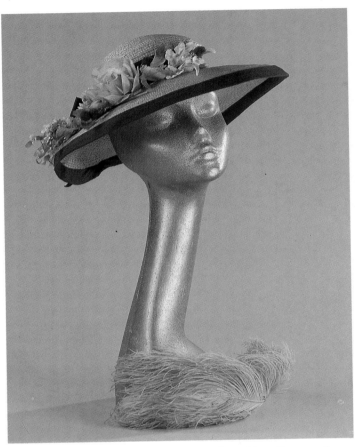

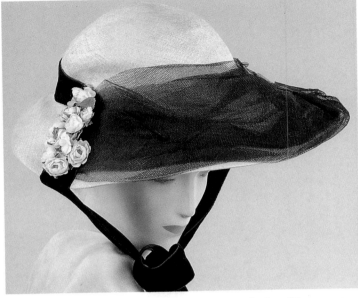

A "Little Bo-Peep" trimmed with gauze netting and velvet ribbon. Label: I. Magnin & Co., Importer. *Courtesy of: Graf's Glitz.* Value: $125-175.

A velvet-banded charmer, highlighted in robin's egg blue. *Courtesy of: Banbury Cross Antiques.* Value: $115-165.

Flights of Fancy

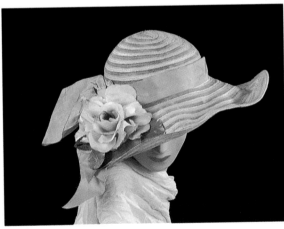

To the garden party in a wavy-brimmed horsehair with cabbage rose accent. *Courtesy of: Banbury Cross Antiques.* Value: $115-165.

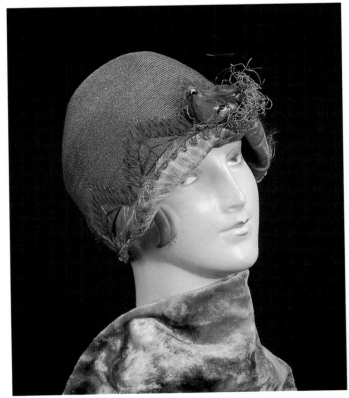

An amusing cloche, its short straw brim serving as a perch for a bird, complete with nest. *Courtesy of: The Way We Wore.* Value: $250-350.

A Day in the Country

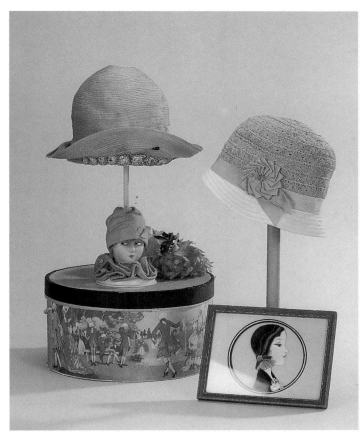

The hat with paper rosettes rests on a doll-faced hatstand, atop a 1920s hatbox. Shown with a two-tone straw trimmed in sage ribbon. The flapper picture is in watercolors and fabric. *Courtesy of (hat, left): Sandra Headley. Courtesy of (all else): Banbury Cross Antiques.* Value (hats, each): $125-175. Value (box): $45-75. Value (picture): $50-75.

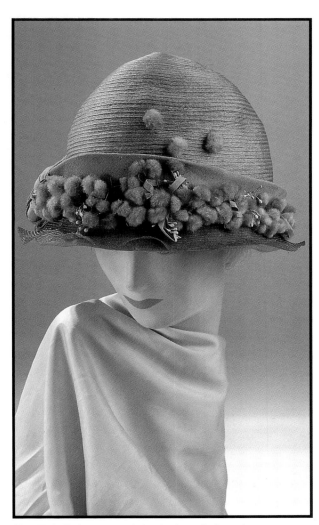

Chenille balls buzz around this beehive cloche in honey-colored straw, for a touch of whimsy. *Courtesy of: Anna's.* Value: $175-250.

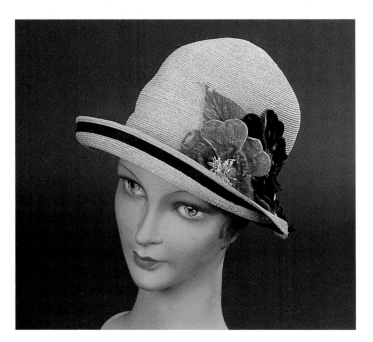

Tall-crowned straw with velvet flowers. *Courtesy of: Sandra Headley.* Value: $125-175.

Delicacies in Lace

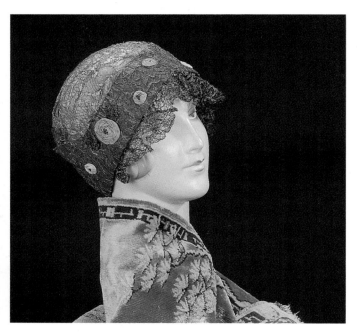

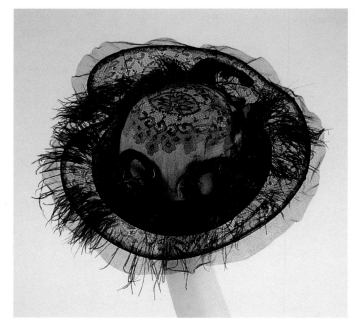

Silver lace cloche gains further glow from its iridescent band, and the twinkle of ribbon flowers. *Courtesy of: The Way We Wore.* Value: $150-225.

An irregular brim in ebony tulle lace, trimmed with horsehair and looped ostrich feathers. *Courtesy of: The Way We Wore.* Value: $200-300.

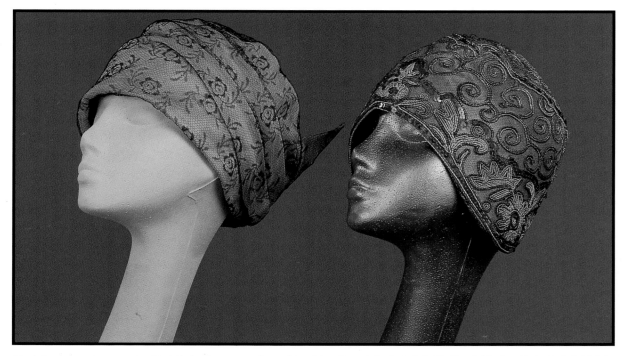

Black lace pleated over nude silk, left. Intricate soutache and hand-beading, right. Label (left): Frank Modes, Paris. Label (right): Marshall Field & Co. *Courtesy of (both): Lisa Carson.* Value (left): $125-175. Value (right): $150-225.

Hatmaker

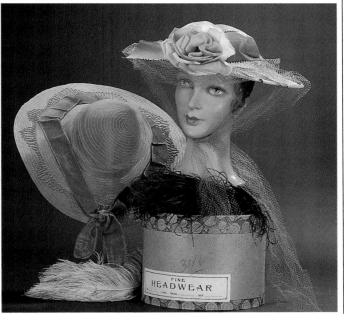

Early wooden hatblocks and vintage hatboxes are shown with lovely golden straw hats. *Courtesy of (hat): Sandra Headley.* Value (hat): $150-250. *Courtesy of (rest): Banbury Cross Antiques.* Value (box, each): $35-65.

Brimming Over

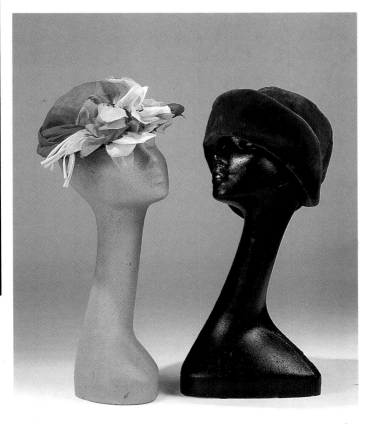

A raspberry beauty, trimmed with silk blooms. With a purple velvet flat-brimmed cloche. Label (left): Original by Woodmere, N.J. *Courtesy of (left): Banbury Cross Antiques. Courtesy of (right): Anna's.* Value (each): $75-125.

Satin Doll

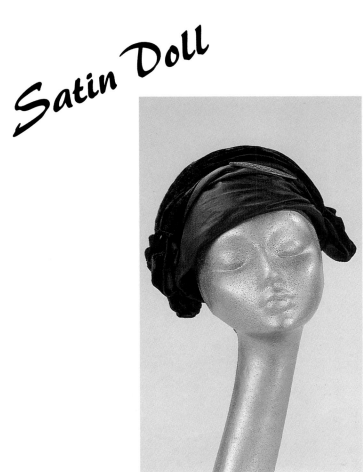

Sleek ebony peau de soie with ruched trim sweeps the brim of this evening cloche with strass ornament, circa 1917. *Courtesy of: Sharon Hagerty.* Value: $150-225.

Evenings in Paris

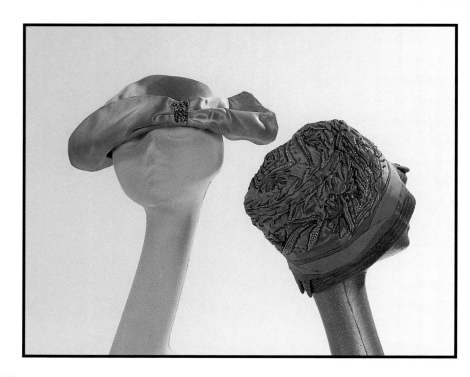

Heavy formed satin with strass buckle, left. Its finely sewn companion, right, is trimmed with glass beads, silk, and chenille. The original price tag of the latter hat was intact: $3.99. *Courtesy of (both): Lisa Carson.* Value (left): $55-95. Value (right): $125-175.

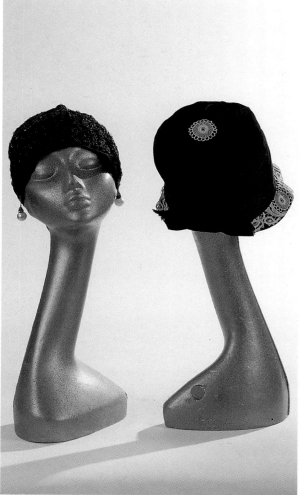

A head-hugger in black satin with pearl eardrops. Paired with a revival bonnet, brimming with lace. Label (right): Alexander Hats, Made in California. *Courtesy of (both): Lisa Carson.* Value (each): $125-175.

Chocolate silk trimmed with French ribbon. *Courtesy of: Anna's.* Value: $150-225.

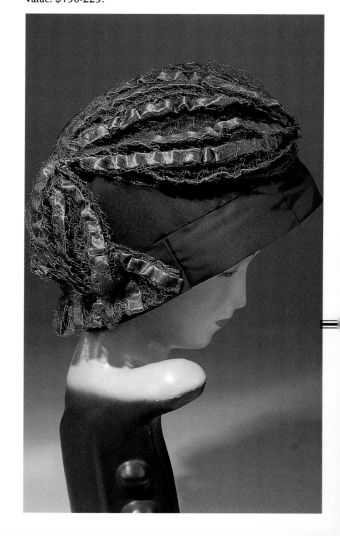

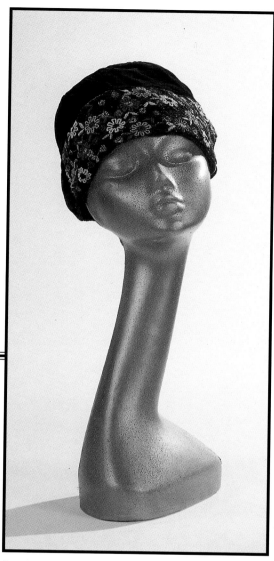

Brown velvet hugger with embroidered flowers on the flat brim. Label: City of Paris. *Courtesy of: Lisa Carson.* Value: $150-225.

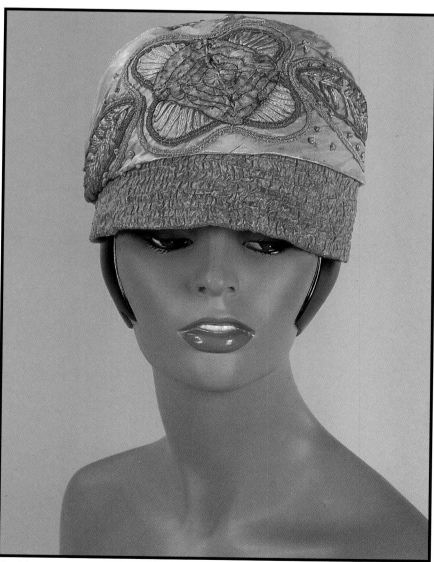

A pink pastry cloche, showing the demi-brim version of this style that continued to be popular in the early 1930s. *Courtesy of: Past Perfect.* Value: $150-225.

Fashionable Flappers

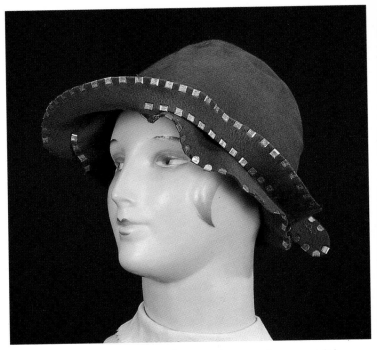

Slate-blue velour to keep warm, with square chrome studs to stay stylish. *Courtesy of: The Way We Wore.* Value: $150-225.

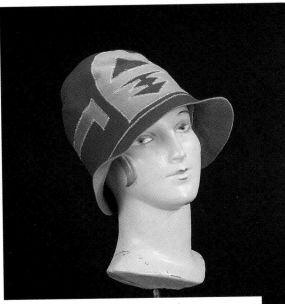

Stunning in magenta, appliqued in lavender felt. Label: Lazarus. *Courtesy of: The Way We Wore.* Value: $150-225.

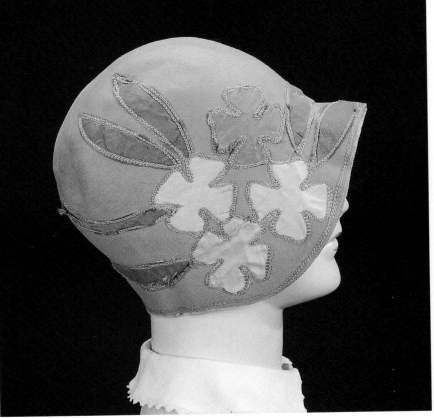

Short-brimmed cloche with appliqued felt daisies. *Courtesy of: The Way We Wore.* Value: $150-225.

Variations
on
a Theme

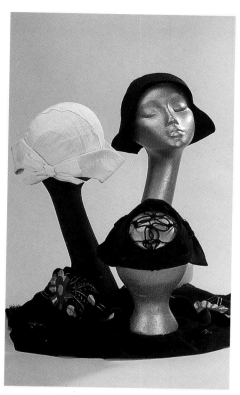

A lemon linen cap bowed at the nape, left. The similar style in black straw, center, is shaped from Milan so fine it folds like a hanky. To its right, a peek-a-boo crown adds interest. Label (left & right): New York Creations. *Courtesy of (all): Sandra Headley.* Value (each): $75-125.

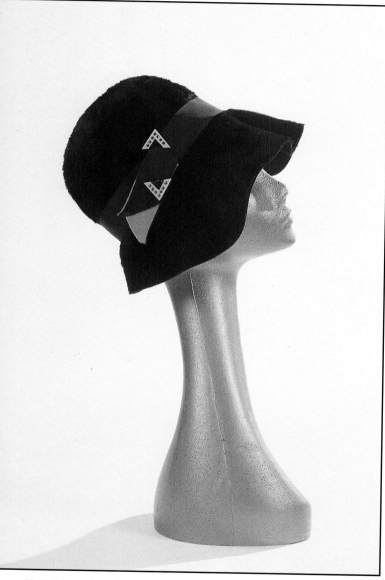

Fur felt hugs the neck, features a celluloid hatpin. Labels: Lilli of California, Duchess—Made in Italy. *Courtesy of: Lisa Carson.* Value: $95-145.

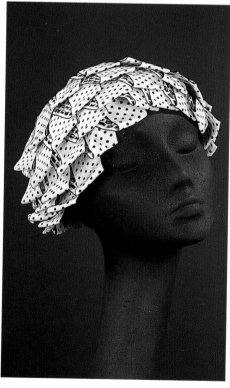

A real "crown pleaser," done entirely in polka-dot ribbon. Label: Mad Caps. *Courtesy of: Banbury Cross Antiques.* Value: $75-125.

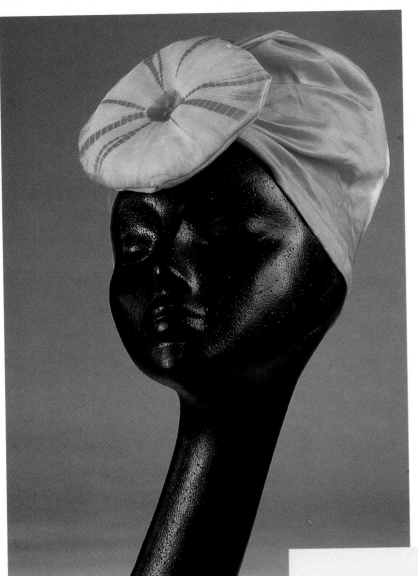

Neon Lights

A stunning turban in tie-died orange silk with large central medallion. *Courtesy of: Anna's.* Value: $125-175.

Light as a Feather

A black straw Pamela with irregular brim, made more eccentric by three large iridescent feathers. *Courtesy of: The Way We Wore.* Value: $150-225.

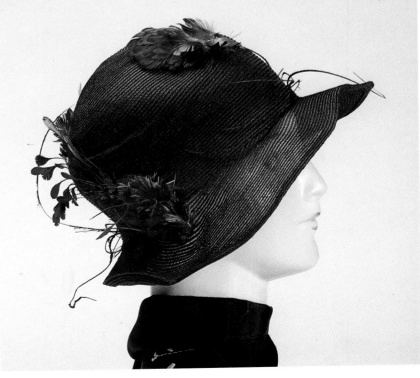

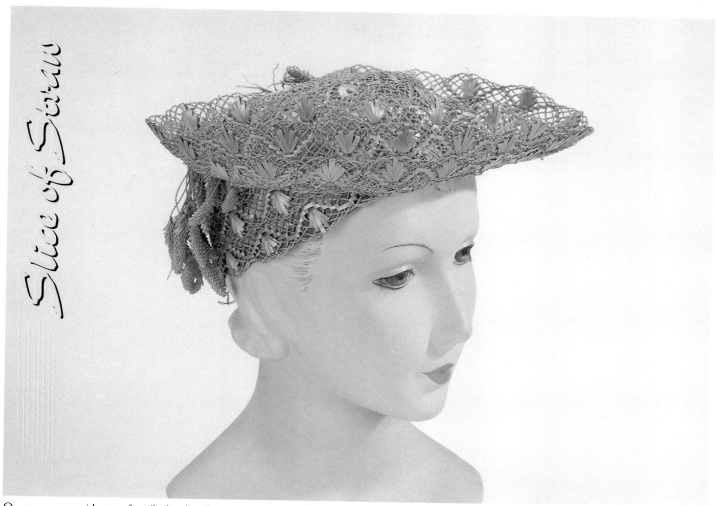

Openweave cap with straw foxtails dangling from a sculpted bill, all in woven raffia. *Courtesy of: The Way We Wore.* Value: $150-225.

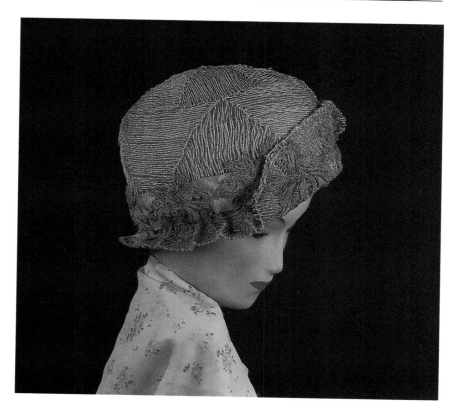

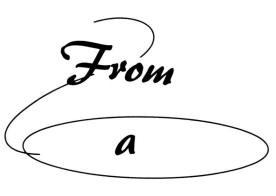

From a Different Angle

Stripped raffia whorls along a cloche with a flapper flap brim on just one side, shown. *Courtesy of: Mary Aaron Museum.* Value: Special.

A transitional cloche, its upswept brim punctuated by a rondele, all in navy straw. Label: M.S. Andree by Bellini. *Courtesy of: Banbury Cross Antiques.* Value: $75-125.

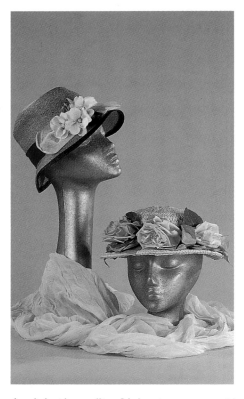

Straw toque, banded with camellias. It's keeping company with an ivory satin-finish boater, trimmed with silk blooms. Label (left): Brucewood; Maurice L. Rothschild, New York. Creation. *Courtesy of (both): Banbury Cross Antiques.* Value (each): $95-145.

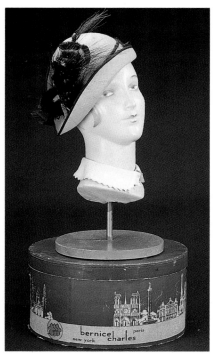

Fine natural straw forms a demi-cloche with large floral feather, on the original hatbox. Label: Bernice Charles. *Courtesy of (both): The Way We Wore.* Value (hat): $125-195. Value (box): $35-65.

A revival bonnet, bedecked with silk flowers and ribbon. It bears the original pricetag: $2.77. Label: Richard Original. *Courtesy of: Banbury Cross Antiques.* Value: $95-145.

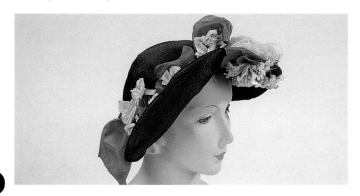

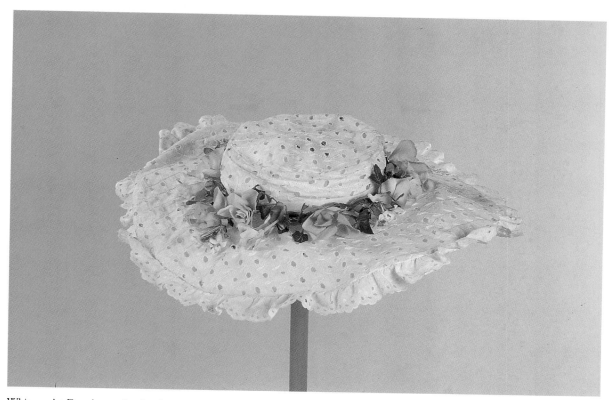

White eyelet Pamela, perfect for that garden wedding. *Courtesy of: Past Perfect.* Value: $125-175.

A Visit to Grandma's

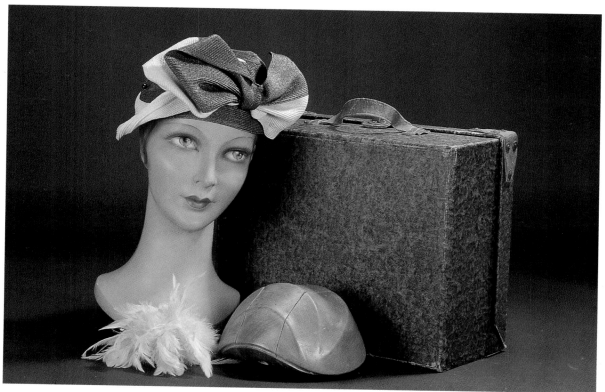

Pink and taupe straw, snugly tied with a front bow. Shown with vintage hatbox and hatblock. Label (hat): Janet. *Courtesy of (hat): Lottie Ballou.* Value (hat): $75-125.

Coming Home

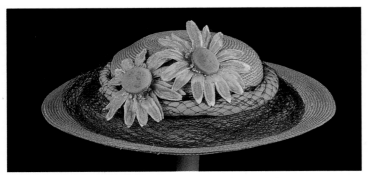

A dilly of a hat in summer straw with fabric daisies, and netting. *Courtesy of: Banbury Cross Antiques.* Value: $75-125.

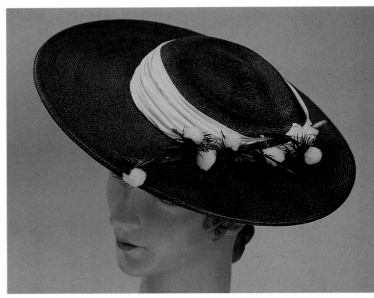

Navy straw banded in chartreuse chiffon, trimmed with a branch of cellophane pussy willows. Label: Dajon Original—New York. *Courtesy of: Banbury Cross Antiques.* Value: $75-125.

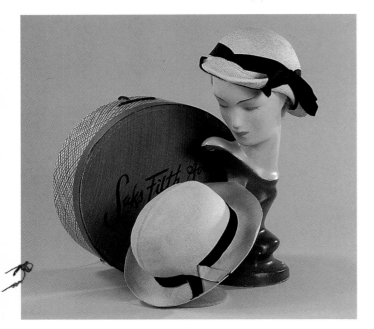

Two sweetly simple styles in straw, banded with black ribbon. Label (left): Lady Stetson, Genuine Panama. *Courtesy of (both): Sheryl Birkner.* Value (left): $75-125. Value (right): $55-75.

Said the Spider to the Fly

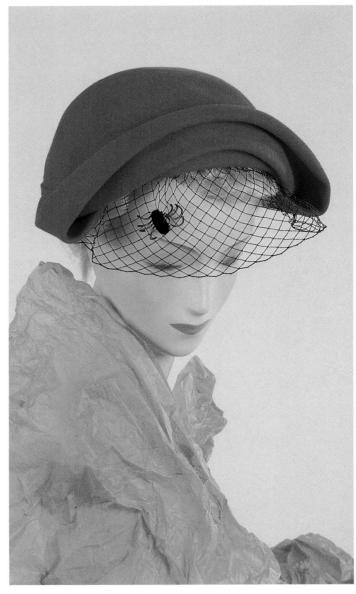

A chenille spider weaves its magic web on the fabulous veil of this poppy-red felt cap. Label: Janet. *Courtesy of: Shirley Birkner.* Value: $125-175.

Two felt cloches with small brims, typical of the early 1930s. Note the large rhinestone buckle on the violet, a bit of glamour during the grim Depression. Label (left): Christine Original, New York. Label (right): Maryse Cegallois, Paris. *Courtesy of (both): Banbury Cross Antiques.* Value (left): $75-125. Value (right): $95-145.

Brim pleated to frame the face, crown shaped to hug the head, all in Kelly green felt. *Courtesy of: Donna McMaster.* Value: $95-145.

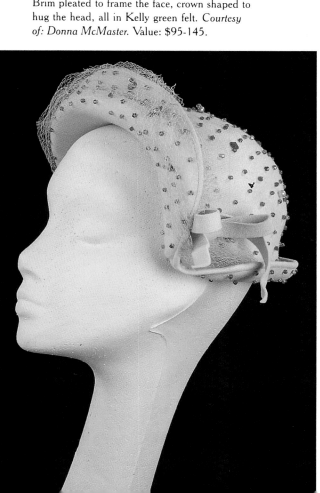

A pert cap with upturned brim, and multicolored crystal beads and pearls. Label: Rickie Original—New York. *Courtesy of: Banbury Cross Antiques.* Value: $55-75.

Spring Chic

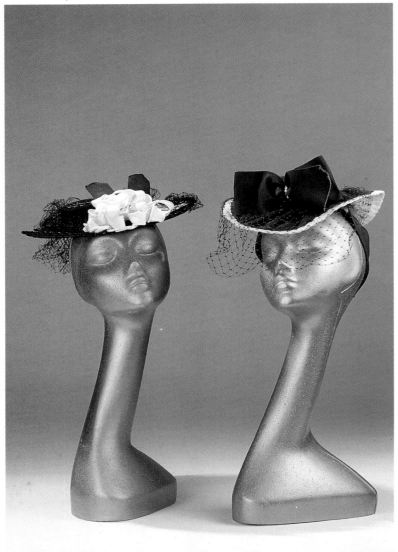

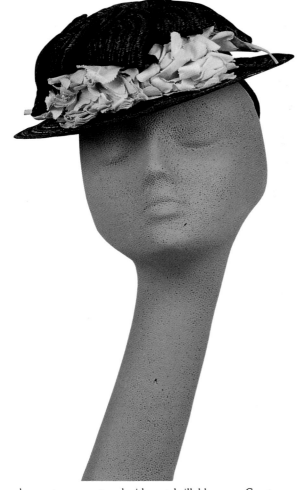

Layered navy straw, sweetened with pastel silk blossoms. *Courtesy of: Lisa Carson*. Value: $75-125.

Black straw in a modified Pamela, with white rayon chou, left. Similar in style, a white straw with black grosgrain bow, right. *Courtesy of (left): Sandra Lagorio. Courtesy of (right): Banbury Cross Antiques.* Value (each): $55-75.

Puttin' on the Ritz

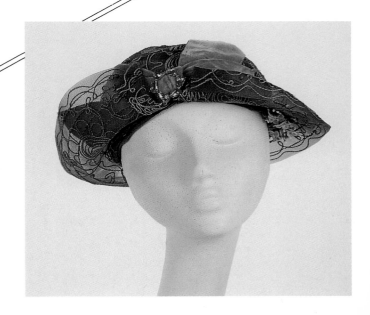

A classic mid-1930s style in lacy, woven horsehair. Note the Deco-inspired trim. *Courtesy of: Lisa Carson*. Value: $125-175.

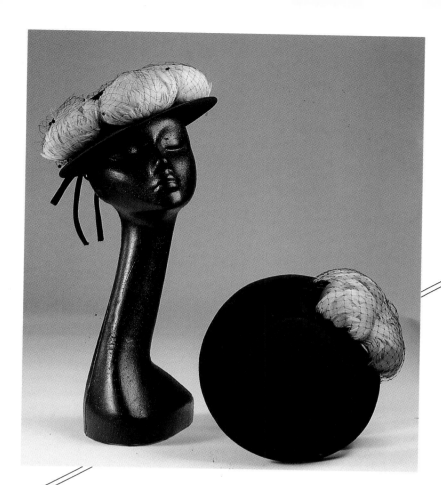

Two similar black boaters lightened with pastel feathers. Label (right): Jeanne Tête; Harriet Short, San Francisco. Label (left): Midinette, City of Paris. *Courtesy of (both): Sandra Lagario.* Value (each): $45-65.

Tailored Toppers

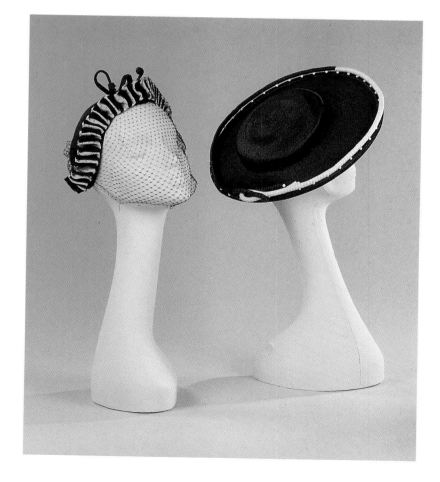

Ruched navy and white grosgrain perks up a cap. The same colors sail cheerfully across a sophisticated sailor. Label (left): G. Henry Ross. Label (right): Marché. *Courtesy of (left): Graf's Glitz. Courtesy of (right): Karen Burrows.* Value (each): $75-125.

Pretty as a Picture

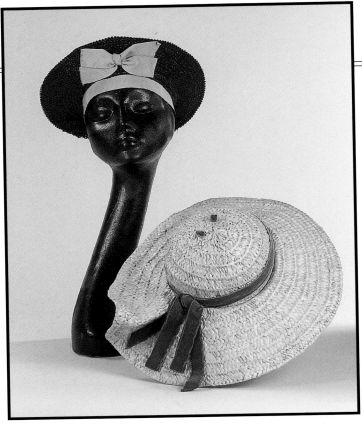

A jaunty beret with avocado grosgrain trim, and an avocado straw picture hat with self-hatpins. *Courtesy of (left): Shirley Birkner. Courtesy of (right): Rich Man, Poor Man.* Value (each): $95-145.

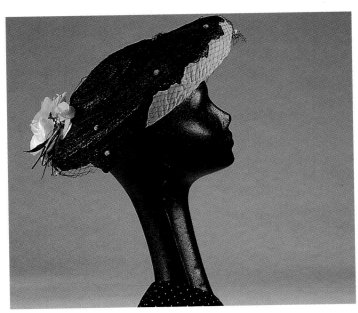

Lacquered black straw picture hat, with buttercup feathers and flowers. *Courtesy of: Graf's Glitz.* Value: $75-125.

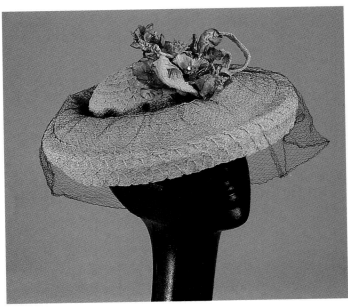

A picture hat in vivid, patterned chartreuse straw. *Courtesy of: The Rag Bag.* Value: $95-145.

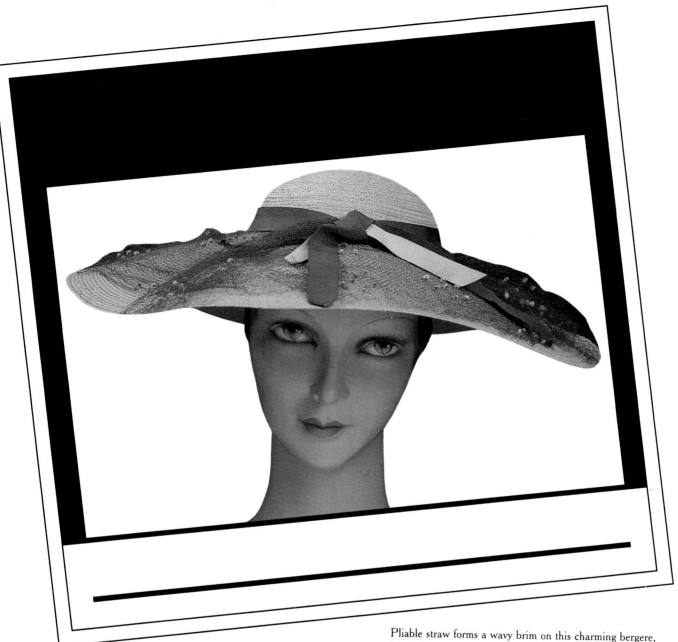

Pliable straw forms a wavy brim on this charming bergere,
banded in two-tone grosgrain. A layer of silky netting is dotted
with chenille. Label: Hale Bros. *Courtesy of: Banbury Cross
Antiques.* Value: $95-145.

Broad-Brim Bergere

Suitable for Framing

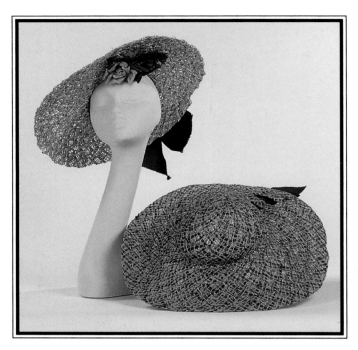

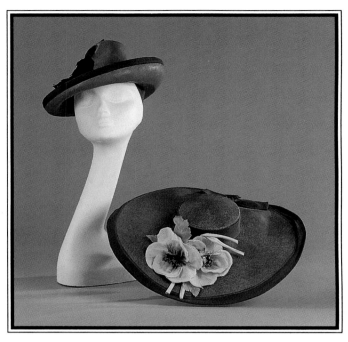

A pretty pair in wide-weave natural straw, one with silk roses and the other with ribbon trim. *Courtesy of (both): Banbury Cross Antiques.* Value (each): $75-125.

A snappy, tall-brimmed Breton with velvet trim. To its right, a fine straw cartwheel, also trimmed in velvet. Label (right): Leslie James. *Courtesy of (left): Sheryl Birkner. Courtesy of (right): Past Perfect.* Value (left): $65-95. Value (right): $75-125

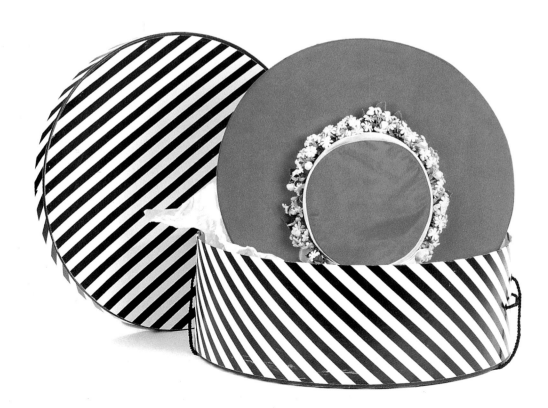

Lipstick-red picture hat trimmed with lilies of the valley, shown with a licorice-whip vintage hatbox. Label (hat): Maisôn Mendesolle. *Courtesy of (hat): Rich Man, Poor Man. Courtesy of (box): Sheryl Birkner.* Value (hat): $75-125. Value (box): $25-45.

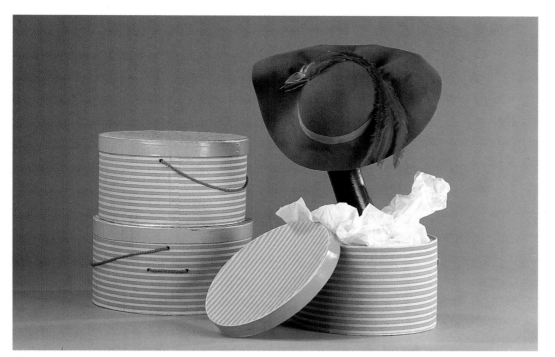

The charcoal felt of this floppy brim is highlighted by a large scarlet bird. Label: Elinor's of San Francisco. *Courtesy of: Connie Beers.* Value: $150-225.

A fur felt fedora in mahogany with malines on the brim. To its right, another felt fedora with ostrich feathers. Label (left): Paris Maid. Label (right): Louis Original, California. *Courtesy of (left): Mary Aaron Museum.* *Courtesy of (right): Graf's Glitz.* Value (left): Special. Value (right): $65-115.

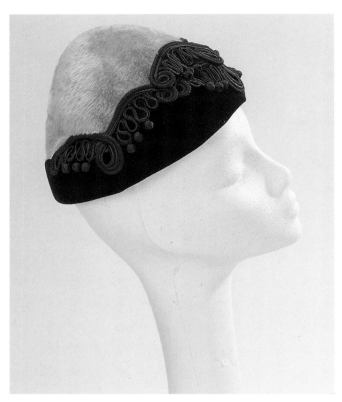

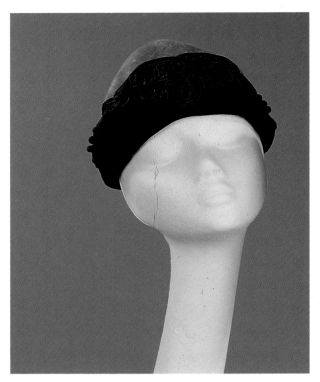

A beautifully-constructed shako in cocoa fur felt, trimmed with black passementerie. Its clean lines are shown in two views. Label: Hattie Carnegie. *Courtesy of: Maureen Reilly.* Value: $125-175.

Cocktails at Seven...

Graceful as a swan, an unknown milliner's custom-made cap, dotted with pearls and rhinestones. *Courtesy of: Banbury Cross Antiques.* Value: $125-175.

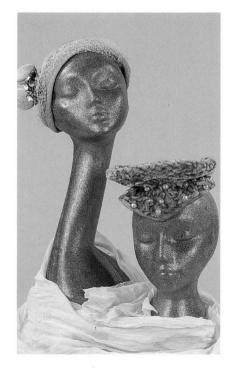

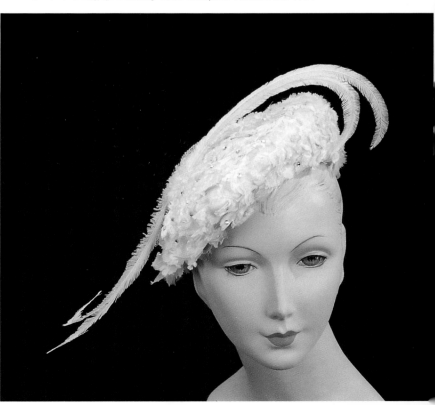

A straw lilac beret is stabbed with pom-pom hatpins and planted in violets. Shown with a chenille "pipecleaner" helmet; its visor-like brim salutes with pearl buttons. Label (left): Leslie James. *Courtesy of (both): Maureen Reilly.* Value (left): $55-75. Value (right): $25-45.

...and Dinner at Eight

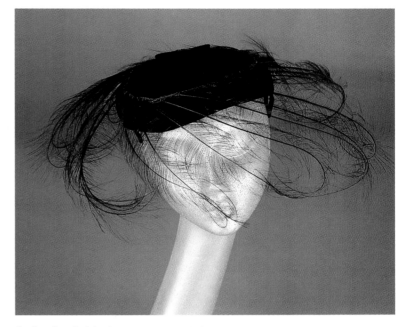

Sculpted curled feathers serve as a veil for this dramatic platter in black velvet. Label: Dorée. *Courtesy of: Connie Beers.* Value: $75-125.

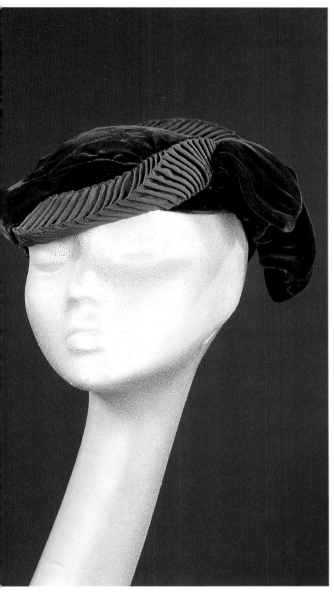

Lustrous blue velvet and ruched satin ribbon create this simple beauty. Label: Livingston Bros. *Courtesy of: Donna McMaster.* Value: $75-125.

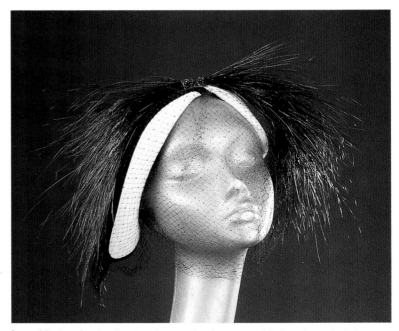

Ivory felt tips steeply, then is sideswept by shimmering black malines. Label: Patrice. *Courtesy of: Maureen Reilly.* Value: $75-125.

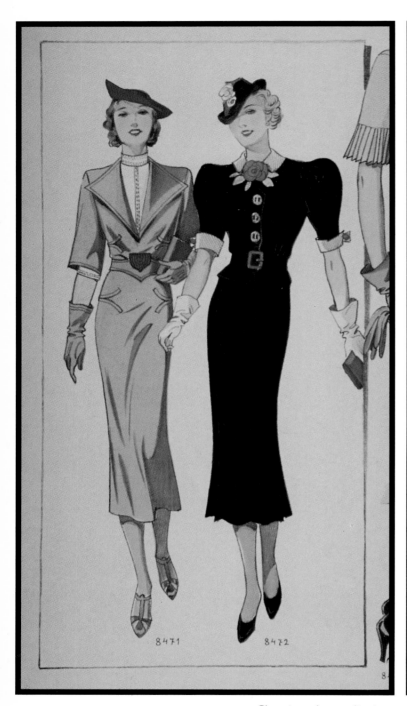

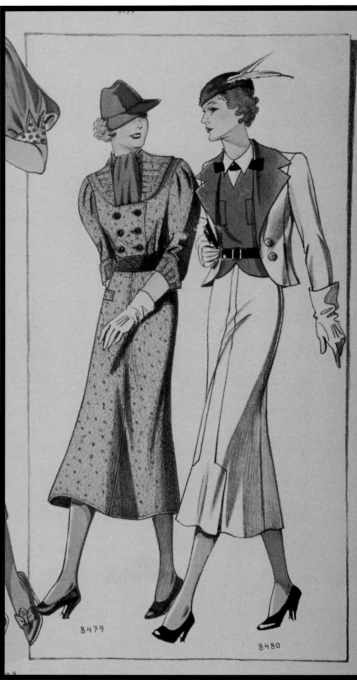

Charming color-coordinating ensembles were very in style
circa 1936, shown in these illustrations from *Chic Parisien*.

VIII. *The Glory Days: 1935-1946*

For a few golden years—after the weary world had pulled itself out of the depths of a Depression and before it plunged into the trenches of a second great war—it seemed as if any dream could be attained by Everyman. As for Everywoman, well, she was able to preen in hats the like of which will never be seen again.

New designers stepped into the spotlight with an array of styles that glowed with wit, charm, and elegance. These were truly the Glory Days of the hat!

The tilt hat or doll hat is emblematic of this era. It rode at rather a steep angle—diminutive and silly and wonderful. The style was flaunted by women, and viewed with some amazement by men. Oftentimes, these styles featured amusing veils.

Veils appeared on collectible vintage hats from the Belle Epoque forward, but were indispensable to styles during the Glory Days. They flew from any hat that could claim a brim, and cascaded over those that couldn't. Some veils were of coarse netting, others, of gossamer silk. Intricate patterns such as the "spiderweb" denote a vintage hat, although it is rare to find one of these delicacies in mint condition.

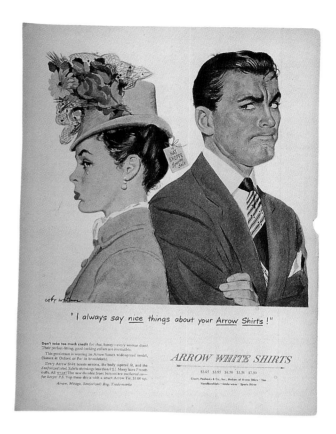

The Arrowshirt man finds fault with his darling's new doll hat! But is the silly veil or the serious pricetag to blame for his reaction?

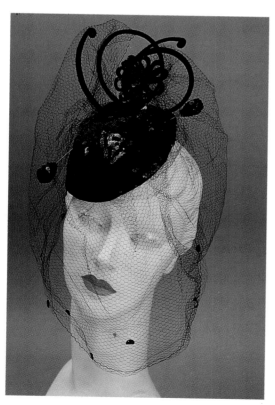

A doll hat in black velvet with velvet-covered wire forming an avant garde design. *Courtesy of: Banbury Cross Antiques.* Value: $65-95

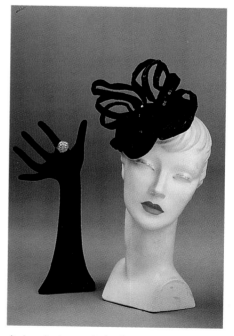

A dot of velvet, a dash of sequins with a dramatic pouf of veil. Label: Monte Rey. *Courtesy of: Banbury Cross Antiques.* Value: $75-125.

If not color-matched to the hat, veils were brown or black. For fun, they might be embellished with pom-poms, patches, or sequins. Typically, they reached one of four standard lengths: eye, nose, chin, and waist. But don't expect to find all veils falling face forward! During the Glory Days, veils were also split and swagged, swooped and swathed, poufed and puffed.

Headwraps were popular for casualwear and sporting events, but could also take on an evening elegance. The American milliner Mme. Paulette created a name for herself with a highly-styled turban and attached snood. The revival of the snood quickly caught on, inspiring other designers to attach hoods and bibs in lieu of veils.

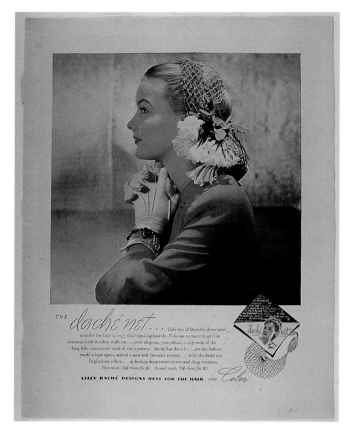

Lilly Daché had a genius for marketing. In 1944, she showed women how to wear two "Daché nets" at one time for a chic swath of snood; not incidentally, doubling her sales volume!

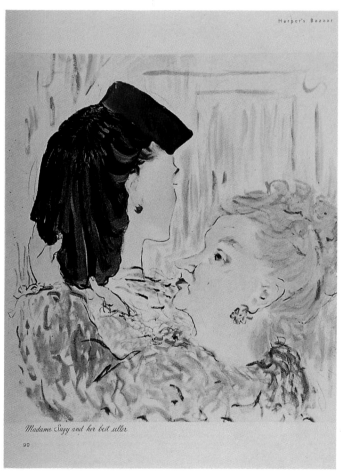

Mme. Suzy's best seller, a Doll Hat with deeply draped velvet snood. As shown in *Harper's Bazaar*, circa 1939.

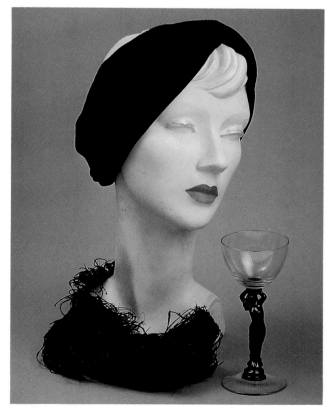

A simple evening style in black velvet, stretched to band the head. *Courtesy of: Banbury Cross Antiques.* Value: $35-55.

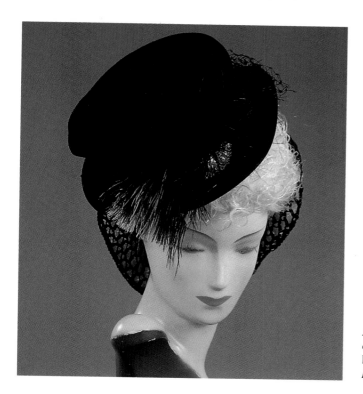

Styles varied widely during the Glory Days. In the late 1930s, the surrealistic influence was strong, and hats were modern in the extreme. Many hats were influenced by Salvador Dali and the surrealist movement in art.

No hat was left without a revival. In the early 1940s, there was great interest in the grandeur of court dress from the Middle Ages and Renaissance. For the sophisticate, there was the turban; and for the working gal, the new boater. But for the ingenue, there was the bonnet.

A chic black derby with metal starburst medallion. This derby may have been worn with a silky snood, as shown here. Label: Fifth Ave. Designer's Group. *Courtesy of: Banbury Cross Antiques.* Value: $55-75.

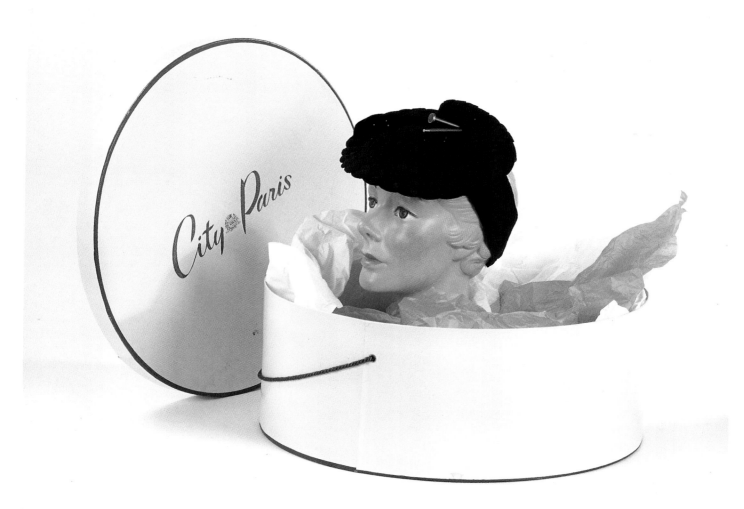

Knitting needles mock hatpins, in this surrealistic style. This photo is styled after one taken by Cecil Beaton. *Courtesy of: Sheryl Birkner.* Value: $75-125.

Menswear-inspired styles were also a major millinery trend during this era. Enter the tufted Tyrolean, adapted for women from an Austrian hunting hat. Its earliest iteration was a flat crown and droopy brim, circa mid-1930s. The true Tyrolean, with peaked crown and snappy brim, tipped into view a few years later.

Several styles were borrowed from the boys, for a look of tailored charm. The top hat was treated to a flared crown and rolled brim. The boater was beautified, with elongated crown and sculpted brim. Not to be outdone, the fedora and Homburg also underwent a millinery transformation with ribbons and plumage.

> In its March 1939 issue, the readership of Vogue was given fair warning of a "new breath of life" from the Paris Openings:
> *"You will tie an 1860 bonnet under your chin."*

The last of the Glory Days were shaped by the tempo of wartime. The Fall of Paris in 1940 brought a temporary end to the influence of haute couture. Despite the best efforts of the French government to keep this important sector of the economy alive, the war effort quickly claimed all of the necessary material and talent.

Certainly, the grim war years brought an end to the whimsical and surrealistic hats that had marked the prior decade. Women were entering the workforce and needed practical clothing that required little maintenance.

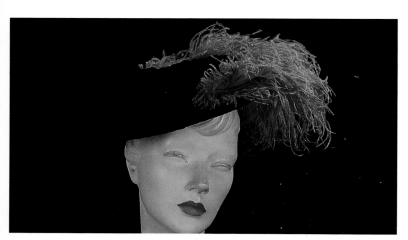

Black velvet is tucked and plumed in the style made famous by Holbein's portrait of King Henry VIII. *Courtesy of: Sandra Headley.* Value: $65-95

Such a sweetie! Fabric flowers and glass grapes nestle in the turned-up straw brim of this revival Sunbonnet. Note the long silk-cord streamers in shades of blue and brown. *Courtesy of: The Rag Bag.* Value: $55-95.

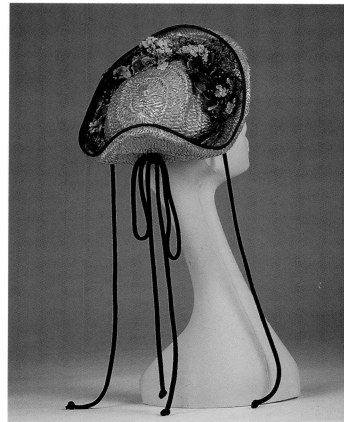

For those who took a factory shift, a simple bandanna served as a hat, also shielding the hair from the dirt and danger of nearby machinery. The tailored influence of mannish styles and fabrics continued in popularity. These were well-suited to the business suits that women began wearing in unprecedented numbers, as they assumed the jobs that had previously been held by men. This is just as well, because luxury hats were soon to become scarce commodities in the wartime marketplace.

Silks were reserved for parachutes, and wool for blankets and uniforms. Felt was rationed, then became unattainable. As a rather odd result, milliners resorted to a flat-nap felt pressed from a formula of fur and skim milk! Sequins were not rationed, and were used to good effect on many hats and veils of this period.

The May 1944 issue of *Vogue* included a brief article on "hat news" and wartime rationing. The editors discussed a rumor that French milliners were lavishly trimming hats "under duress, (as) a joke on the Germans." The passage of time proved it true.

To keep up morale, Parisiennes flaunted fantastic hats during the Occupation. In the face of shortages, these were crafted from offcuts of pre-war fabrics and trimmed with scraps of cellophane, twine, and carpet felt.

In America, fabric was not rationed for millinery by the rationing regulation No. L-38 that ruled the garment industry. Still, our designers made it a point of honor to match the British yard-for-yard. The long run in popularity of the doll hat on both sides of the Atlantic is attributed to fabric rationing during the war years.

Seven Rules of Rationing

In 1944, *Vogue* commended "...the American millinery designers (who) are definitely determined to abide by their own voluntary code in conserving materials." *Vogue* went on to publish a list of "government-approved measurements" for milliners.

These seven rules show the detail and scope of shortages that taxed the creativity of milliners on both sides of the Atlantic during the war years. We reprint them verbatim below:

1. Maximum circumference of hat brims on felt bodies (this means felt hats all of one piece) shall not exceed 48 inches. No limitations on crowns.

2. Berets are not to exceed 38 inches in circumference when made out of felt bodies or any other materials.

3. Hats made of fabric shall not consume more than 6 yards of material, 36 to 39 inches wide (or its equivalent), for one dozen hats.

4. The maximum use of (fur) felt skirtings (yardage) shall not exceed 8 strips per dozen of 15 to 18 inches wide and 45 inches long (or its equivalent).

5. The (wool) felt yardage, 72 inches wide, shall not exceed 3 yards per dozen hats.

6. The maximum amount of ribbon to be used is 1 1/2 yards per hat, not including the head-size band.

7. Veiling of 19-inch width shall not exceed 1 yard per hat or its equivalent.

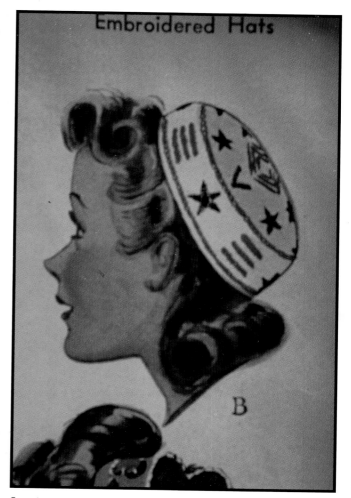

From the cover of a Butterick pattern for hats published in 1942, simple styles to make at home in patriotic colors.

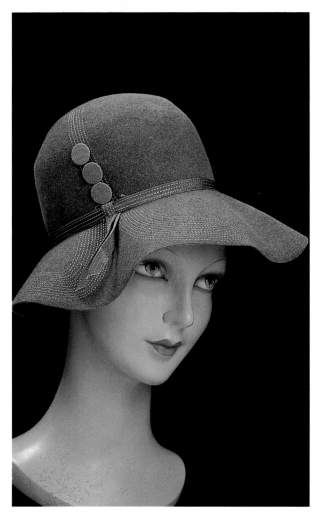

A variation on the fedora, in buttoned-up steel-grey felt. *Courtesy of: Banbury Cross Antiques.* Value: $45-75.

As the war progressed, and fabric became even scarcer, American women resorted to cutting down the civilian suits shed by their men in uniform. In doing so, they were inspired by the British "Make Do and Mend" campaign that encouraged the frugal use of old clothes.

The same patriotism that sold war bonds for Uncle Sam was used to market products by Madison Avenue. Milliners incorporated military insignia, and flew flag colors on all manner of hats. For women who stitched their hats at home, patriotic themes were illustrated in sewing patterns.

With the end of World War II in 1945 came a pent-up desire for consumer goods. As soon as raw materials and labor could catch up with this demand, manufacturers were glad to oblige. These forces were to explode on the fashion scene, in the New Look of 1947.

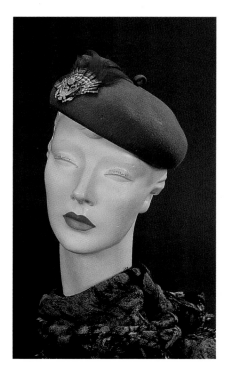

The American eagle struts on this military-style beret, circa 1940. *Courtesy of: Maureen Reilly.* Value: $25-45.

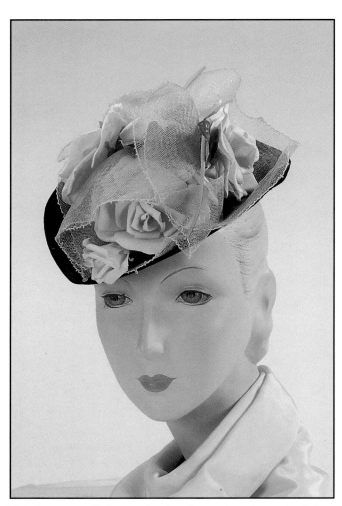

This little posy was likely a wartime remake, cut down into a chic doll hat. An almost identical hat was thus attributed by the Philadelphia Museum of Art in its fashion retrospective of 1993. *Courtesy of: Banbury Cross Antiques.* Value: $65-75.

Tudoresque

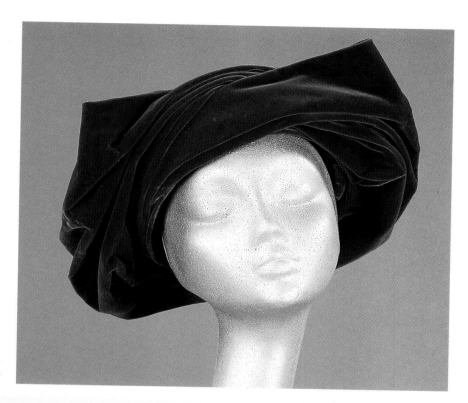

The skill of an expert milliner is apparent in this soft burgundy velvet. Label: Lilly Daché. *Courtesy: Donna McMaster.* Value: $95-145.

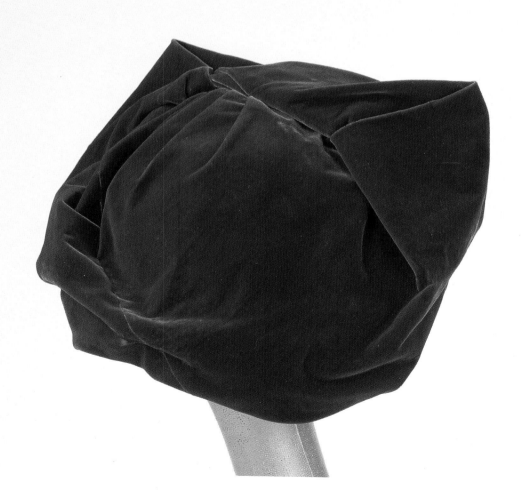

With a Twist

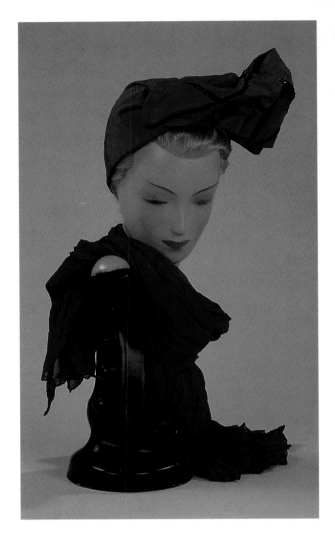

The ever-popular turban, here, in cherry satin edged with sapphire sequins. Label: Betty Co-ed. *Courtesy of: Maureen Reilly.* Value: $95-125.

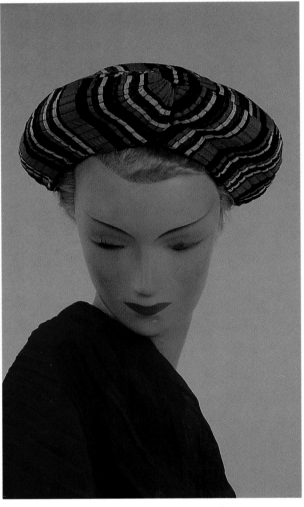

Crayola stripes on a sunny silk demi-turban. *Courtesy of: Maureen Reilly.* Value: $65-95.

Cover Girl

A similar bicorne showed on the cover of *Vogue* in October 1934, the year of the "forward-looking brim." By Lilly Daché in roughened navy straw. *Courtesy of: Banbury Cross Antiques.* Value: $75-125.

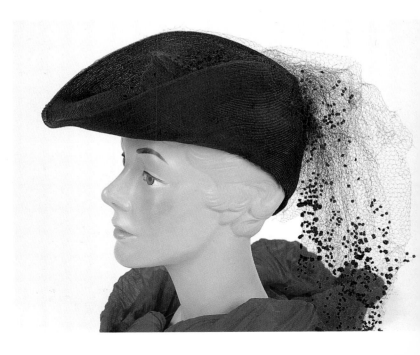

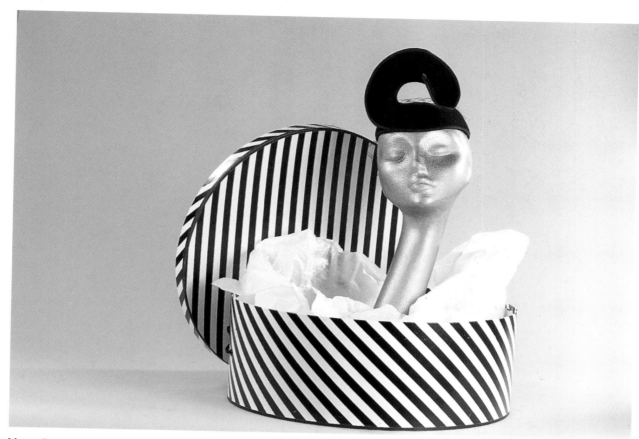

Hattie Carnegie's dream noir, a statement in black felt. *Courtesy of: Banbury Cross Antiques.* Value: $95-145.

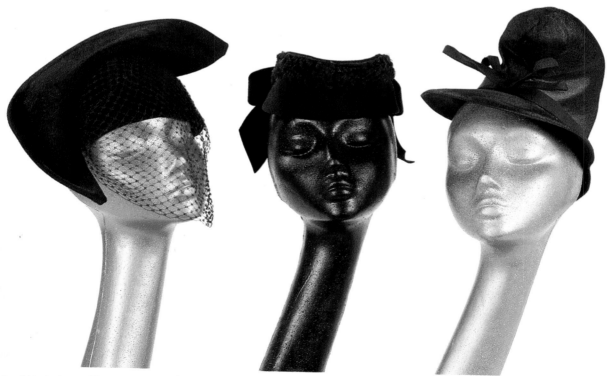

A trio of black shapes. To the right, stiffened fabric stumbles forward, reminiscent of Schiap's "shoe hat."
Courtesy of (all): Maureen Reilly. Value (each): $75-125.

Fit for a Trousseau

Brown felt with dyed feathers and a matching feathered muff, custom-made for a bride's wedding day. *Courtesy of: Sheryl Birkner.* Value: $200-300.

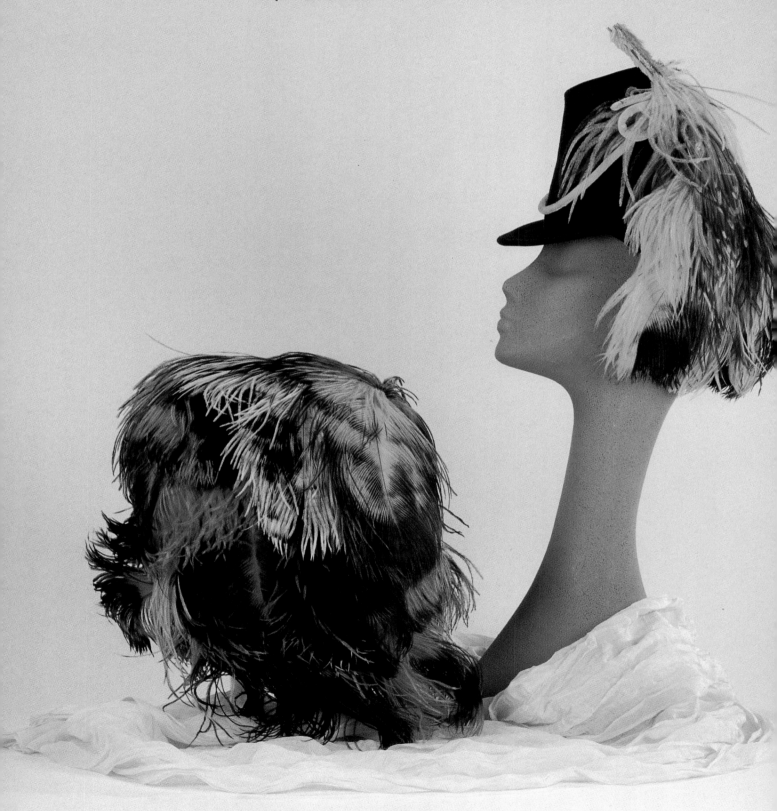

Smart and Sassy

A pat of red, a stab of green, two revival boaters make the scene. *Courtesy of (both): Maureen Reilly.* Value (each): $65-95.

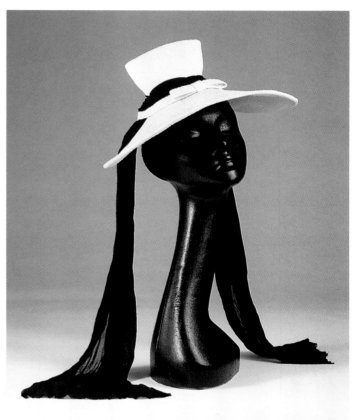

A quirky crown and chiffon ties give personality to ivory fabric picture hat. The brim is stiffened with concentric seaming. Label: Melbourne Original. *Courtesy of: Maureen Reilly.* Value: $95-145.

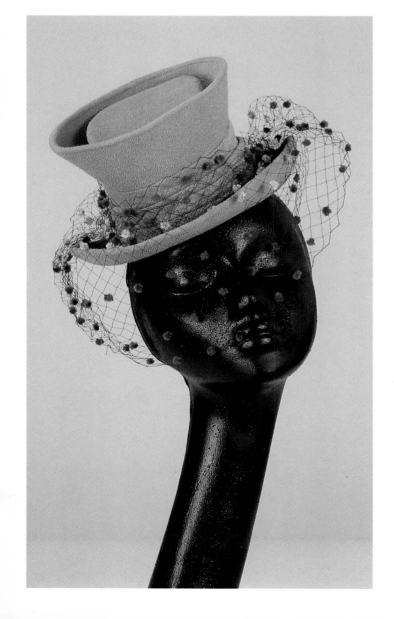

Turquise barkcloth in an amusing top hat, veiled in chenille confetti-colored poms. *Courtesy of: Maureen Reilly.* Value: $95-145.

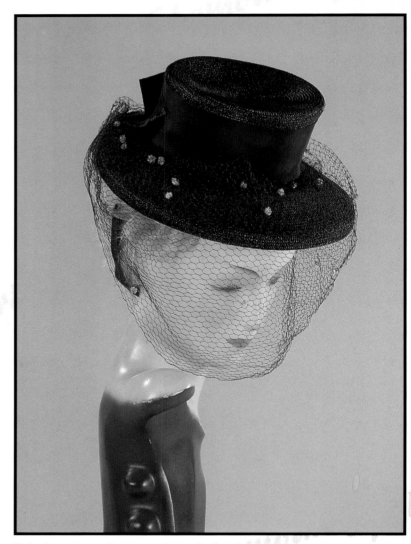

Fudge-brown straw, flirtatious with a pink pom-pom veil. Label: Martha Gene. *Courtesy of: Sheryl Birkner.* Value: $75-125.

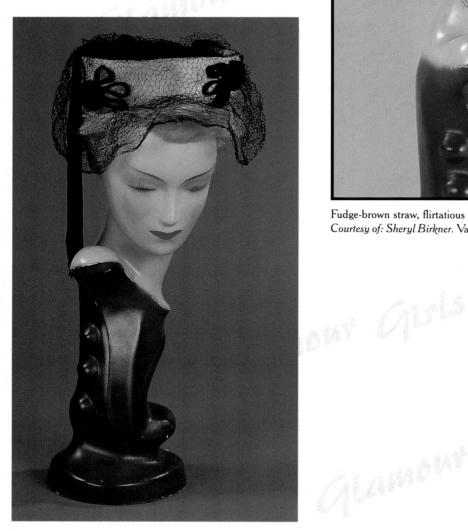

Ivory satin fez with tassel tossed over the right shoulder, in accordance with the "millinery rule." *Courtesy of: 57th Street Antique Mall.* Value: $95-145.

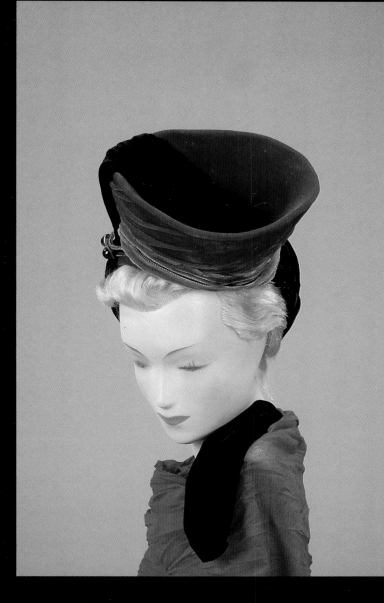

Superb tri-color silk velvet crown, trimmed with a "ruby" clip. *Courtesy of: 57th Street Antique Mall.* Value: $125-175.

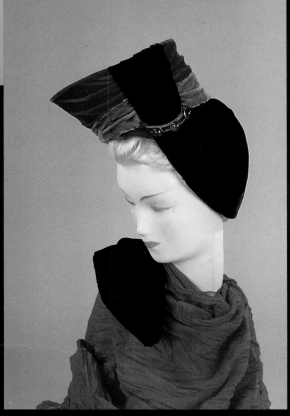

Crowning Glories

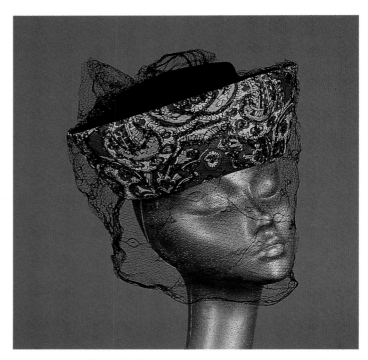

An exaggerated Breton in black felt with the exotic influence of paisley silk and sequins. *Courtesy of: 57th Street Antique Mall.* Value: $95-145.

Wine crepe frames the face. Label: Swank Shop—Brooklyn. *Courtesy of: Barbara Griggs Vintage Fashion.* Value: $125-175.

Two black felt toques are treated to different veiling. One, hooded in shimmering paillettes; the other, draped in front and swagged in back. Label (right): Del Marie Models. Label (left); Mr. Monroe. *Courtesy of (right): Maureen Reilly. Courtesy of (left): Barbara Griggs.* Value (each): $75-125.

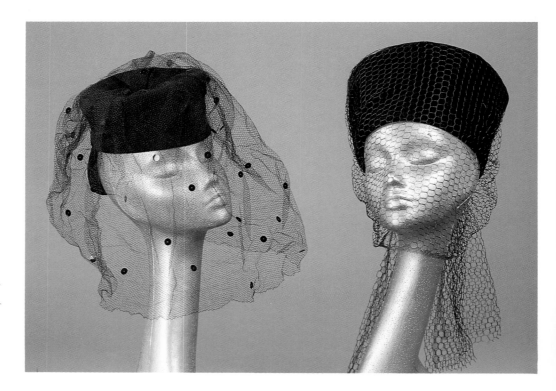

Making an Entrance ....

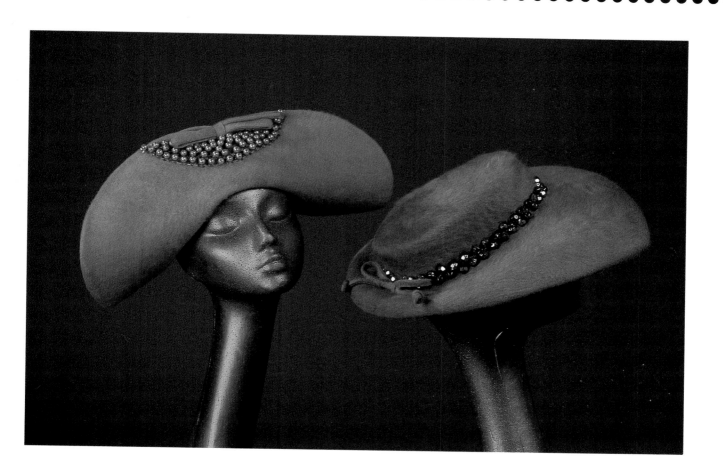

A whisper-pink tricorne, embellished with cut-steel beads, and a powder-blue platter with glittering headband. The pair, in fur felt. *Courtesy of (both): Connie Beers.* Value (each): $95-145.

Birds of a Feather

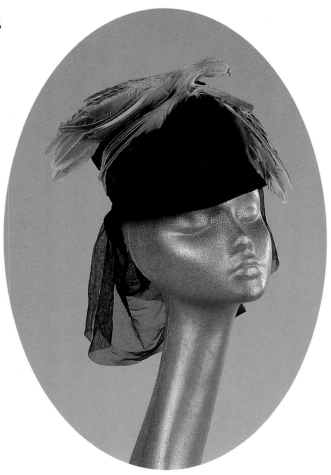

A sweet bird wings its way across a black felt toque. Label: George Mander's Hats, Designed by Laura—New York. *Courtesy of: Maureen Reilly.* Value: $95-145.

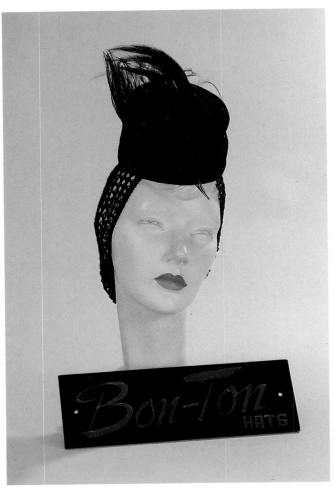

This black felt fez seems about to take flight, until caught by a silken snood. *Courtesy of: It's About Time.* Value: $75-125.

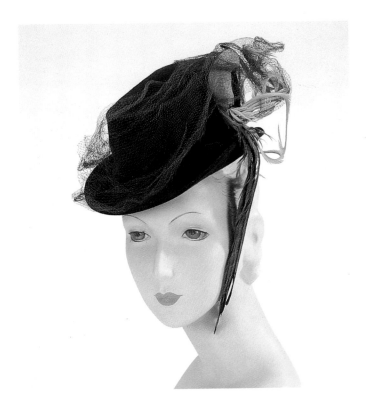

Gold feathers nest in the net of this charming tilt hat. *Courtesy of: Banbury Cross Antiques.* Value: $75-125.

Tawny felt, banded in burgundy velvet. The full veil is boldly trimmed with matching velvet cording. *Courtesy of: Maureen Reilly.* Value: $75-125

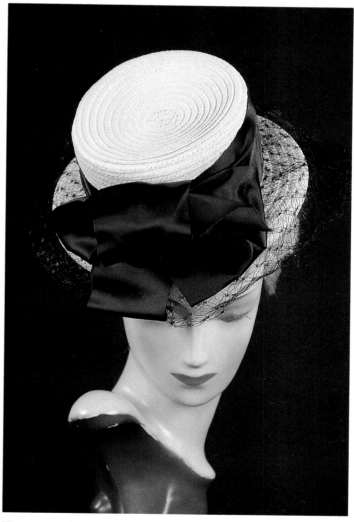

The contrast of cream straw and plum satin, dishing up a sweet tilt hat. Label: Evelyn Varon—Model. *Courtesy of: Maureen Reilly.* Value: $75-125.

The halo-brimmed hat is swagged in fishnet, its companion is draped in a similar veil. *Courtesy of (left): Maureen Reilly. Courtesy of (right): Anna's.* Value (each): $75-125.

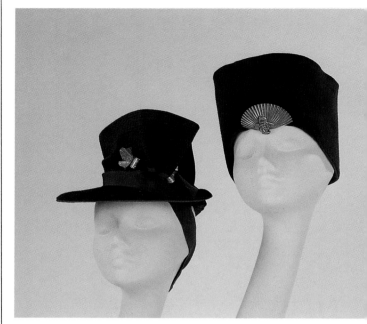

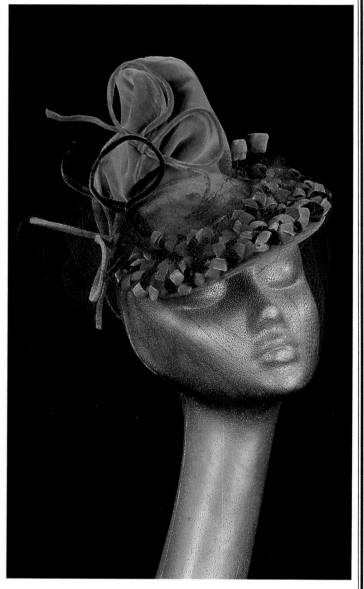

Olive-green velvet, looped and braided in a riot of color. Label: A Marion Vallé Original. *Courtesy of: Maureen Reilly.* Value: $95-145.

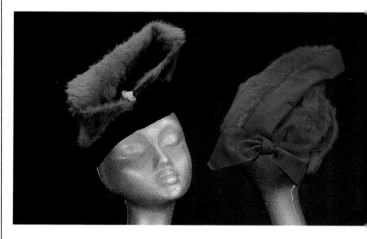

Top right:
Two highrise felts with brass Deco decor. Label (left): Tulip Model—San Francisco. Label (right): Mallory Fur Felt—New York. *Courtesy of (left): Banbury Cross Antiques. Courtesy of (right): Graf's Glitz.* Value (each): $75-125.

Center right:
Two plush fur velours sculpted in brilliant jade and deep cinnamon. Label: (left): New York Creation. *Courtesy of (both): The Way We Wore.* Value (each): $95-145.

Bottom right:
A light brown straw with grosgrain trim, next to a brown-sugar straw with honeyed braid. Label (right): N.L. Court. *Courtesy of (left): Banbury Cross Antiques. Courtesy of (right): Maureen Reilly.* Value (each): $75-125.

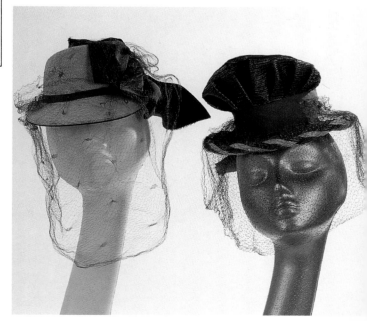

Sensuality

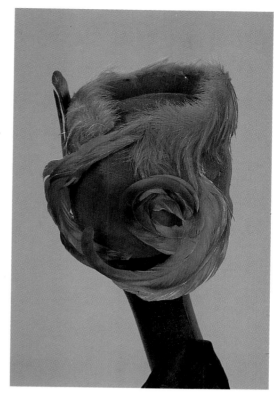

A soft swirl of feathers for a cranberry-crested lovebird.
Courtesy of: Connie Beers. Value: $95-145.

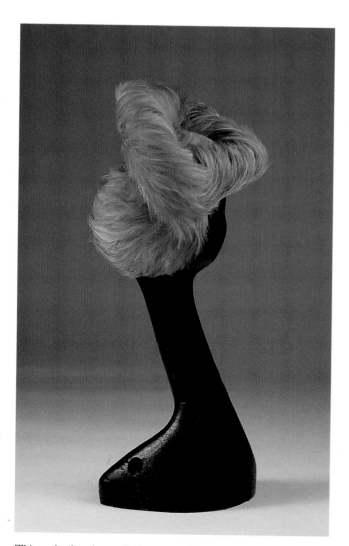

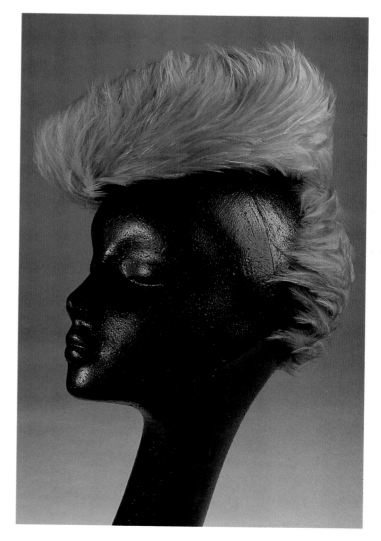

This cocktail cockatoo displays magnificent turquoise plumage, shown
here in two views. *Courtesy of: Graf's Glitz.* Value: $95-145

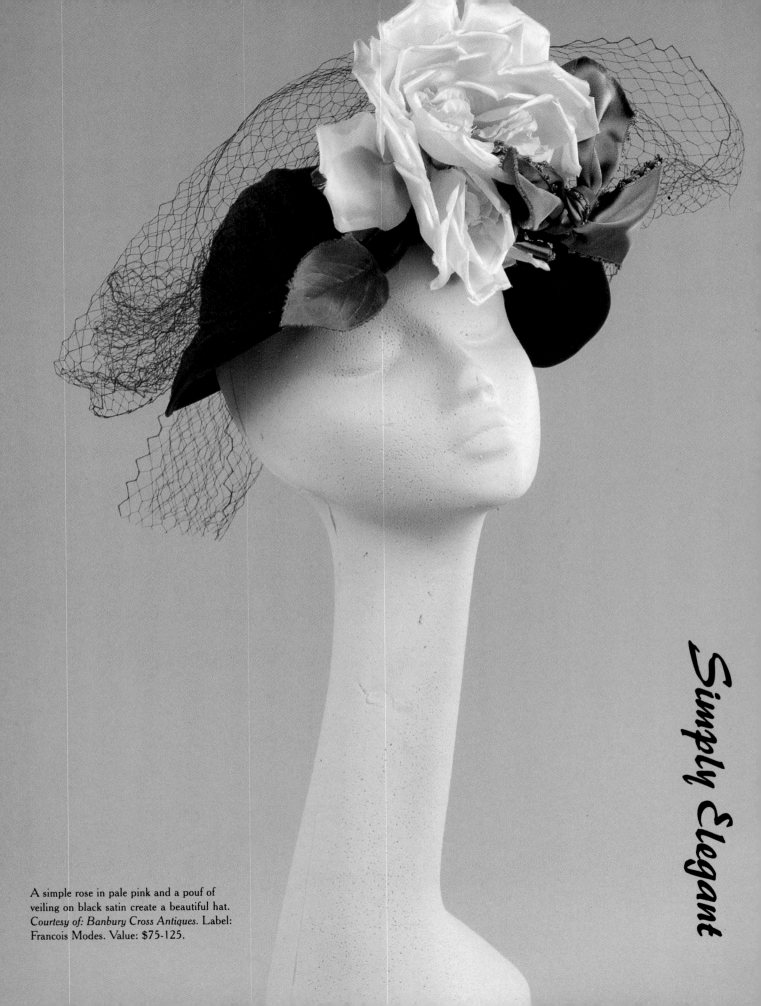

A simple rose in pale pink and a pouf of
veiling on black satin create a beautiful hat.
Courtesy of: Banbury Cross Antiques. Label:
Francois Modes. Value: $75-125.

Simply Elegant

Easter Parade

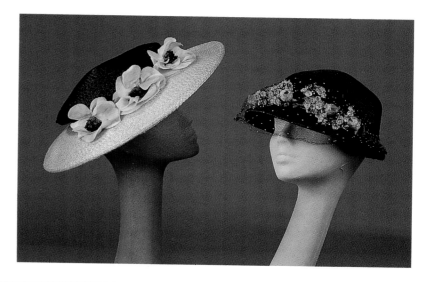

Navy and ivory Milan straw with a circlet of gardenias. Shown with a pert navy straw with pink flowerettes and beautymark veiling. Label (left): Gertrude Menczer. *Courtesy of (left): Lisa Carson. Courtesy of (right): Laurie Newman.* Value (left): $75-125. Value (right): $35-55.

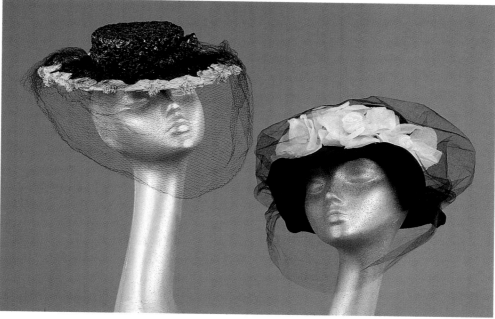

A black straw boater graced with white petals. It is paired with a floppy black bombazine, brightened with large white roses and a swath of veiling. Label (left): Addie Ann of California—Hale Bros. Label (right): Eva Mae Modes. *Courtesy of (both): Banbury Cross Antiques.* Value (each): $65-95

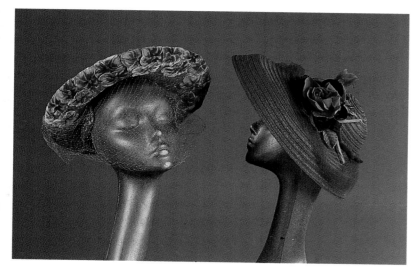

An appealing Breton, ladylike in soft peach straw with matching velvet flowers. Pictured with a Pamela in lilac Milan, punctuated by a rose of magenta silk. Label (left): Trêt Moulin. *Courtesy of (left): Maureen Reilly. Courtesy of (right): Rich Man, Poor Man.* Value (each): $65-95

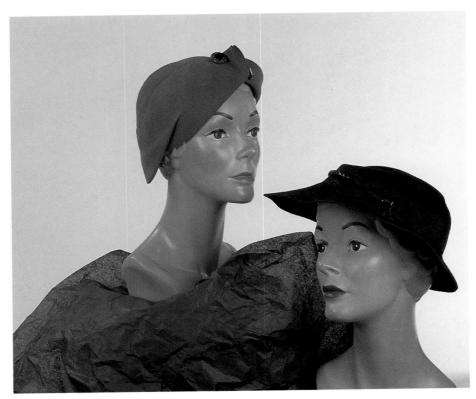

A taupe head-hugger by Hattie Carnegie. Shown with a fedora in bark brown with a leather hatband, by Agnés of Paris. *Courtesy of (both): Sheryl Birkner.* Value (each): $95-145.

Designer Duo

A Soft Palette

By its provenance, the ivory satin boater banded in pearls was worn by a bride circa 1945. The Breton, netted in pom-poms, would have been perfect for her maid of honor! Label (right): Agnés. *Courtesy of (left): Maureen Reilly. Courtesy of (right): C.J. Granados.* Value (left): $75-125. Value (right): $95-145.

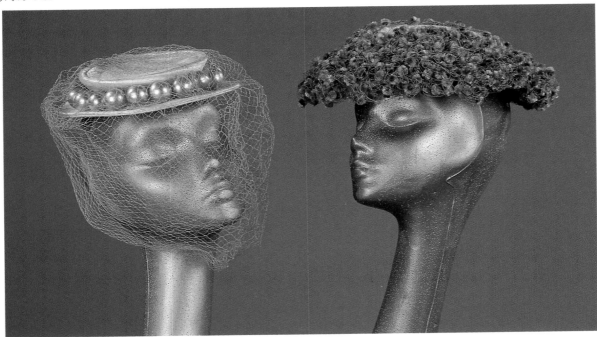

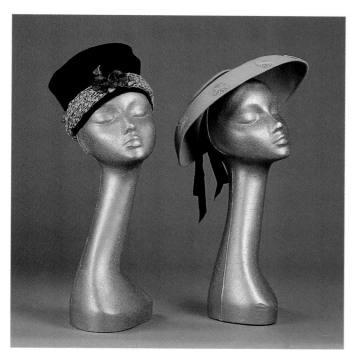

A brown felt toque with paprika posy, secured by its own celluloid hatpin (not visible) and a chartreuse felt picture hat, its brim spinning with raffia pinwheels. Label (right): Earl R. Lindberg Co. *Courtesy of (both): Banbury Cross Antiques.* Value (each): $45-65.

In fawn velvet, a new boater with backswept veil. In button-tufted velvet, a cap references the Renaissance. Label (right): Custom Made by Vivian—California. *Courtesy of (left): Banbury Cross Antiques. Courtesy of (right): Barbara Griggs Vintage Fashion.* Value (left): $25-40. Value (right): $50-75.

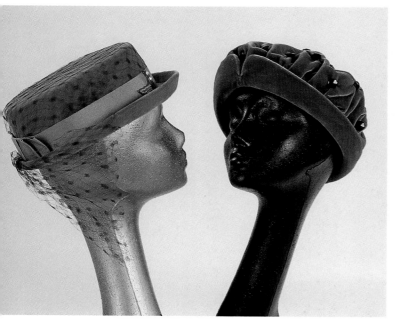

Lady of Luxury

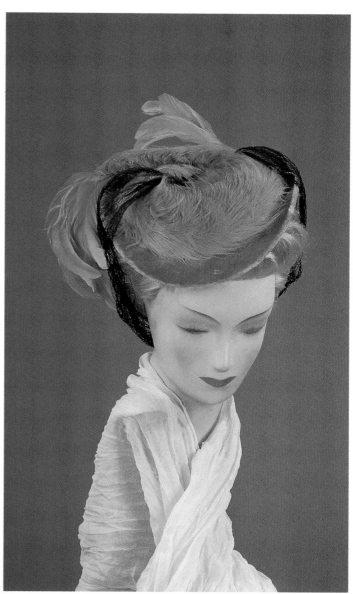

Goldenrod feathers nestle on a tilt hat of gold velvet. Its split veil was designed to be swagged under the chin, or tied in back as shown. *Courtesy of: Julia Moore.* Value: $75-125.

Back in Time

A pink velvet cap, cute as a button with sequin trim. Shown with a tulle-brimmed cap with topstitched crown, in turquoise. Label: hats, Carolyn Kelsey—San Francisco. *Courtesy of: (both): Maureen Reilly.* Value: $45-65.

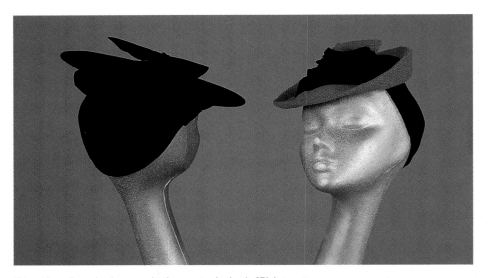

Felt with a tilt to the front, and a hugger in the back. With it, a jaunty vermilion straw, banded in back by black jersey. Label (left): Mitzi's Hats, Los Angeles. *Courtesy of (left): Karen Burrows. Courtesy of (right): Maureen Reilly.* Value (each): $75-125.

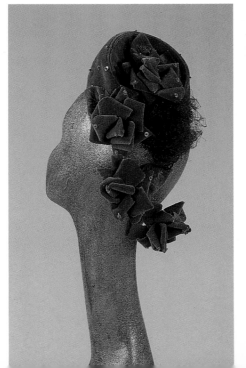

Violet velveteen bows stream down the back like a kite's tail, and would have provided the perfect accent for a soaring French twist. Label: Veola-Model. *Courtesy of: Maureen Reilly.* Value: $35-55.

Grandmother's Special Hat

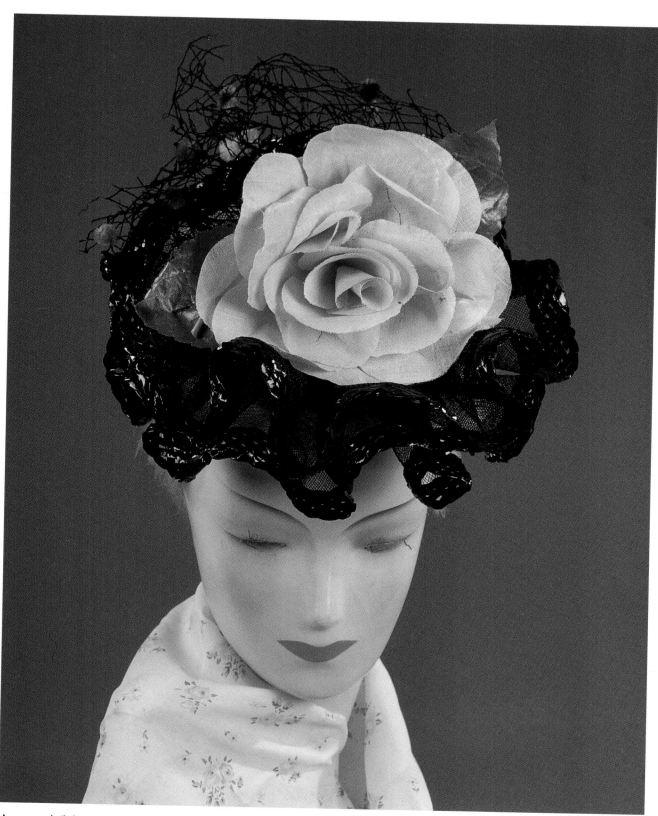

A treasured tilt hat, saucy as a French parlormaid's. The rose and veil are designed for flirting. Altogether alluring, it was a favorite of the owner's grandmother. *Courtesy of: Karen Burrows, curator of the Mary Aaron Museum.* Value: Special.

Tilt Tops

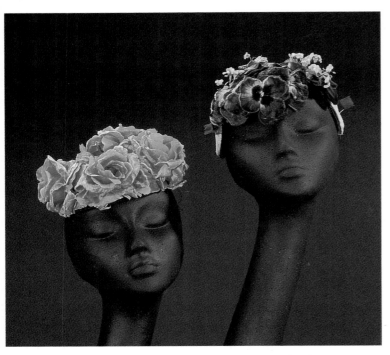

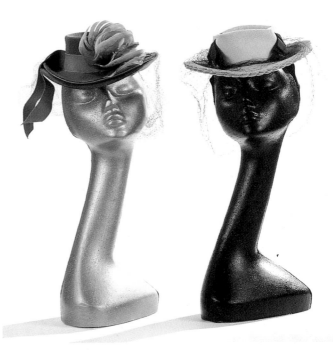

To be worn tilted down or at a slant, a dove-grey felt with rose accents. Paired with a similar design in curry and black felt. Label (left): Studio Styles by Warner Bros. Label (right): Monte Rey of California. *Courtesy of (both): Sheila Parks.* Value: $75-125.

A pink faille cap abloom with silk and velvet roses, paired with a pansy-sprigged bandeau. Label (right): Snellenberg's. *Courtesy of (both): The Way We Wore.* Value (each): $75-125.

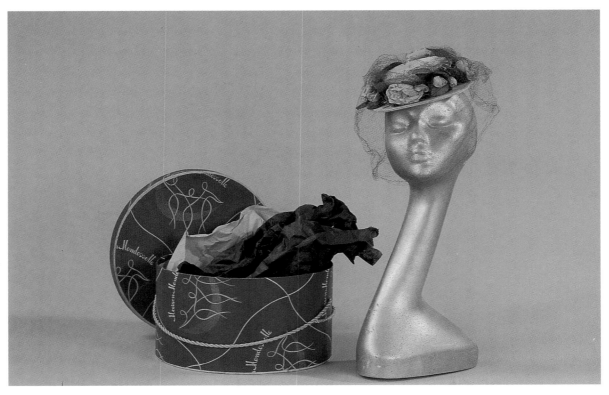

A cocktail boater in pale apple-green satin, rimmed in ivory roses. Shown with its original hatbox. *Courtesy of (all): Banbury Cross Antiques.* Value (hat): $75-125. Value (box): $35-55.

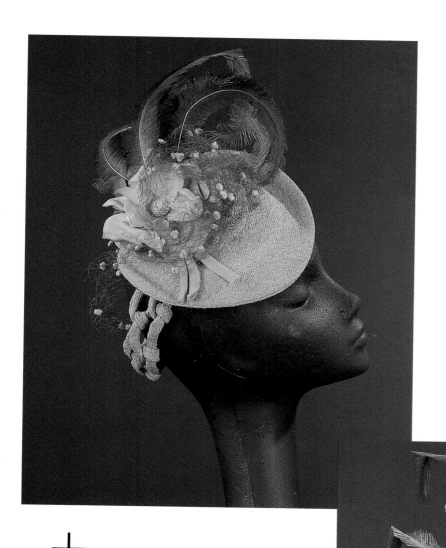

Artful
by
Design

An artfully-executed tilt hat in honey-toned fabric, with a swirl of veiling. Feathers and flowers trim it, and braiding holds it. Label: Yvonne Millinery—California. *Courtesy of: Banbury Cross Antiques.* Value: $95-145.

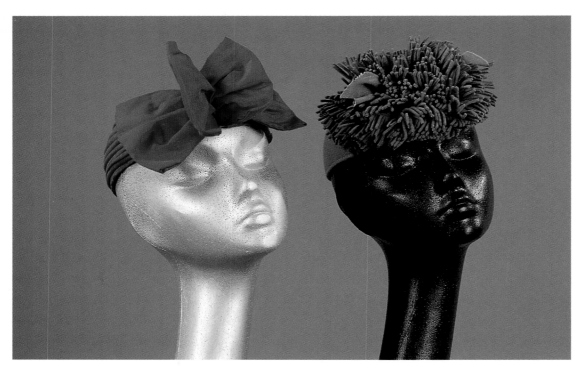

Candy-apple red grosgrain tied in a candy-box bow. With it, taupe felt is curled to form a chou. *Courtesy of (left): Graf's Glitz. Courtesy of (right): Barbara Mosca.* Value (each): $35-55.

Sweet *Nothings*

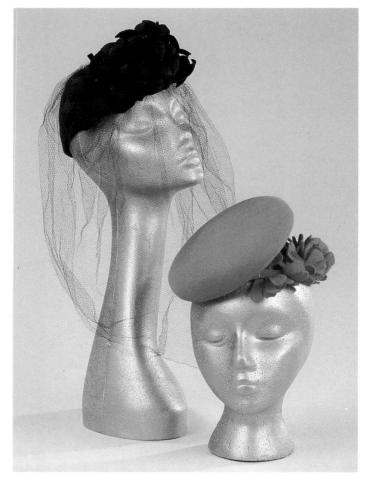

Felt petals and dramatic veiling distinguish a cocktail hat, left. A shocking pink demi-beret tilts to the right, with the aid of a hoop covered in felt petals. Label (left): Saks Fifth Ave, Debutante. *Courtesy of (all): Maureen Reilly.* Value (left): $65-95. Value (right): $55-75.

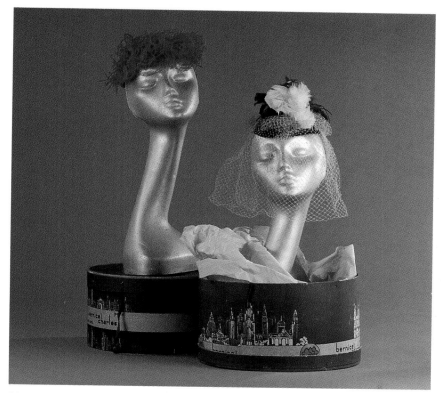

Hot-pink ostrich plumage whispers around a felt toque. Shown with a cap highlighted by blue and pink ostrich feathers, and a sweeping pink veil. Label (left): Julie Clare Shop. *Courtesy of (both): Rich Man, Poor Man.* Value (each): $55-75.

Make Mine a Double

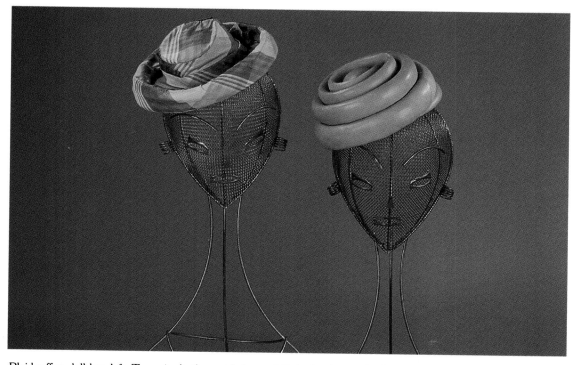

Plaid taffeta doll hat, left. Turquoise leather swirls into a doll-sized turban, right. Label (right): Schiaparelli. *Courtesy of (both): Sharon Hagerty.* Value (left): $55-75. Value (right): $95-145.

A Class Act

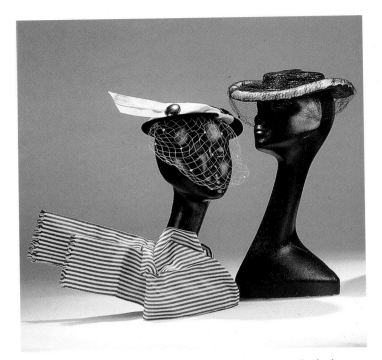

A pink grosgrain ribbon is styled to the side, in the manner of a feather plume. Padded pink satin circles a brim, on its companion. Label (left): Jeanne Tête. Label (right): Midinette. *Courtesy of (left): Banbury Cross Antiques. Courtesy of (right): Maureen Reilly.* Value (each): $65-95.

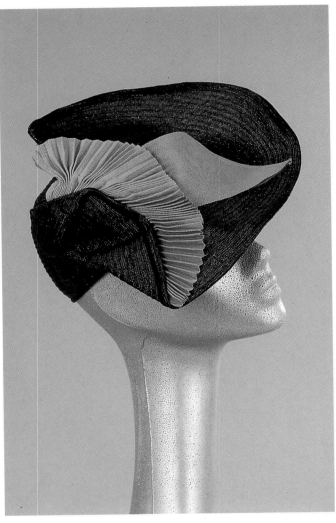

Black cellophane straw and pink pleated grosgrain shape a Deco-inspired cap. *Courtesy of: Banbury Cross Antiques.* Value: $55-75.

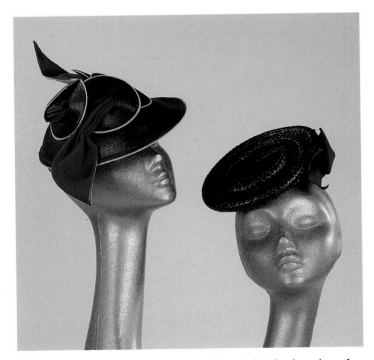

Chestnut straw circles around a crown. It's paired with a honeybun of a hat, in cellophane straw. *Courtesy of (left): Sheryl Birkner. Courtesy of (right): Maureen Reilly.* Value (each): $55-75.

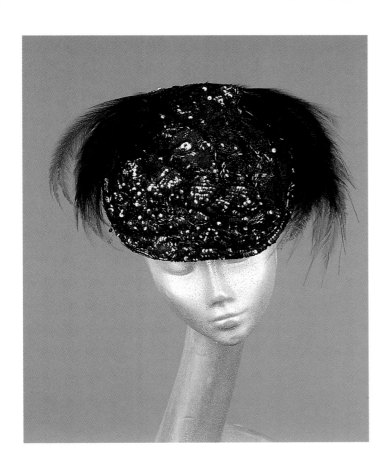

Opening Night

Black sequins pave this beret, with its fabulous bird perched mid-flight on the crown. *Courtesy of: Barbara Griggs Vintage Fashion.* Value: $95-145.

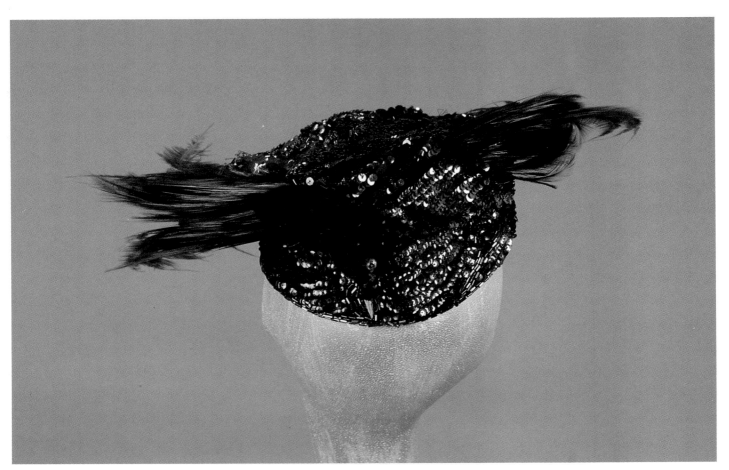

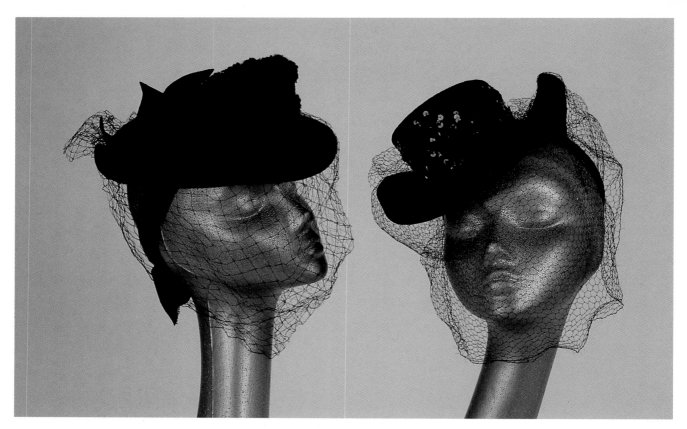

Mouton trims a fedora, left. Sequins sparkle a boater, right. Label (left): Betty Co-ed. Courtesy of (left): *Maureen Reilly. Courtesy of (right): Barbara Griggs Vintage Fashion.* Value (each): $75-125.

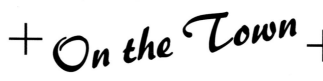

On the Town

A show-stopper swathed in sequins, with aigrette sidewings. Label: G. Howard Hodge. *Courtesy of: Barbara Griggs Vintage Fashion.* Value: $125-175.

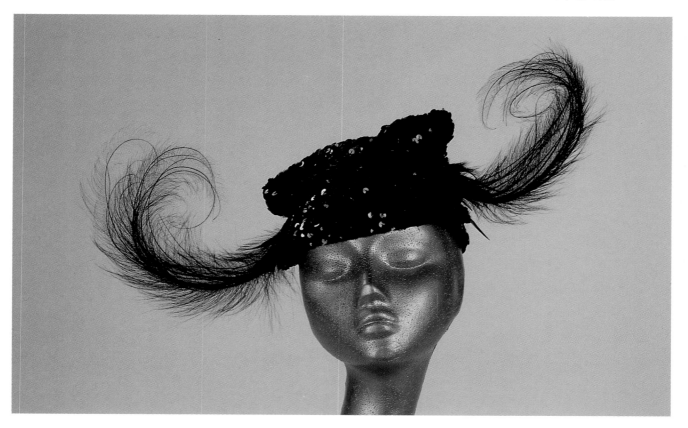

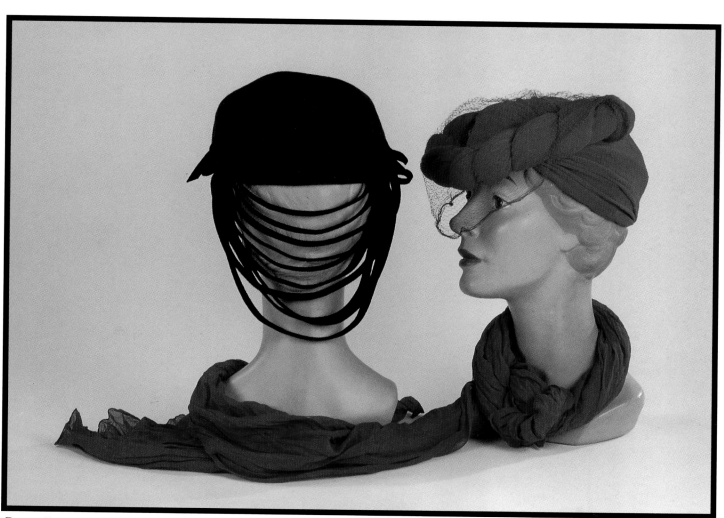

Ropes of brown felt skip across the back, making a playful hat. Shown with a raspberry rayon crepe turban. Label (left): Martha Gene. Courtesy of (left): Sheryl Birkner. Courtesy of (right): Rich Man, Poor Man. Value each $75-125.

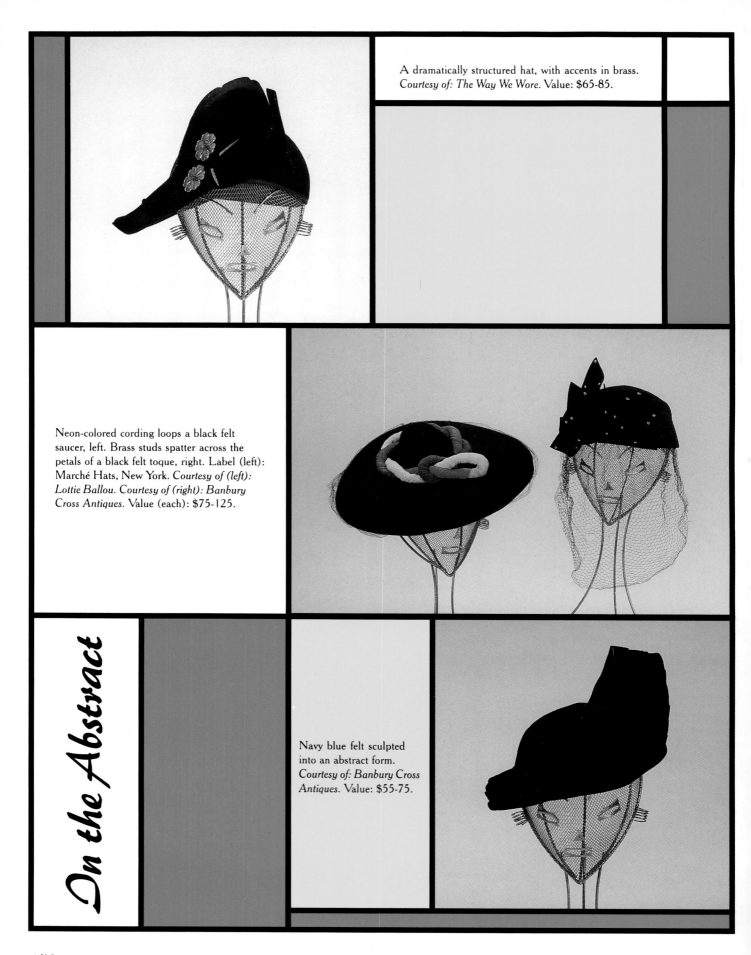

A dramatically structured hat, with accents in brass. *Courtesy of: The Way We Wore.* Value: $65-85.

Neon-colored cording loops a black felt saucer, left. Brass studs spatter across the petals of a black felt toque, right. Label (left): Marché Hats, New York. *Courtesy of (left): Lottie Ballou. Courtesy of (right): Banbury Cross Antiques.* Value (each): $75-125.

In the Abstract

Navy blue felt sculpted into an abstract form. *Courtesy of: Banbury Cross Antiques.* Value: $55-75.

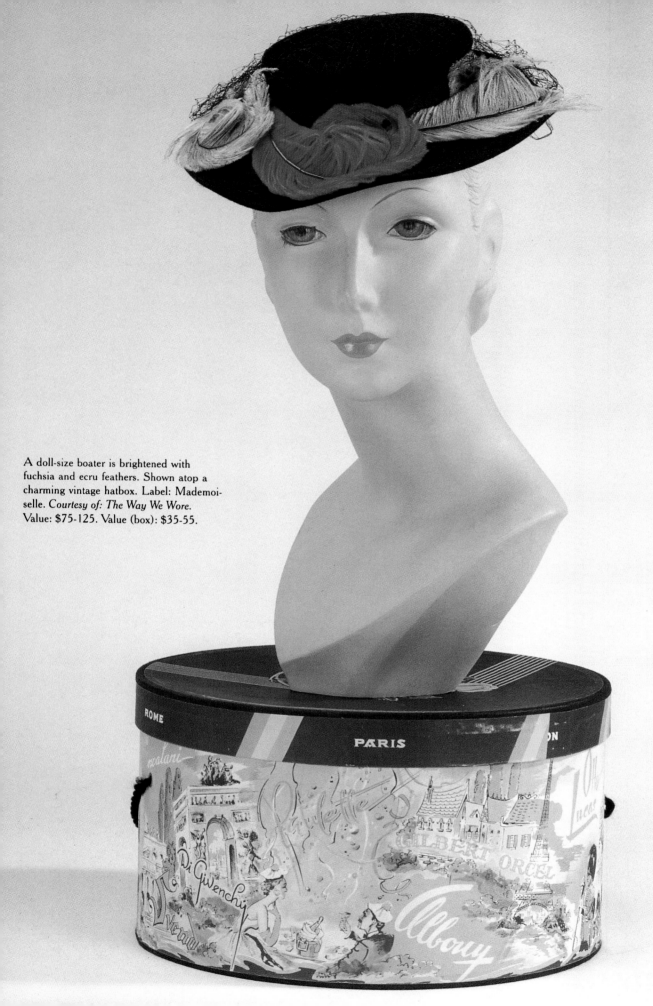

A doll-size boater is brightened with fuchsia and ecru feathers. Shown atop a charming vintage hatbox. Label: Mademoiselle. *Courtesy of: The Way We Wore.* Value: $75-125. Value (box): $35-55.

Felts with Flair

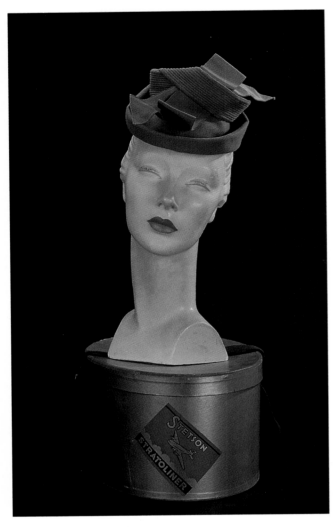

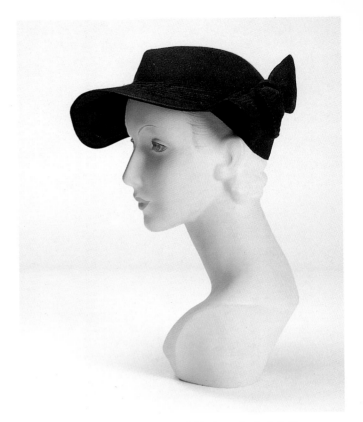

A stiff bow tie gives this simple wool felt city style. Label: Rumar Hats. *Courtesy of: Banbury Cross Antiques.* Value: $55-75.

A chic felt cap with turned-up brim, gift-wrapped in felt ribbons. A Stetson hatbox forms the platform. *Courtesy of (both): It's About Time.* Value (hat): $55-75. Value (box): $25-55.

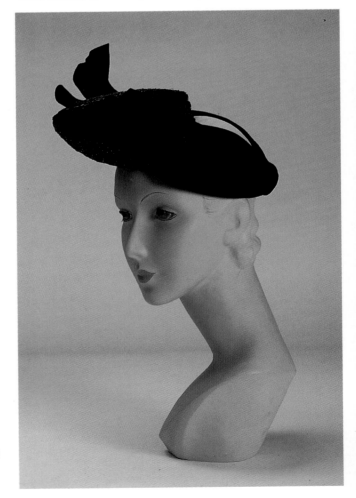

This flirty little hat presents a dashing bow to your beau! Label: Louie Miller. *Courtesy of: The Way We Wore.* Value: $95-145.

Daché Delight

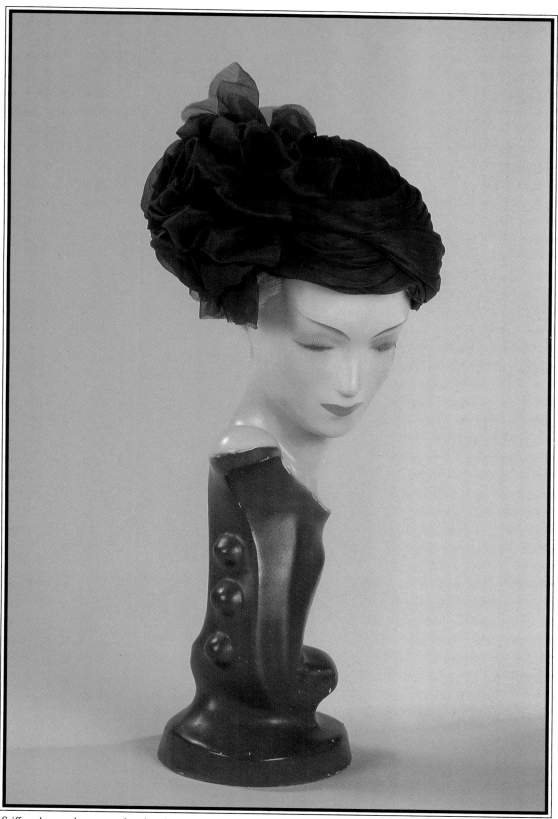

Stiffened organdy, wrapped and tied in a chocolate kiss. Label: Lilly Daché. *Courtesy of: Banbury Cross Antiques.*
Value: $95-145.

All the Trimmings

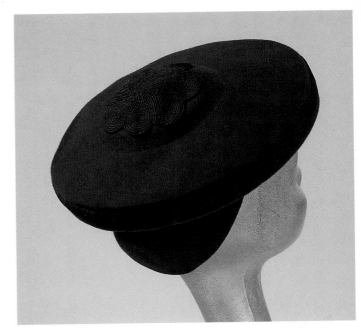

A nape-hugging tam o'shanter with a petal design in place of the usual button or tassel. Label: Dobbs. *Courtesy of: Donna McMaster.* Value: $75-125.

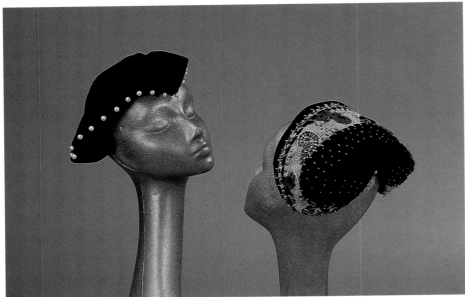

A Mary Stuart cap in black velvet, dripping with pearls. Shown with a cap in black felt with paisley-print banding. *Courtesy of (left): Banbury Cross Antiques. Courtesy of (right): Maureen Reilly.* Value (each): $35-55.

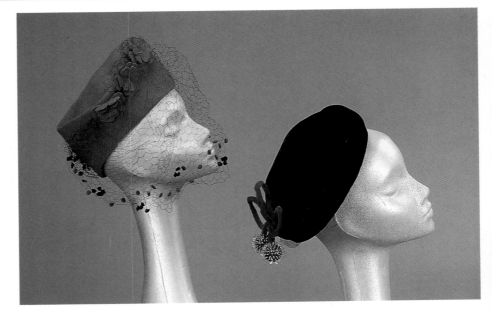

Rose-red felt petals form a vintage toque, but the navy and red pom-pom veil was added. Navy blue velvet forms a demi-beret, tied with a scarlet bow and sparkly accents. *Courtesy of (both): Maureen Reilly.* Value (each): $45-65.

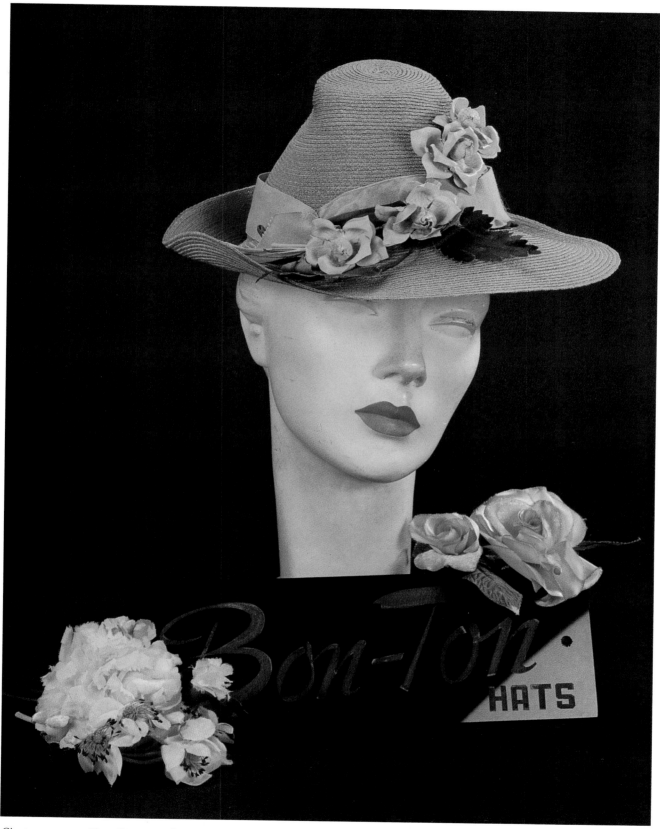

Chartreuse straw with trailing roses, the type of hat that may have been featured in the window of the "Bon Ton" hat shoppe.
Courtesy of (hat): Lottie Ballou. Courtesy of (sign): Banbury Cross Antiques. Value (hat): $75-125. Value (sign): $75-125.

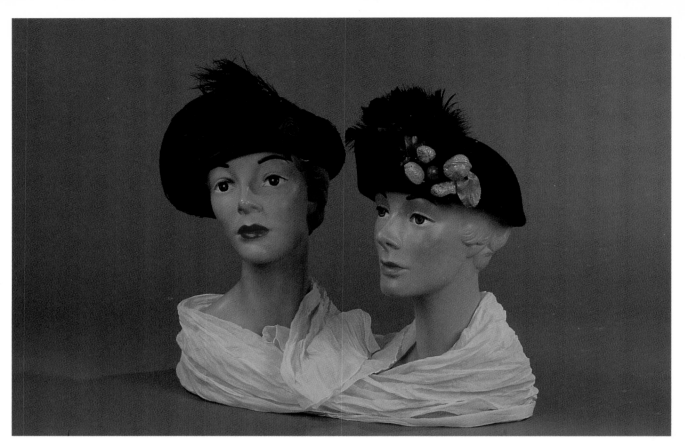

Two wool felt berets, hunter green and nut brown. The trim is inexpensive but amusing. *Courtesy of (both): Maureen Reilly.* Value (each): $25-45.

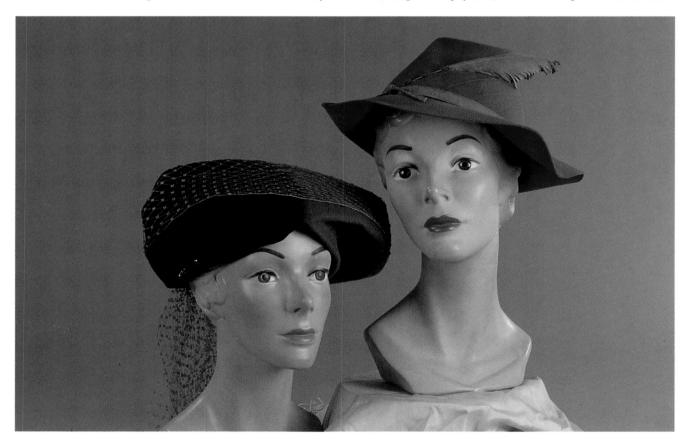

Styled after a medieval headdress, in two tones of grey-green felt. Shown with a paprika Tyrolean, with pistachio feather. Label (left): Tulip Model, San Francisco. *Courtesy of (both): Sheryl Birkner.* Value (each): $65-95.

Top Knotch

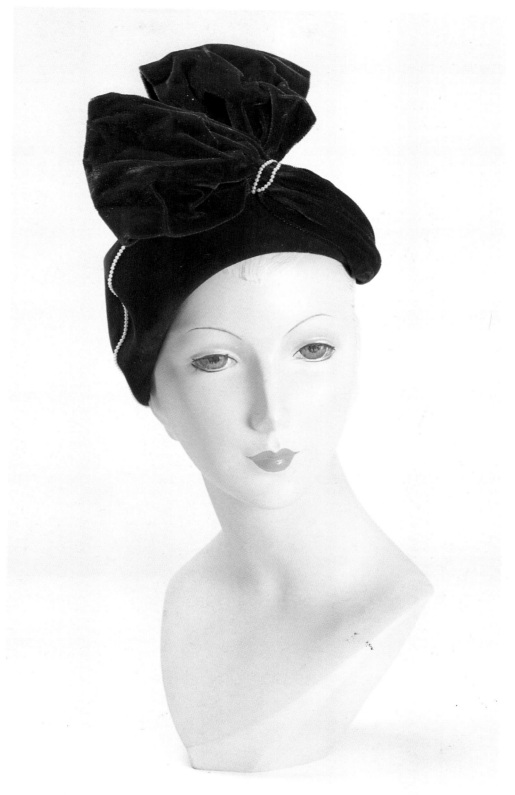

For evening, blue velvet is enhanced by a large bow outlined in seed pearls. Label: Carolyn Kelsey.
Courtesy of: The Way We Wore. Value: $95-145.

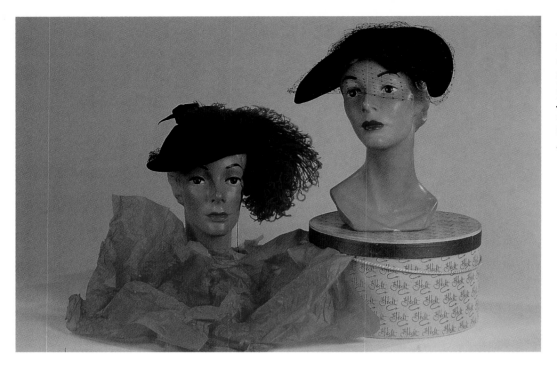

A jaunty russet ostrich plume flies from a brown felt beanie. The brim of its companion scoops up to reveal a shiny satin bow. Label (right): Noreen, Reproduction of Original Jacques Costet—Paris. *Courtesy of (left): Rich Man, Poor Man. Courtesy of (right): Banbury Cross Antiques.* Value (each): $45-75.

A dramatic navy blue felt with Aureole brim, left. A sassy velvet with pinwheel aigrette, right. Label (left): Lydia—Livingston Bros. Label (right): DuBarry French Adaptations. *Courtesy of (both): Sheryl Birkner.* Value (each): $45-75.

Cosmopolitan Chic

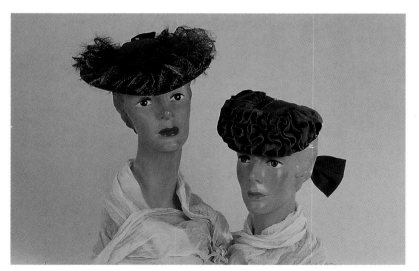

Pistachio and nut-brown feathers scurry across the brim of a felt boater. Joined by another charmer in nutmeg grosgrain with ruching around the crown and a "follow me lads" streamer in back. *Courtesy of (left): Karen Burrows. Courtesy of (right): Maureen Reilly.* Value (each): $45-75.

Brimming Over

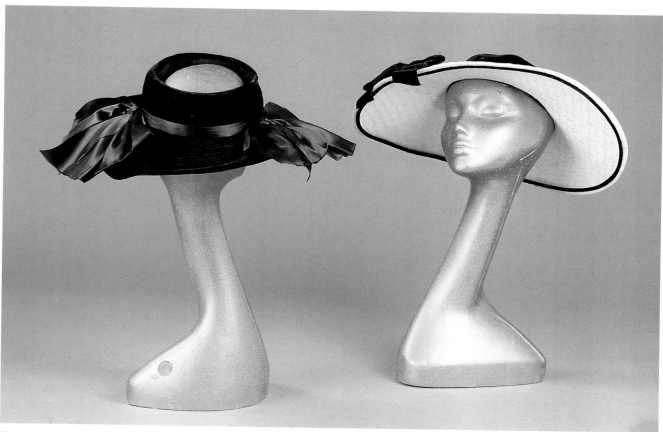

Two picture hats, one in black velvet with peek-a-boo crown, from Hale Bros. in Sacramento. The other in white eyelet, punctuated by black velvet. *Courtesy of (left): Banbury Cross Antiques.* Value (each): $45-75.

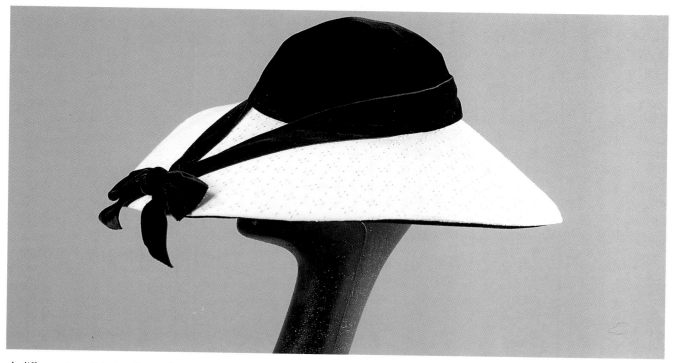

A different view of the hat shown above right. It's the very "picture" of motion-picture chic. Label: An Original Studio Style designed by Caspar Davis of Hollywood. *Courtesy of: Maureen Reilly.* Value: $95-145.

Picture Perfect

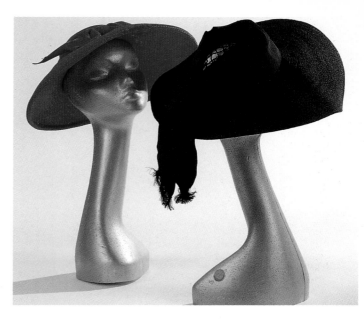

Two straws, in flame-red and navy blue. The latter style keeps cool with an open-air crown. Label (left): J. Magnin. *Courtesy of (left): Lisa Carson. Courtesy of (right): The Sheepish Grin.* Value (each): $75-125.

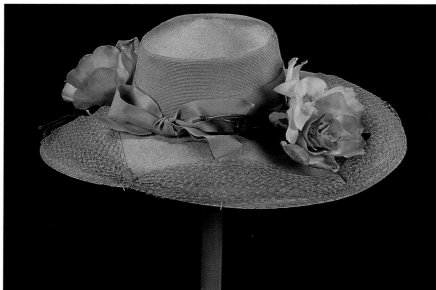

Pale lilac straw with twin frosted blue roses. Label: Gage Bros. & Co. *Courtesy of: Maureen Reilly.* Value: $95-135.

The navy straw features a latticed crown, while its ivory companion is trimmed in navy feathers and netting. Label (left): J. Hudson Co. *Courtesy of (both): Connie Beers.* Value (each): $75-125.

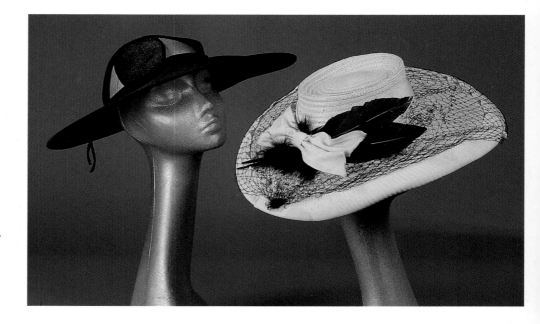

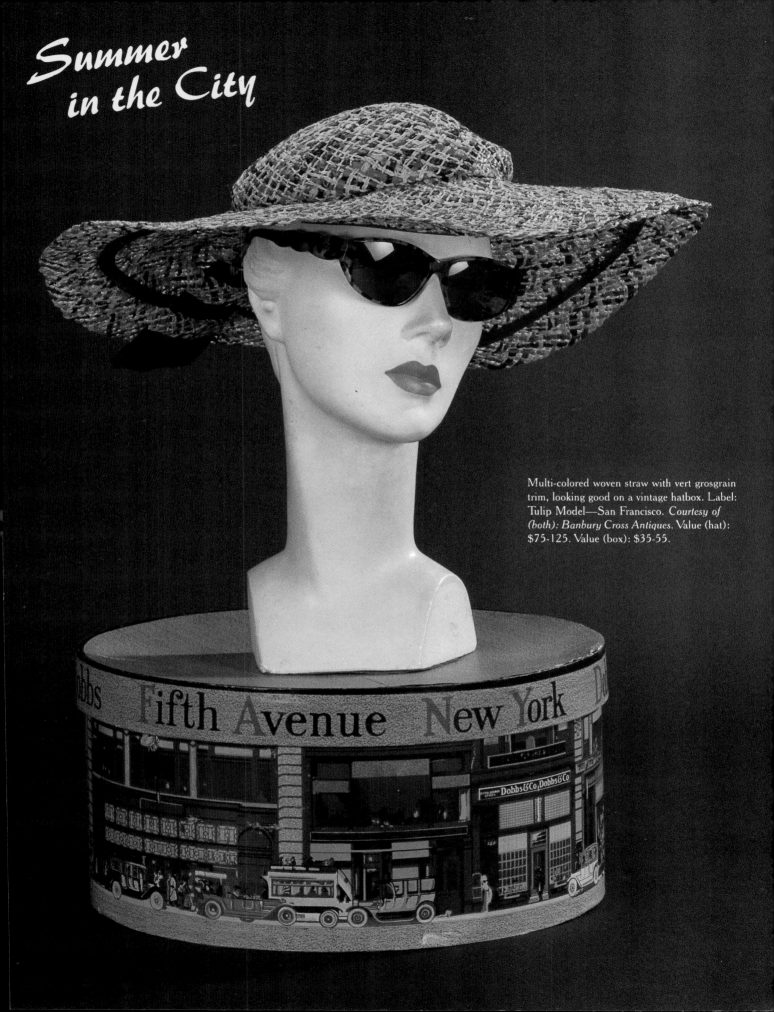

Summer in the City

Multi-colored woven straw with vert grosgrain trim, looking good on a vintage hatbox. Label: Tulip Model—San Francisco. *Courtesy of (both): Banbury Cross Antiques.* Value (hat): $75-125. Value (box): $35-55.

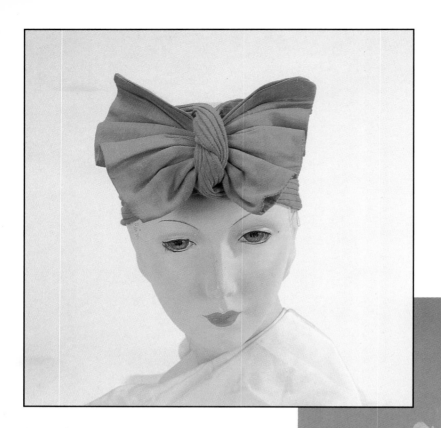

On the Boardwalk

A butterfly bow alights on this coral silk headband. *Courtesy of: The Way We Wore.* Value: $55-75.

Two open-crown picture hats in the roughest natural straw; one trimmed with a garden of linen flowers, the other banded with grosgrain ribbon. Label (bottom): Kaufmann, 5th Ave—Custom Made. *Courtesy of (top): Banbury Cross Antiques. Courtesy of (bottom): It's About Time.* Value (top): $65-95. Value (bottom): $55-75.

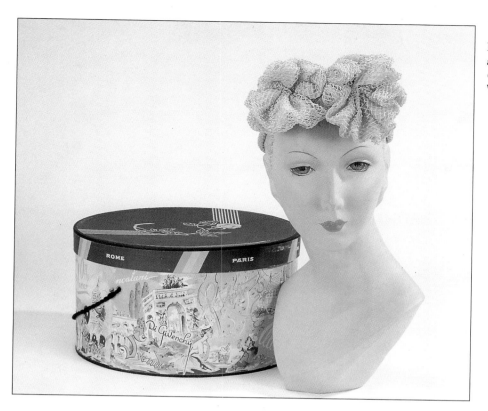

Flesh-colored cotton pinwheels pair up in front, and a matching snood completes the look in back (not visible in photo). *Courtesy of: The Way We Wore.* Value: $55-75.

Fun in the Sun

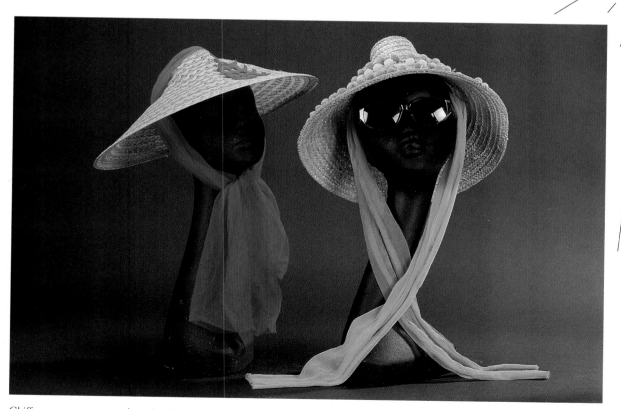

Chiffon scarves wrap up these fun beach hats, circa 1945. The pagoda is trimmed with a red felt Chinese character. Its companion has multicolored chenille pom-poms on a spiral brim. *Courtesy of (both): Banbury Cross Antiques.* Value (each): $55-75.

IX. The New Look: 1947-1959

Soldiers returned from the South Pacific in 1945, and America entered an age of economic expansion. England and France were slower to recover, due to the loss of natural resources on the battlefield. Still and all, the mood was one of exuberance and optimism. The byword of this era was "return to normalcy." It was a time of industrial and political re-tooling, as the Allied nations and their defeated enemies struggled to stabilize.

As couples who had married during the chaos of war were reunited, wives quit their wartime jobs. It was the "baby boom" when growing families migrated to the suburbs in droves, seeking lives of well-ordered tranquility. Wives became mothers, with busy schedules. But they still wore hats and gloves to shop in the new supermarkets, attend PTA meetings or assist at the Junior League.

Fashion's pendulum had swung in a wide arc by the end of World War II. Away from the tailored look made necessary by fabric rationing—on to the ultra-feminine New Look! It is generally agreed that this look was launched by Christian Dior in 1947. It called for a "wasp waist" to show off crinolined skirts, and once again women subjected themselves to corsets for the sake of fashion.

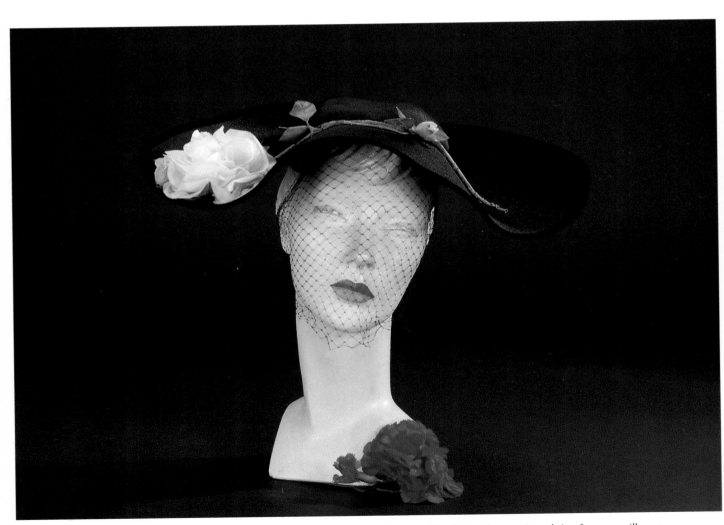

A double scoop of navy rimmed in velvet, graced by one perfect rose. Note how the crown blends into the prominent brim, for a new silhouette. Label: Noreen Fashions. *Courtesy of: Sandra Headley.* Value: $75-125.

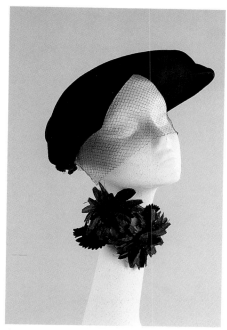

Hats were necessary to complete the structured lines of Dior's elegant designs, and the legions of knock-offs. Dior accessorized to good advantage with long gloves, high heels and a type of broad-brimmed hat nicknamed the Dior Dish. Its structural design included an inner brim, to situate it squarely on the crown of the head.

A coolie hat was introduced in the couture collections of Dior and Balenciaga in the mid-1950s. Also called the pagoda (or pagodine if diminutive), it was an amusing style that worked well, depending on fabrication, with either cocktail dress or capri pants.

Dior dominated "hat couture" for a full decade. There were the usual berets, turbans, and pillboxes, but we must credit Dior with the newest and smartest styles of each season. He introduced not only the dish, but a sort of inverted bowl that could be used to good effect with cascading trim.

In the late 1950s, he introduced three new dresses described by their resemblance to letters of the alphabet: H, S, and A. These were just as chic, but certainly more relaxed, than the wasp waisted New Look. Indeed, the H revived the flattering lines of Poirot's chemise.

A knock-off of the Dior Dish in plush black felt. Label: Du Barry French Adaptions. *Courtesy of: Sheryl Birkner.* Value: $55-75.

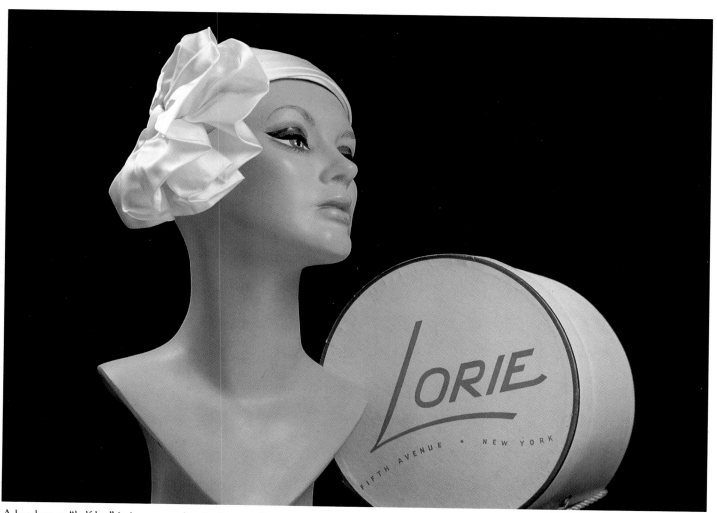

A bandeau or "half hat" in ivory peau de soie. Its curvy lines went with the swingy A-shape dress by Dior. *Courtesy of: Banbury Cross Antiques.* Value (hat): $65-95. Value (box): $25-45.

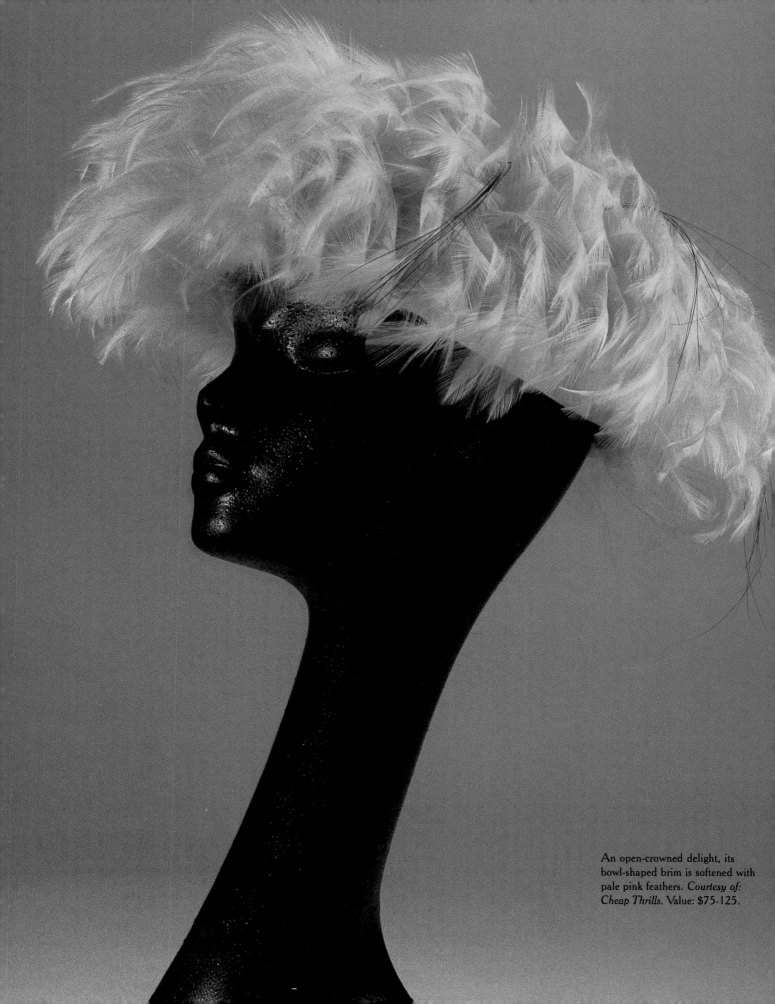

An open-crowned delight, its bowl-shaped brim is softened with pale pink feathers. *Courtesy of: Cheap Thrills.* Value: $75-125.

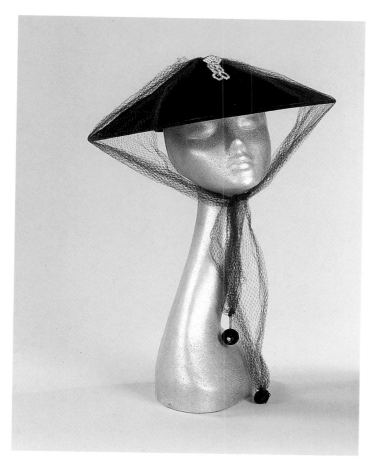

A velvet coolie with rhinestone clip, for evening. Like the Dior Dish, it features an inner brim. *Courtesy of: Rich Man, Poor Man.* Value: $55-75.

The alphabet collection debuted in the late 1950s, themed to new styles of hat: platter (for the chemise-like "H"), bandeau (for the flared "A"), and lampshade (for the fitted "S"). On both sides of the Atlantic, retailers rushed to interpret these hats for their own salon and ready-to-wear labels.

Throughout the New Look era, flowered hats were extremely popular. If the ads are to be believed, women might purchase several each year, to freshen up a spring wardrobe. When crafted by the couture, floral hats were highly becoming and charming. However, collectors should choose from this genre with care, as their very popularity led to overproduction. As a result, some floral hats are of poor quality and uncertain design.

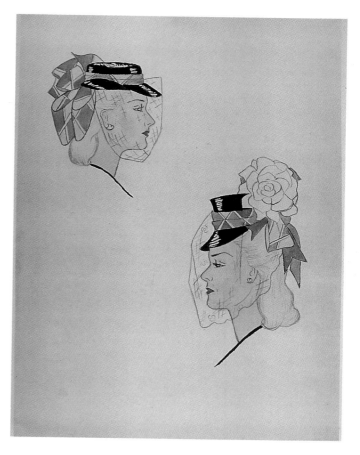

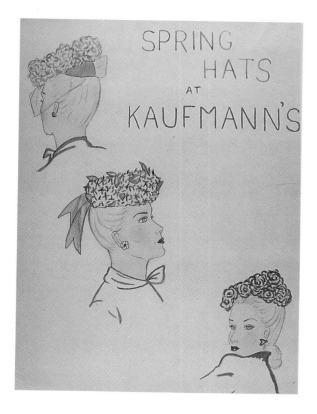

These advertising sketches were a student project, showing the type of spring hat that would be popular for over a decade.

During the 1956 Olympics in London, a discus thrower for the Russian women's team was unable to resist the hats on display in the department stores. Nina Ponomareva must have been low on ruples, because she resorted to shoplifting—and was caught. Nina was built like a tank, but favored the most dainty flowered hats.

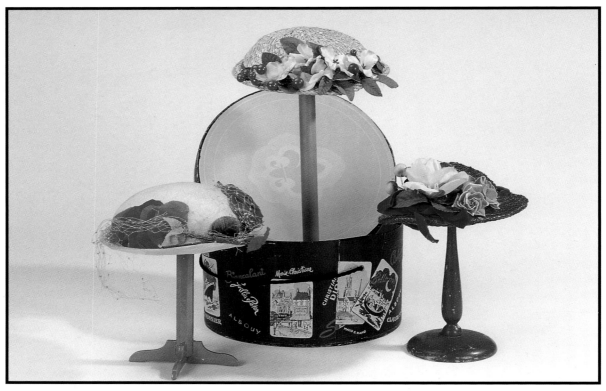

Hats of the type that caught Nina's eye. Three boaters in red and cream, trimmed with an assortment of fruit and flowers. Label (left): Eve Nouvelle, N. Y. Label (right): G. Howard Ross Original—New York—Paris. *Courtesy of (all): Banbury Cross Antiques.* Value (each hat): $45-65. Value (box): $25-45.

As an era, the 1950s have variously been described as fun, fabulous, and faddish. Certainly, as relates to fashion, the era was all three. New scientific developments brought miracle fibers to the fashion marketplace, such as elasticized caps that were planted with Nylon flowers. A revival of the mobcap, they stretched over a headful of curlers—which was a matter of necessity before the invention of the blow dryer!

Once the curlers came off on a Saturday night, the chiffon went on. The wrap of choice? Indisputably, a mink stole. Mink was a universal symbol of status, in the same class as Cadillacs and Champagne. Women wore mink on their sweaters, gloves, handbags, belts, jewelry—and of course, their hats.

For evening, the world of fashion was enjoying the return of the many luxury fabrics that had been restricted during the war years. Sequins, brocade, velvet, beading, feathers and other fancy trim were favorites for the cocktail hour.

These new cocktail hats were a perfect topnote to the ubiquitous "little black dress." Although some were oversized, in the manner of the Dior dish, others were miniscule and strongly reminiscent of doll hats from the previous era.

Space exploration began in 1957 with the launching of Sputnik, a Soviet satellite the size of a large beachball. It started the "space race" and a fascination with the sleek forms of spacecraft in the fine and applied arts. (Picture the concentric circle architecture of Frank Lloyd Wright's design for the Guggenheim Museum in 1959!) Even fashion was caught up in the excitement, with designs for hats, bags, and jewelry that could have been worn by Judy Jetson.

Many design themes of the late 1950s would carry over into the next decade, as shown in the fashion magazines. For example, in 1960 *Vogue* described a "beret with pouffed UFO shape" by Mr. John. In 1964, *Vogue* featured an allover anemone "bubble hat" on the cover.

The styles favored by mainstream America would change but gradually, until the baby boomers came of age and began exploring alternative lifestyles which all but excluded traditional notions of fashion and millinery.

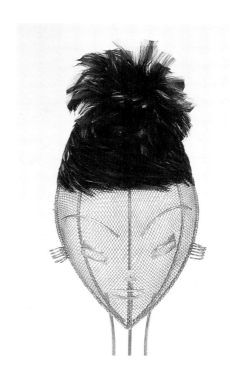

A little black cocktail hat in allover feathers, to top off a favorite "little black dress." Label: Madcap—Paris, New York. *Courtesy of: The Way We Wore.* Value: $75-125.

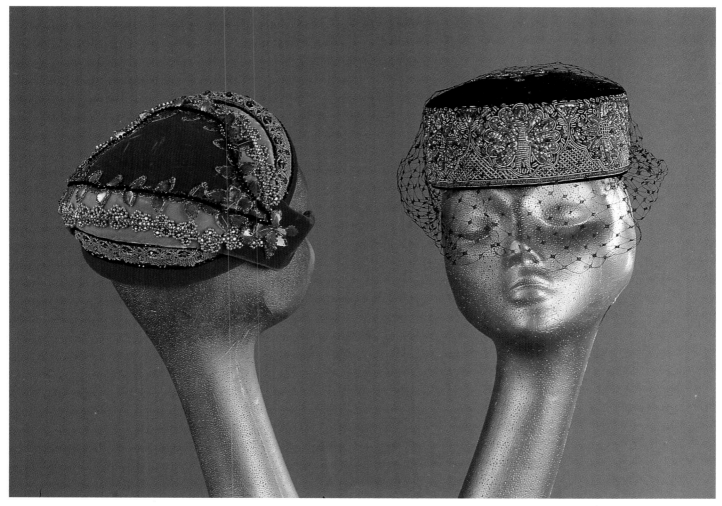

Luxurious fabrication creates a darling duo for evening wear. Wine red velvet banded in sequins and fancy beadwork, by Lilly Daché. Shown with an ornately brocaded pillbox. *Courtesy of (left): Maureen Reilly. Courtesy of (right): Barbara Griggs Vintage Fashion.* Value (left): $95-145. Value (right): $75-125.

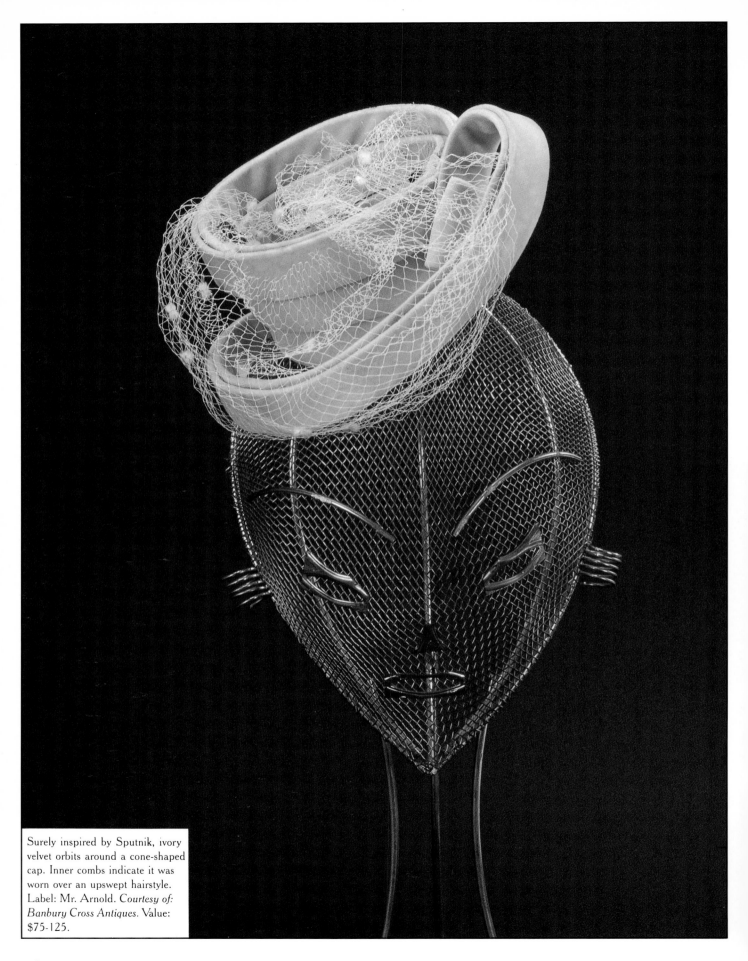

Surely inspired by Sputnik, ivory velvet orbits around a cone-shaped cap. Inner combs indicate it was worn over an upswept hairstyle. Label: Mr. Arnold. *Courtesy of: Banbury Cross Antiques.* Value: $75-125.

Opening Night

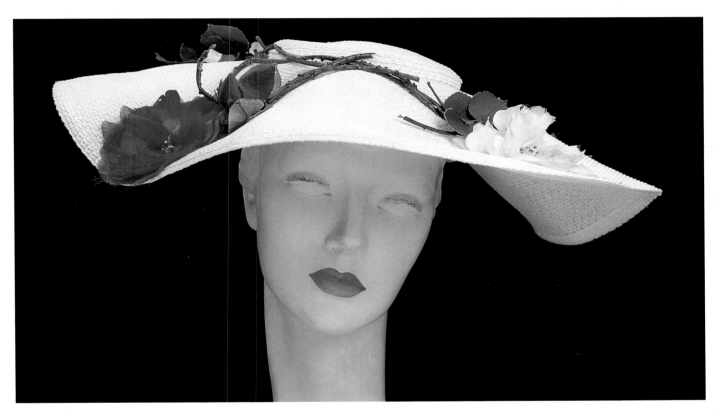

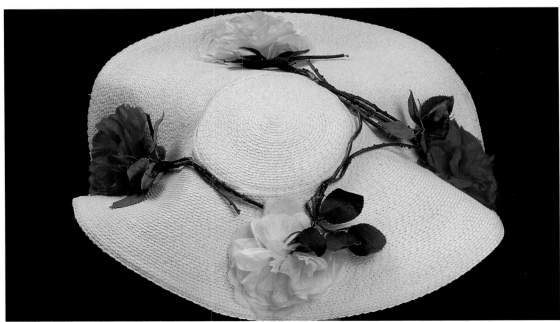

A straw cartwheel planted with rose-red and snow-white silk flowers. *Courtesy of: Banbury Cross Antiques.* Value: $95-145.

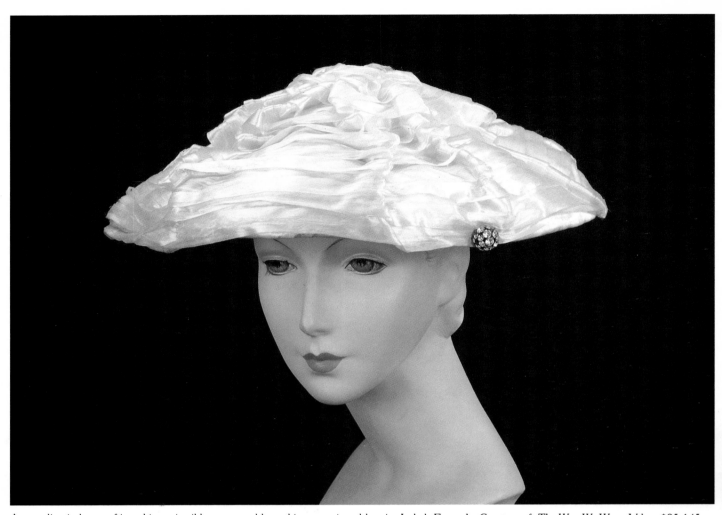

A pagodine in layers of ice-white satin ribbon, speared by a rhinestone-tipped hatpin. Label: Fannye's. *Courtesy of: The Way We Wore.* Value: $95-145.

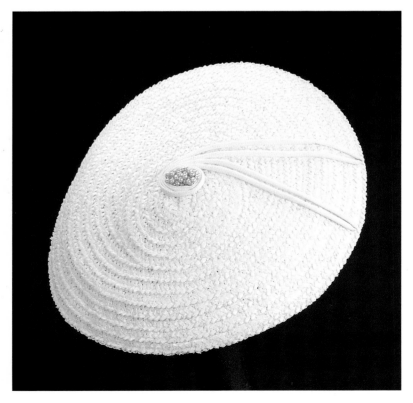

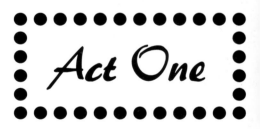

Act One

Rough straw is finely seamed into a spiral, to form this cartwheel with a single pearl as decoration. Label: Original by Sherman. *Courtesy of: Banbury Cross Antiques.* Value: $65-95.

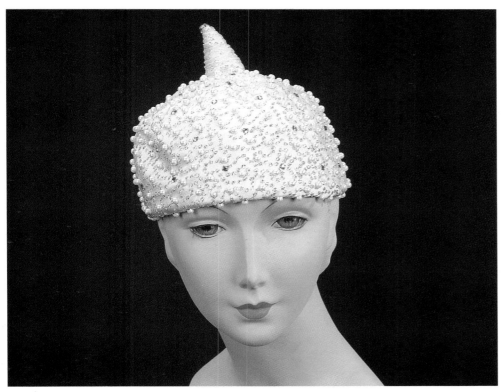

A rhinestone dangles from the tip of a white toque, clustered with pearls and more rhinestones. Label: Dachétte. *Courtesy of: The Way We Wore.* Value: $95-145.

Act Two

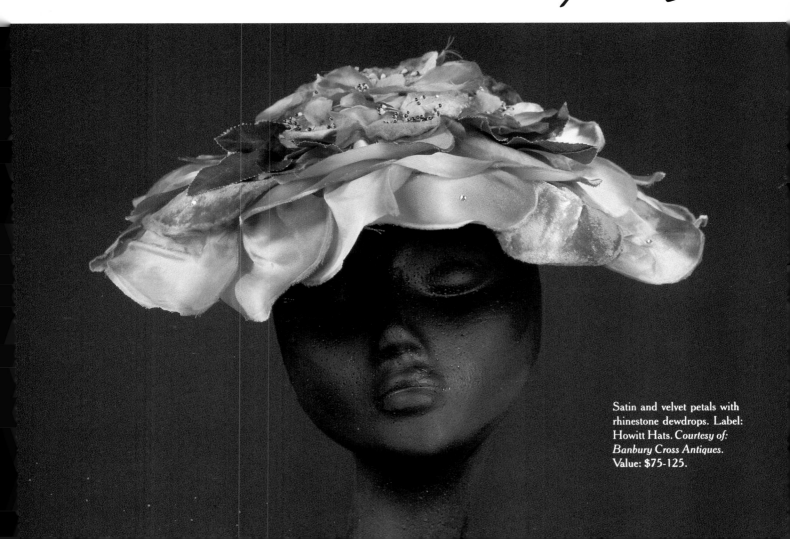

Satin and velvet petals with rhinestone dewdrops. Label: Howitt Hats. *Courtesy of: Banbury Cross Antiques.* Value: $75-125.

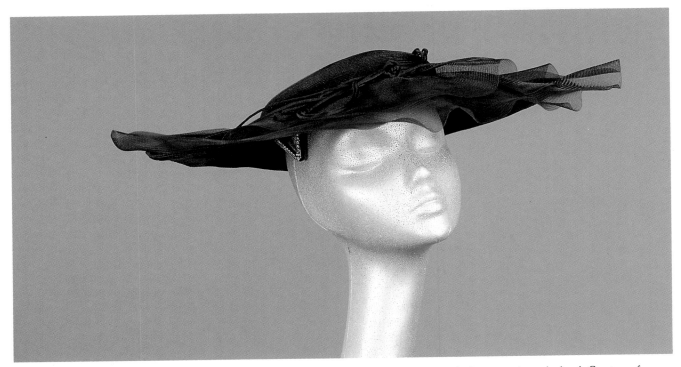

Black horsehair skirts this straw cartwheel. The bottom view shows how rhinestone clips position the hat squarely on the head. *Courtesy of: Barbara Griggs Vintage Fashion.* Value: $75-125.

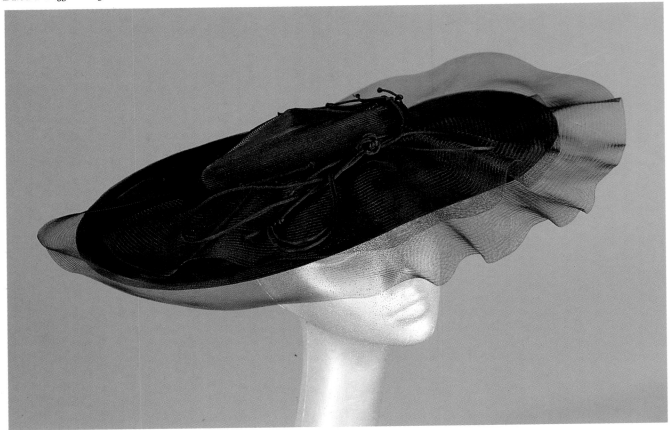

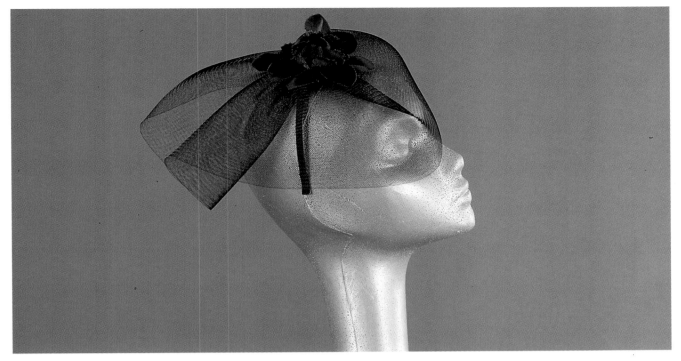

Horsehair net and not much more on a cocktail headband. *Courtesy of: Barbara Griggs Vintage Fashion.* Value: $35-55.

Applause

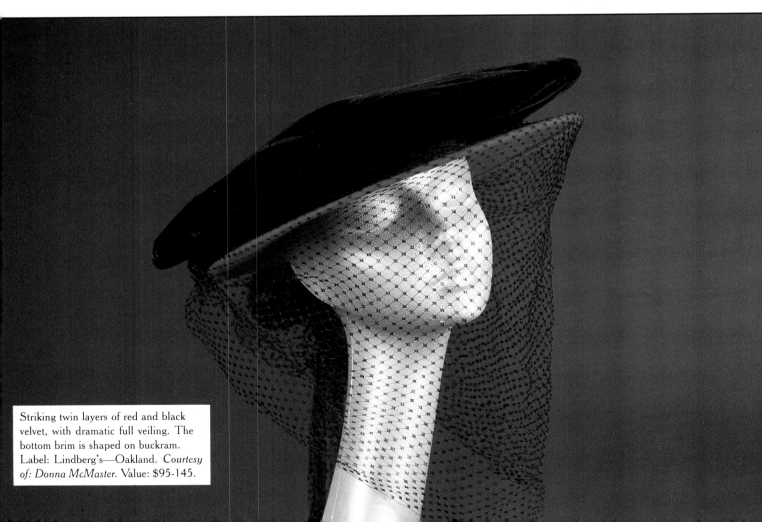

Striking twin layers of red and black velvet, with dramatic full veiling. The bottom brim is shaped on buckram. Label: Lindberg's—Oakland. *Courtesy of: Donna McMaster.* Value: $95-145.

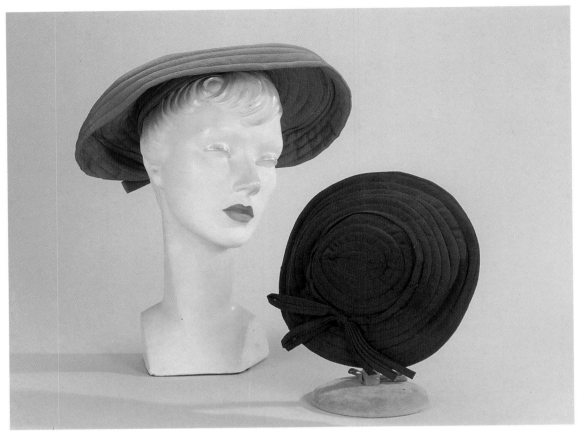

Sewn strips of rayon cording swirl around a floppy-brimmed dish and a simple beret. Label: Ripple Rounders—Lee Reading. *Courtesy of (both): Banbury Cross Antiques.* Value (each): $35-55.

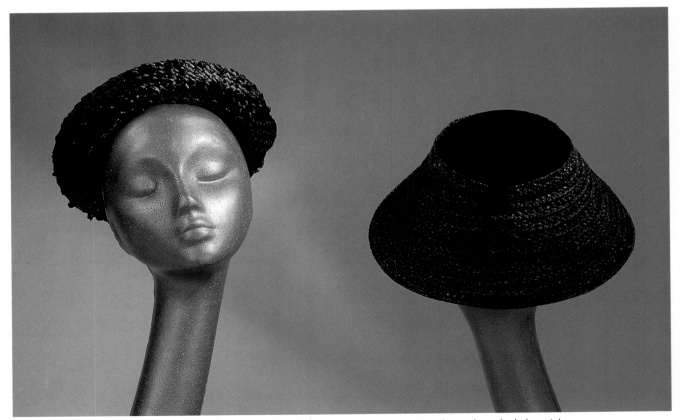

A Breton in rough black straw with black velvet buttons, left. The same materials are used to form a lampshade hat, right. Label (left): Leslie James. *Courtesy of (both): Maureen Reilly.* Value (left): $55-75. Value (right): $35-55.

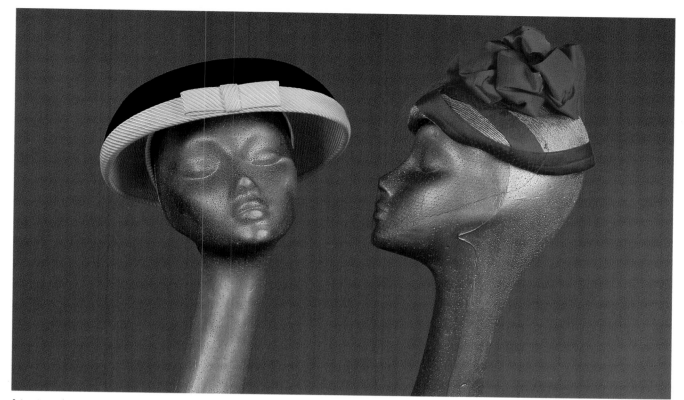

Licorice velvet and vanilla satin "take the cake" on the dish, while a strawberry satin bow gift-wraps the cap. Label (left): G. Howard Hodge; Roos Bros. Label (right): Dayne. *Courtesy of (both): Maureen Reilly.* Value (each): $55-75.

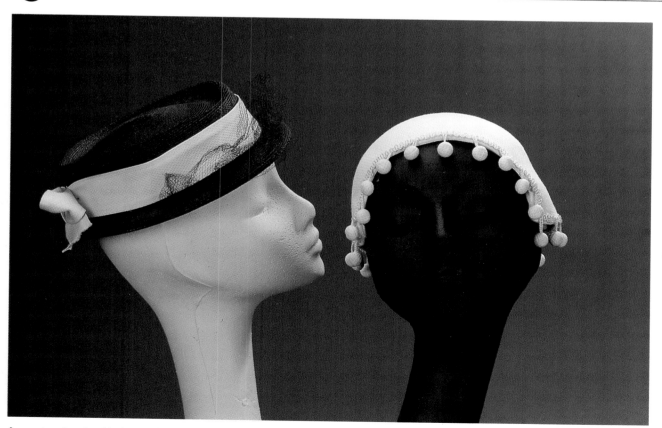

Ivory pique bands a black straw boater, and forms a Juliet cap with ball fringe. Label (left): I. Magnin. *Courtesy of (left): Maureen Reilly. Courtesy of (right): Sandra Headley.* Value (each): $35-55.

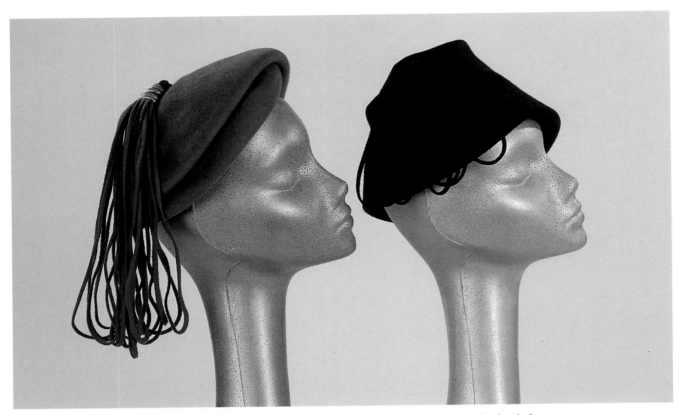

Loopy tassels fall from a Kelly green beret, and swing to the side of a navy blue fez. *Courtesy of (left): La Cat & Co. Courtesy of: Maureen Reilly.* Value (each): $35-55.

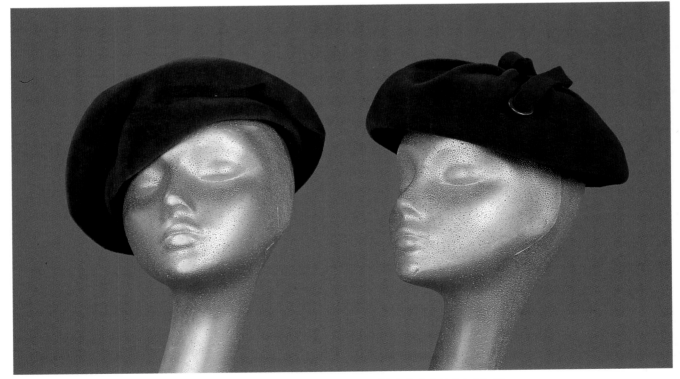

The enduring beret and tam, in royal purple velour. Label (left): Dorée of New York. Label (right): Mr. Dave. *Courtesy of (both): La Cat & Co.* Value (each): $35-55.

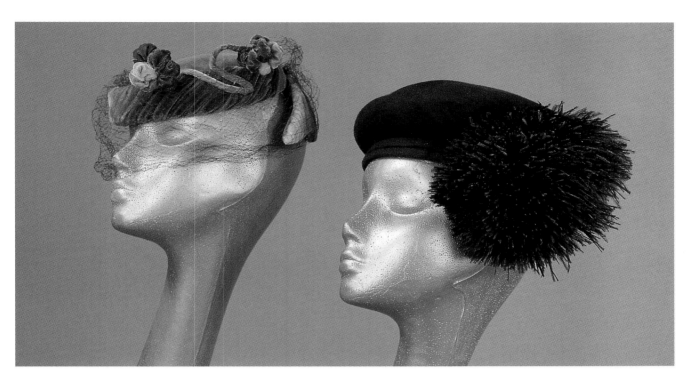

An unusual tie-dyed velvet in tones of wine and rose. Shown with a small black tam, feathered at the side. *Courtesy of (left): Banbury Cross Antiques. Courtesy of (right): 57th Antique Mall.* Value (each): $35-55.

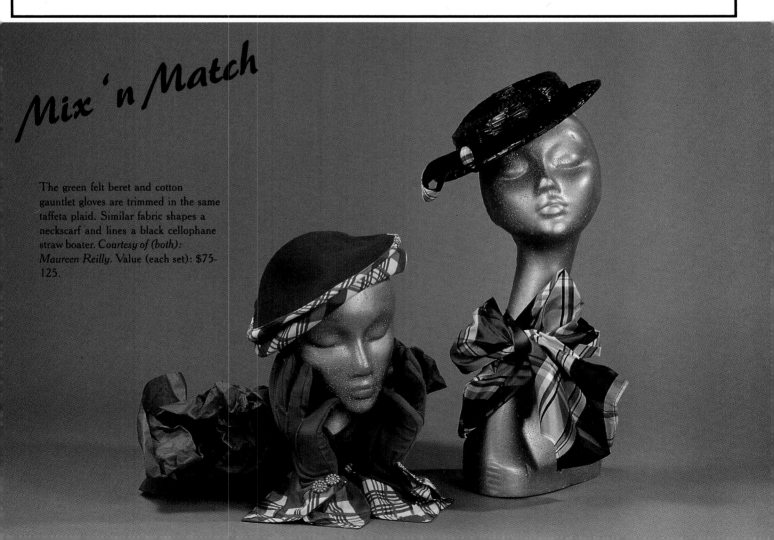

Mix 'n Match

The green felt beret and cotton gauntlet gloves are trimmed in the same taffeta plaid. Similar fabric shapes a neckscarf and lines a black cellophane straw boater. *Courtesy of (both): Maureen Reilly.* Value (each set): $75-125.

Duets

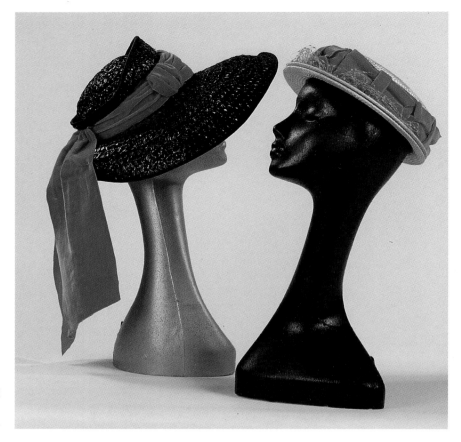

Rough black straw shapes a picture hat, softened with velvet streamers. The double-brim ivory straw boater is banded in velvet bows, of a similar peachy shade. Label (left): G. Howard Hodge. Label (right): Robinson's. *Courtesy of (both): Maureen Reilly.* Value (left): $55-75. Value (right): $25-45.

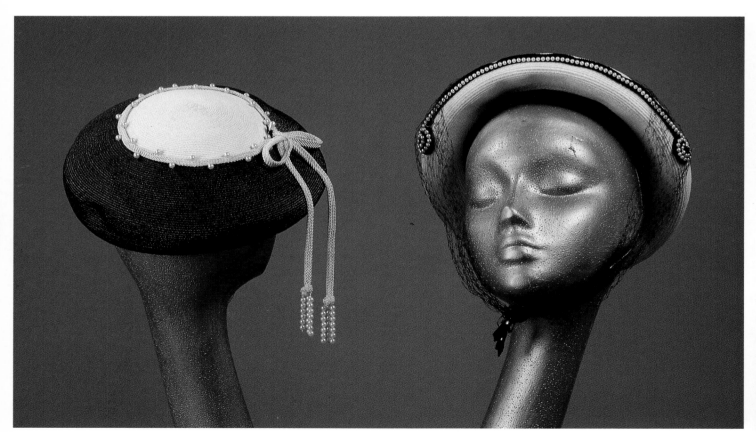

A "twin set" in navy and cream straw, each graced with a strand of pearls. *Courtesy of (both): Maureen Reilly.* Value (each): $25-45.

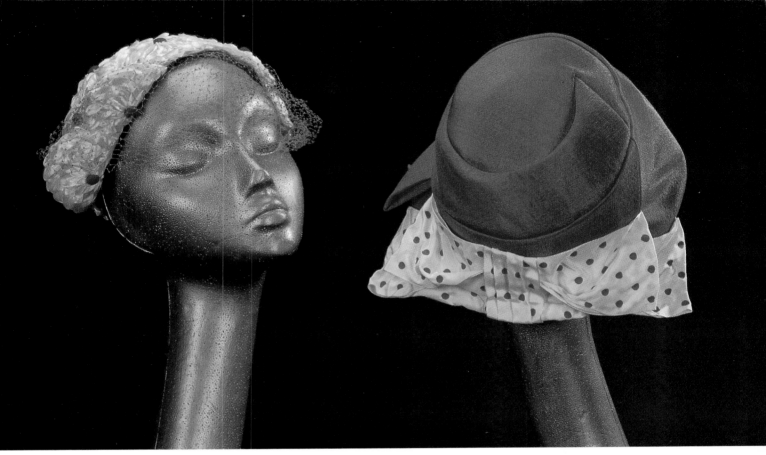

Raspberry dots dance across a straw bandeau, and polka on the satin bow of the cap to its right. *Courtesy of (both): Sandra Headley.* Value (each): $55-75.

Fruit Cocktail

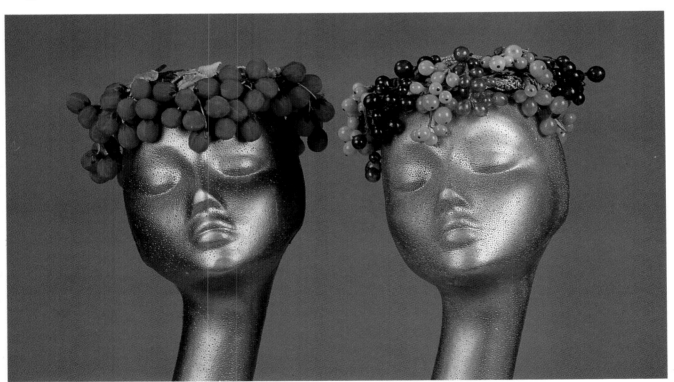

A pair of fabulous fruit hats, one in velvet cherries and the other in hollow plastic grapes. Label (right): Bernard Workman. *Courtesy of (both): Sheila Parks.* Value (each): $55-75.

Fruit Salad

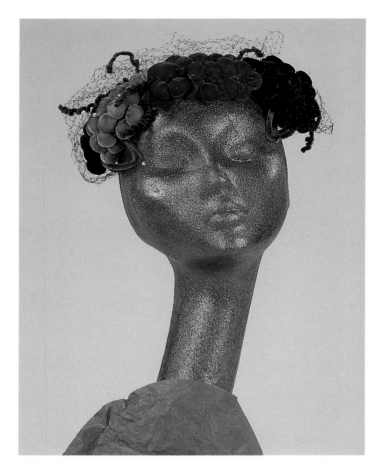

Velvet grapes are a summertime treat. *Courtesy of: Graf's Glitz.* Value: $35-55.

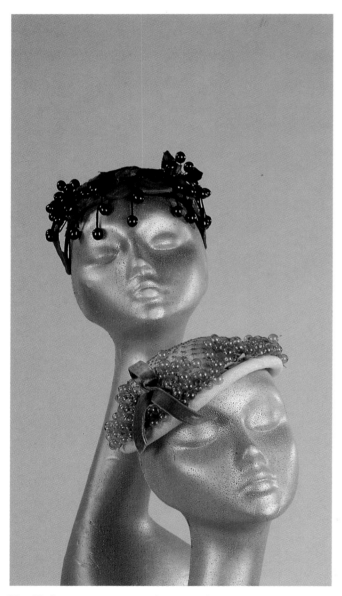

Top, black composition grapes cluster on a bandeau. Bottom, green glass grapes glow against white straw. Label (bottom): Roos\Atkins, CA. *Courtesy of (top): Banbury Cross Antiques. Courtesy of (bottom): Maureen Reilly.* Value each: $35-55.

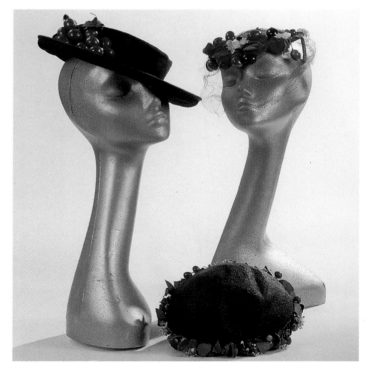

Red cherries cheer a navy boater, freshen a bandeau. *Courtesy of (left): Lisa Carson. Courtesy of (right): Maureen Reilly.* Value (each): $35.55.

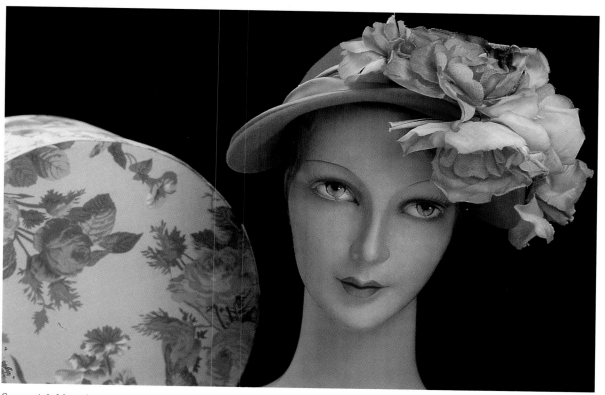

Sweet pink felt and satin cap, romanced with roses. Label: Muller Modes-California. *Courtesy of: Banbury Cross Antiques.* Value: $75-125.

The New Sophisticate

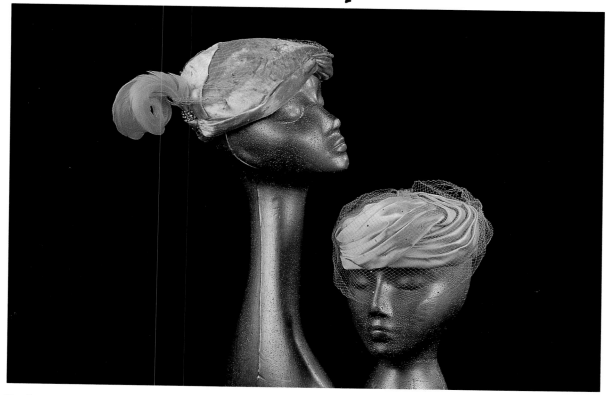

Powder pink satin for feminine allure, in two cocktail caps. Label (bottom): Sonni. *Courtesy of (both): Graf's Glitz.* Value (each): $35-55.

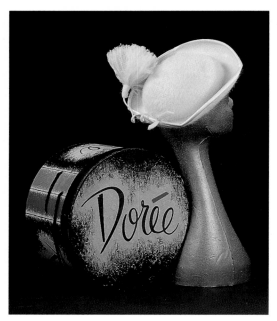

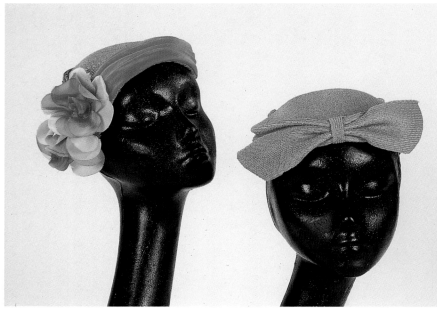

Ivory fur felt, rimmed in satin and dusted with a feather tuft. Note the unique square brim. Shown with its original hatbox. Label: Dorée. *Courtesy of (both): Maureen Reilly.* Value (hat): $35-55. Value (box): $25-35.

A straw duo, the color of watermelon. One with floral flair, the other banded with a self-straw bow. Label (right): New Era. *Courtesy of (both): The Sheepish Grin.* Value (each): $25-45.

Cascades

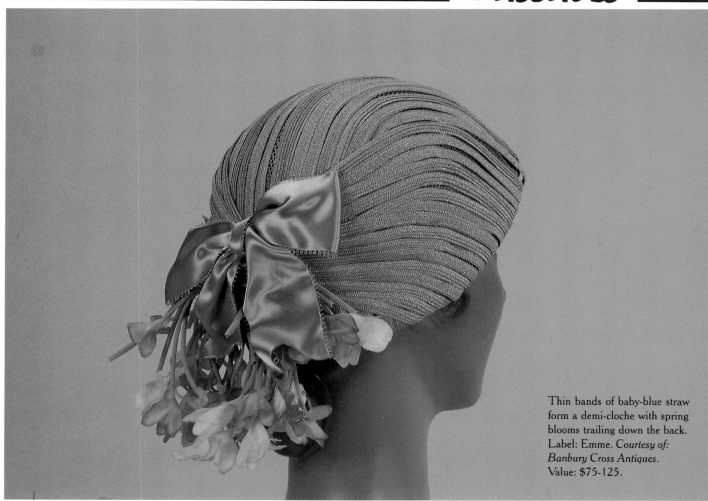

Thin bands of baby-blue straw form a demi-cloche with spring blooms trailing down the back. Label: Emme. *Courtesy of: Banbury Cross Antiques.* Value: $75-125.

Springtime

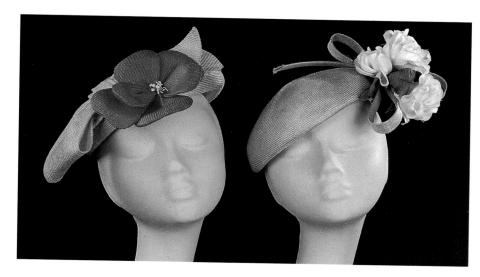

Two natural Milan straw berets, pinned with perky corsages. Label (right): Adolfo II. *Courtesy of (both): Banbury Cross Antiques.* Value (left): $25-45. Value (right): $45-75.

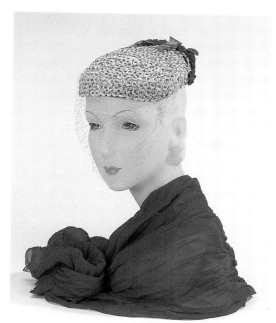

Tiny scarlet beads embedded in natural straw, punctuated with a red velvet flower. Label: Dece Original. *Courtesy of: Banbury Cross.* Value: $45-75.

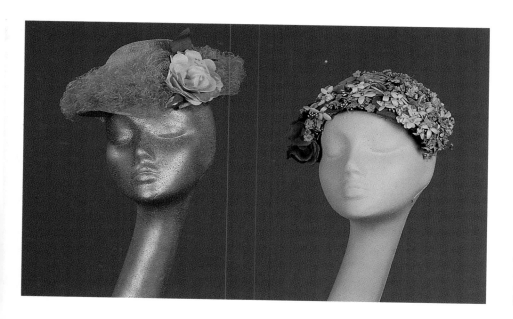

Frills of dusty pink horsehair make an unusual hat, left. Various dainty flowers are planted in silk, right. Label (left): Evelyn Varon—Model. Label (right): Hattie Carnegie. *Courtesy of (both): Banbury Cross Antiques.* Value (each): $45-75.

Fancy Free

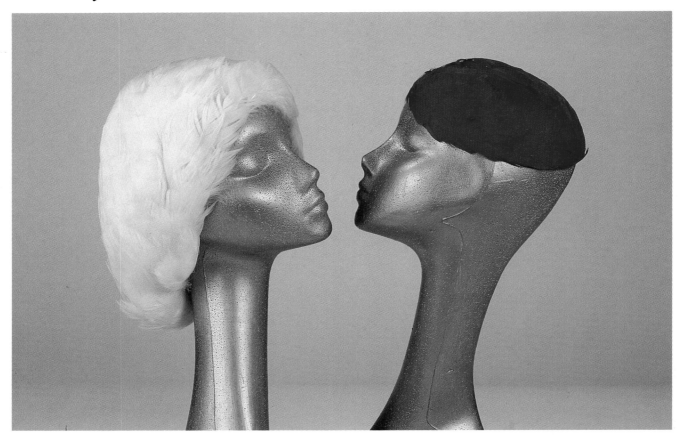

Snowy feathers drape loosely on a net snood, elegant as a swan. Vermilion feathers on a buckram cap, perky as a robin. Label (left): Made in Yugoslavia. *Courtesy of (both): Barbara Griggs Vintage Fashion.* Value (left): $45-75. Value (right): $25-45.

A Winsome Pair

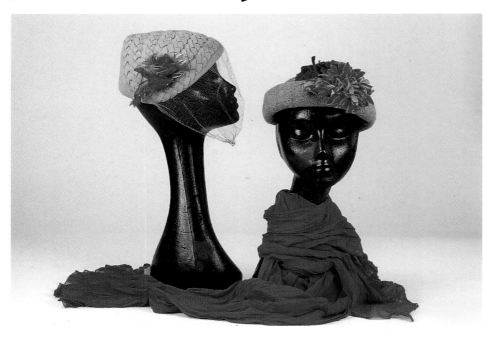

Soft grey felt is braided into a cap, shaped into a Breton. Both styles are livened with crimson, in a feathered birdie and a velvet mum. *Courtesy of (left): The Sheepish Grin. Courtesy of (right): The Rag Bag.* Value (each): $35-55.

Fine-Feathered Friends

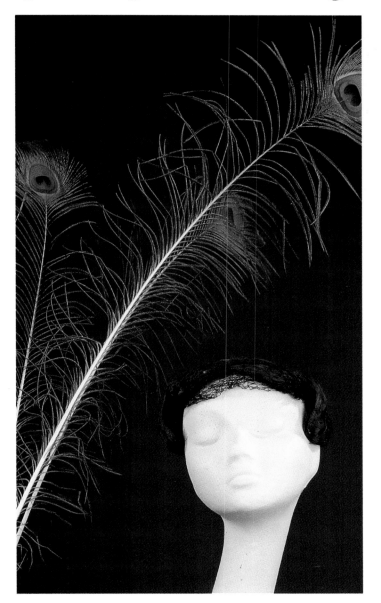

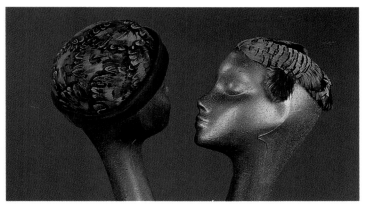

Autumn colors captured in feathers under net, a finely detailed toque with velvet banding. Its friend is a "made" pheasant, shaped on a buckram bandeau. Label (left): Noreen. Label (right): Patrice. *Courtesy of (both): Maureen Reilly.* Value (each): $35-55.

Faux peacock plumage is swirled on a felt cap, in a style that was typical of the mid-1950s. Label: Chapeaux by Roze; Ransohoff's. *Courtesy of: Maureen Reilly.* Value: $25-45.

Two feathered caps in tones of green and gold. Label (left): I. Magnin. *Courtesy of (both): Maureen Reilly.* Value (each): $35-55.

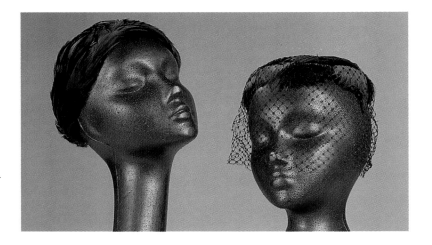

Fall Splendor

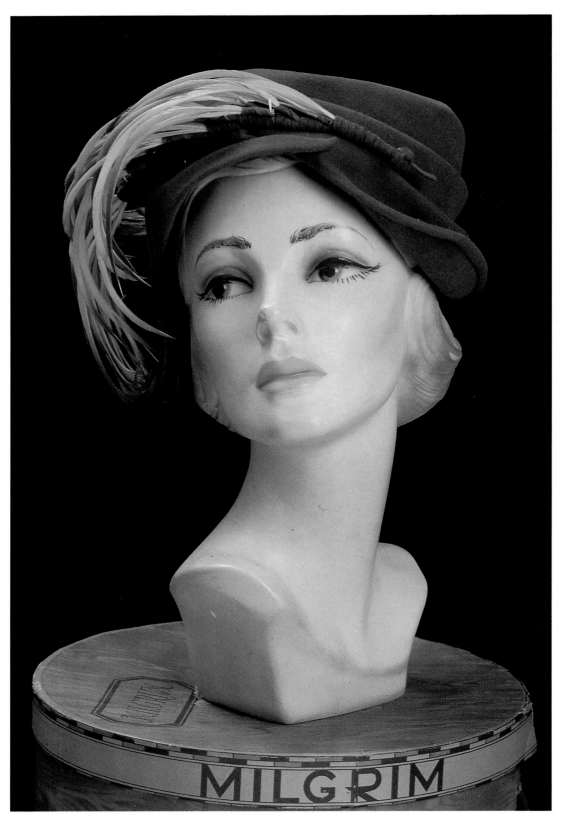

A well-constructed coffee-brown felt hat with an arch of dramatic golden plumes. *Courtesy of: Banbury Cross Antiques.* Value: $65-95.

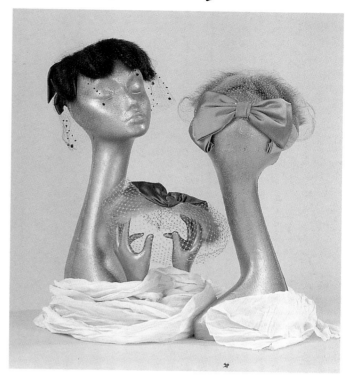

Snuggle Up

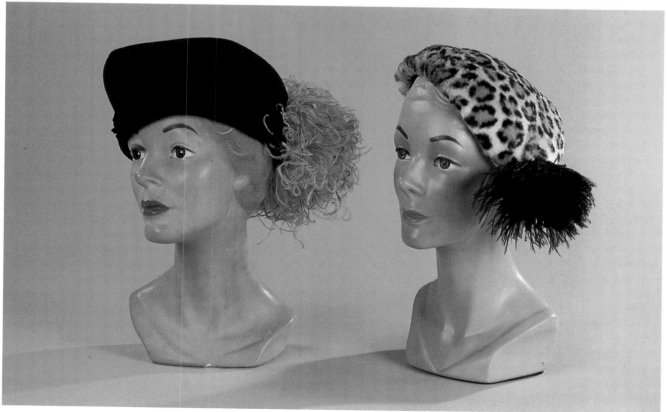

Think mink, three more times. Top left, a fudge-brown felt Breton is rimmed in cocoa-brown mink. Bottom, a swirl of mink, just right to wear over a bun. The felt cap shown upper right boasts a mink "tail" over its beautymark veil. *Courtesy of (all): Maureen Reilly.* Value (each): $35-55.

Three little mink bandeaux, all with plump satin bows, all from Sonni. *Courtesy of (all): Maureen Reilly.* Value (each): $25-45.

Berets are better in fun fur! One, in deep brown with a whisper of ostrich. The other, in fabulous faux leopard with a feathery tuft. Label (left): Velda Original. Label (right): Robinaire. *Courtesy of (left): Sheryl Birkner. Courtesy of (right): Banbury Cross Antiques.* Value (each): $35-55.

A midnight rose perched on a satiny cap, sparkled with sequins, at left and right. A satin ribbon chou tilts forward in a toy hat, center. *Courtesy of (all): Barbara Griggs Vintage Fashion.* Value (each): $45-75.

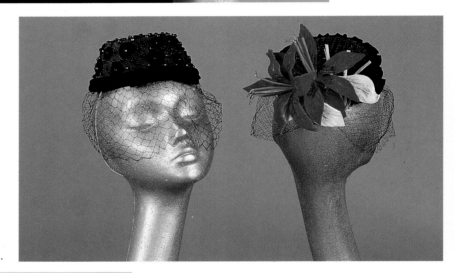

A stiff black fez sparkles with paillettes, left. Shown with a flowering cocktail cap, right. *Courtesy of (both): Maureen Reilly.* Value (each): $45-75.

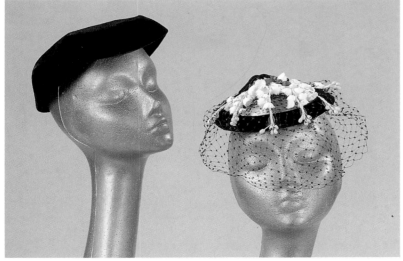

Black velvet on a buckram frame forms a horseshoe-shaped cap, while white lilies-of-the-valley spray over a black velvet diadem. Label (left): Phil Starr. Label (right): Sally Victor. *Courtesy of (both): Maureen Reilly.* Value (left): $25-45. Value (right): $45-75.

Dramatic Flair

White and black feathers dramatize a deeply-piled felt toque. The same idea is interpreted in a revival bonnet, with a white curled ostrich plume peeking out from an upturned black velvet brim. *Courtesy of (both): Banbury Cross Antiques.* Value (each): $55-75.

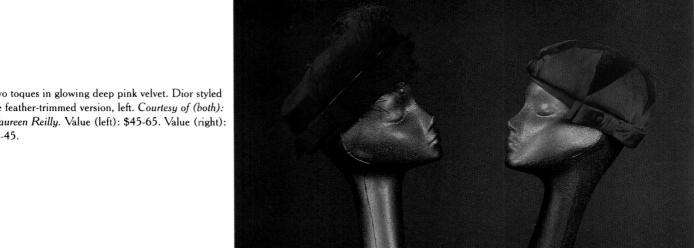

Two toques in glowing deep pink velvet. Dior styled the feather-trimmed version, left. *Courtesy of (both): Maureen Reilly.* Value (left): $45-65. Value (right): 25-45.

Gem Quality

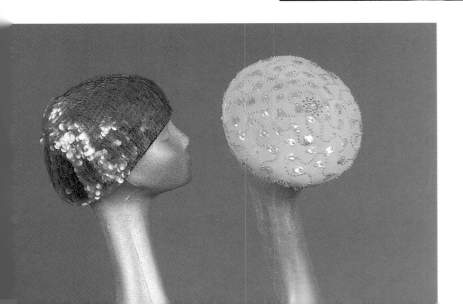

Two sequined berets. Dripping in silvery pink, left; studded in pearly white, right. *Courtesy of (both): Banbury Cross Antiques.* Value (each): $25-45.

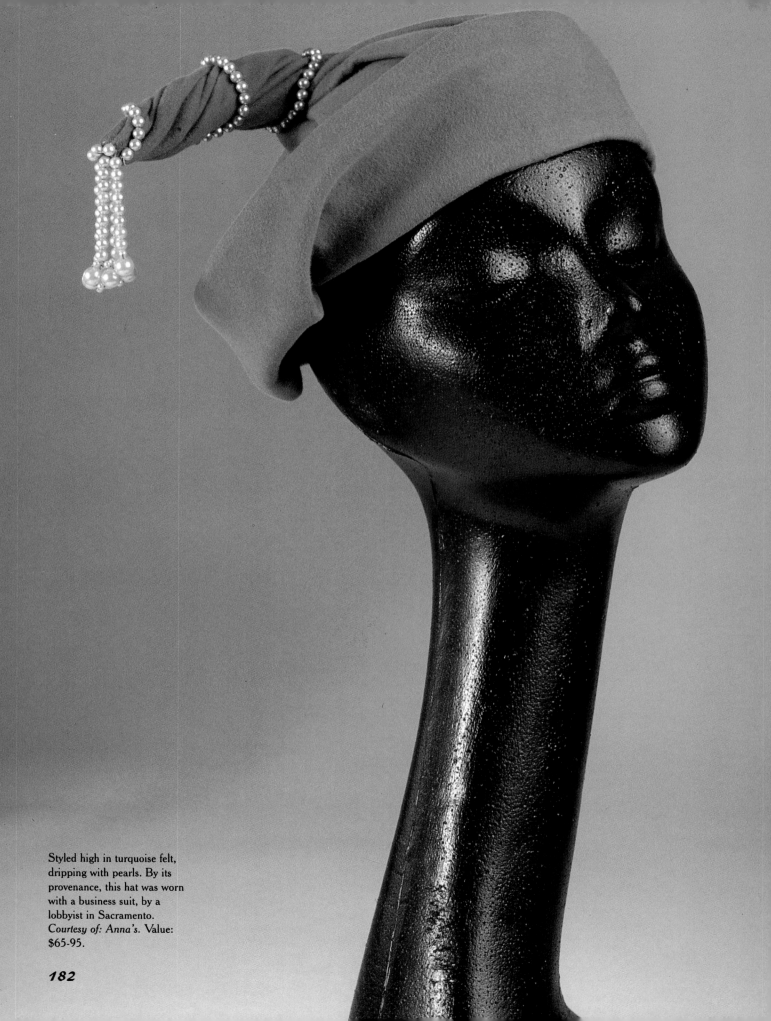

Styled high in turquoise felt,
dripping with pearls. By its
provenance, this hat was worn
with a business suit, by a
lobbyist in Sacramento.
Courtesy of: Anna's. Value:
$65-95.

Hearts
and
Flowers

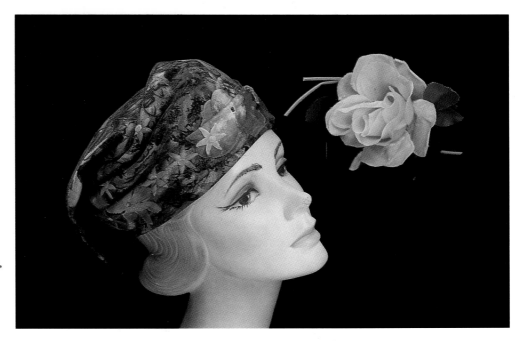

Incredible detailing. This hand-painted draped silk is decorated with velvet hearts, silk and velvet flowers, peacock feathers and sequins under a fine gauze netting. Label: I. Magnin. *Courtesy of: Banbury Cross Antiques.* Value: $75-125.

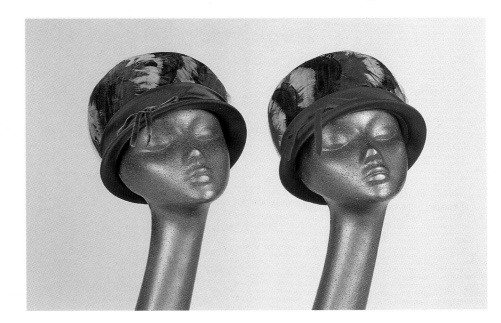

Twin toques, feathers under net on a velvet brim. The similarity of design from different labels indicates that both were knock-offs from the couture. Label (left): Patrice. *Courtesy of (both): Maureen Reilly.* Value: (each): $35-65.

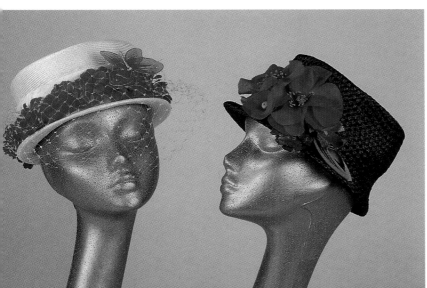

Lady in Red

Red silk poppies bloom on white and navy straw toques. The hat shown at right is an original design by a friend of the authors, Sheila Parks. *Courtesy of (both): Banbury Cross Antiques.* Value (left): $25. Value (right): Special.

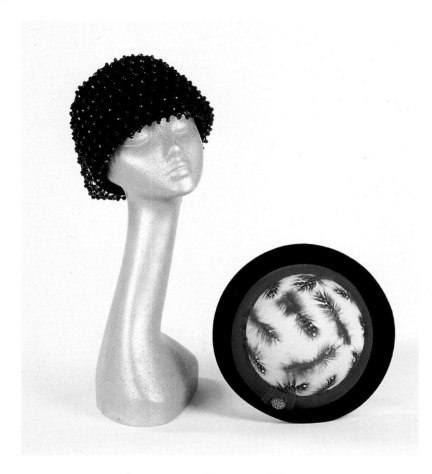

Jet beading dazzles on black fez, top. Red velvet and feathers spark a white and black Breton, bottom. Label (bottom): G. Henry Ross. *Courtesy of (both): Banbury Cross Antiques.* Value (each): $45-75.

In Black and White

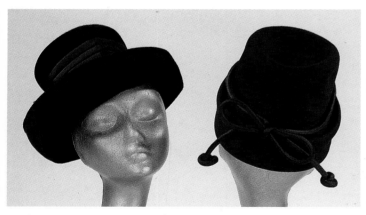

A derby crown with Breton brim on the hat at left. A lampshade hat banded in quirky satin, right. Label (left): Amy, New York. Label (right): Casper Davis. *Courtesy of (both): Maureen Reilly.* Value (left): $35-55. Value (right): $45-75.

White leather and black felt team up in this unusual design by Lilly Daché. Label: Dachéttes. *Courtesy of: Sheryl Birkner.* Value: $45-75.

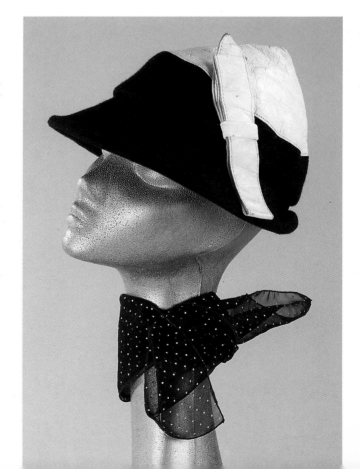

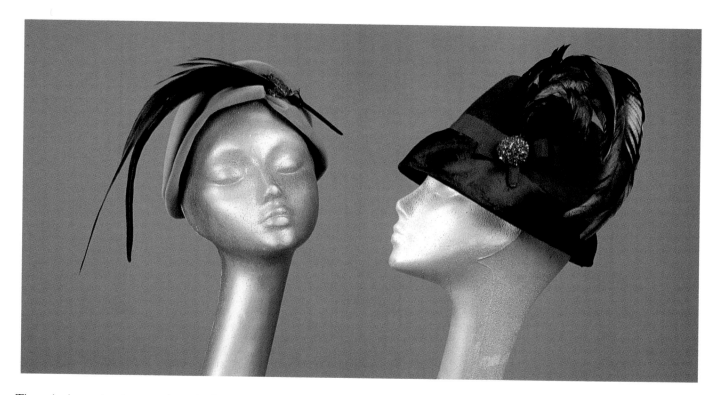

The author's grandmother wore the greige beret with roostertail plumage, circa 1949. Shown with a black beaver toque, boasting bushier plumage, from the same era. Label (left): G. Howard Hodge. *Courtesy of (left): Maureen Reilly. Courtesy of (right): The Rag Bag.* Value (left): Special. Value (right): $45-75.

Top Toques

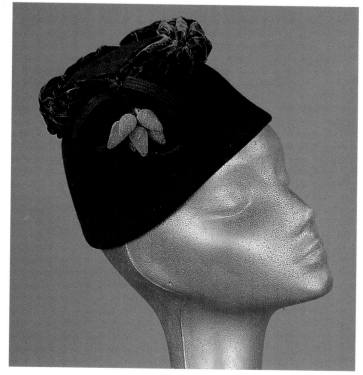

Nutmeg brown fur felt forms a fez, decorated with a velvet ruche at the crown and dangling gold-dusted almonds. *Courtesy of: 57th St. Antique Mall.* Value: $35-55.

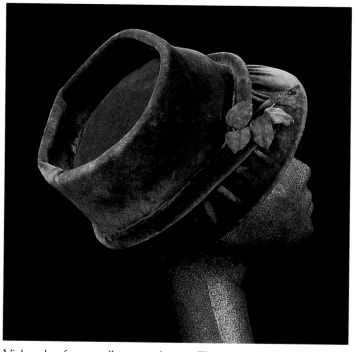

Violet velvet forms a tall structured toque. This was a custom-made hat, with a rhinestone-studded velour pansy sewn in place of a label. *Courtesy of: Maureen Reilly.* Value: $35-55.

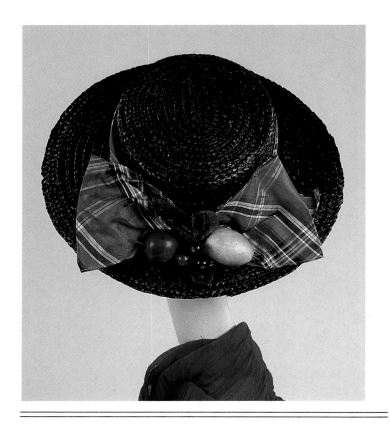

Fresh navy straw boater with oversize plaid taffeta bow. Note the papier maché fruit, an amusing throwback to the Belle Epoque. *Courtesy of: Banbury Cross Antiques.* Value: $65-95.

Picture This

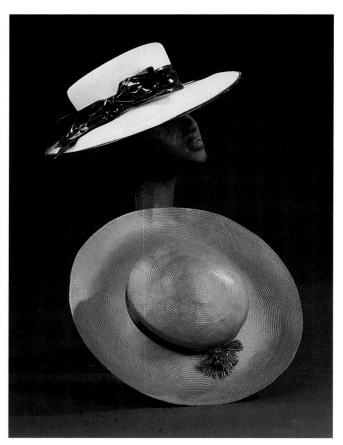

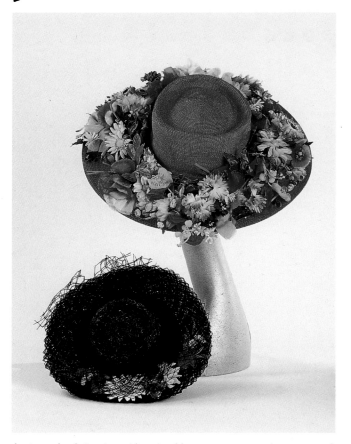

A smart ivory straw with patent-leather hatband, and a red Milan with patent-leather flowers. Label (top): Suzi of California. Label (bottom): Jordan Marsh Co. *Courtesy of (both): Banbury Cross Antiques.* Value (each): $25-50.

A picture hat brimming with spring blooms on tomato-red straw, top. A boater with daisies pressed into net for a ruffled brim, bottom. Label (top): Delle Donne. Label (bottom): *Courtesy (top): Rich Man, Poor Man): Courtesy (bottom): Maureen Reilly.* Value (top): $45-75. Value (bottom): $75-125.

Stardust

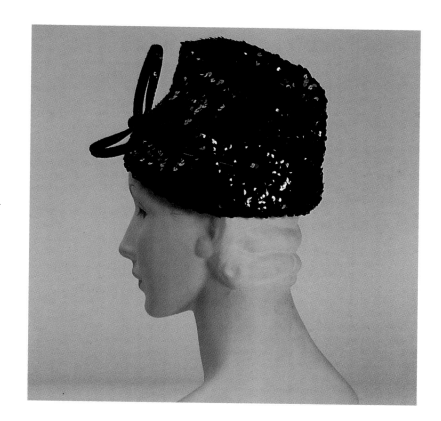

A couture toque, in allover silvered black sequins. Label: Evelyn Varon-Model. *Courtesy of: Banbury Cross Antiques.* Value: $75-125.

Closing Act

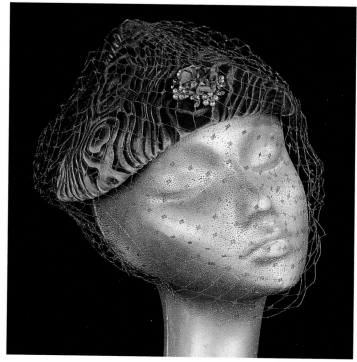

Jacquard velvet with a rhinestone brooch, in a cocktail beanie by Mr. John. *Courtesy of: Maureen Reilly.* Value: $75-125.

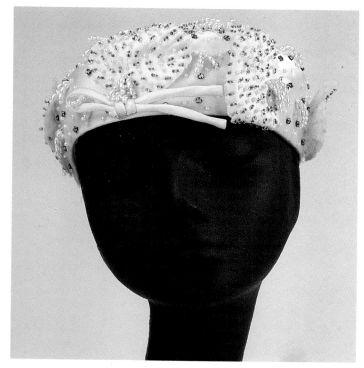

Satin appliques covered with pearls and rhinestones. Label: Wm. Silverman—Marshall Field & Co. *Courtesy of: The Way We Wore.* Value: $75-125.

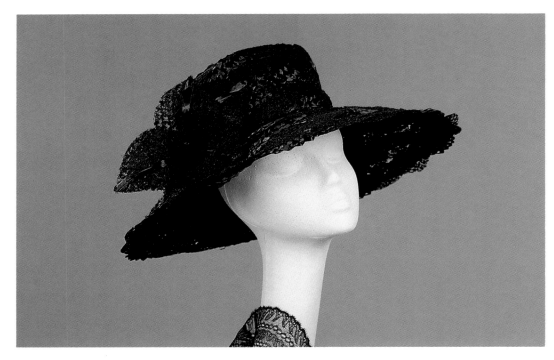

Lacy black straw in a revival Edwardian style hat, from the genius of Jack McConnell. *Courtesy of: Barbara Griggs Vintage Fashion*. Value: $75-125.

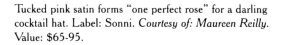

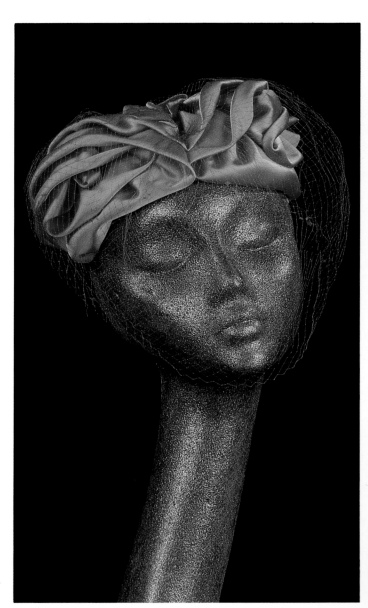

Tucked pink satin forms "one perfect rose" for a darling cocktail hat. Label: Sonni. *Courtesy of: Maureen Reilly*. Value: $65-95.

X. End of an Era: 1960-1975

"Perhaps the biggest style note is 'hats.' The fashionable woman is actually wearing a hat, a real hat!" In these glowing terms, fashion historian R. Turner Wilcox chronicled the fashion trends of his own time, when he published *The Mode in Costume* in 1958.

Wilcox gleefully described the full range of these new hats:

> *"Many are tall and have feathery ornaments rising to surprising height. Feathers, flowers, ribbons, velvets, tulle, jewels, buckles, felts and straws are once more on the shelves of the milliner. The modiste is again designing hats for each season of the year and for every occasion..."*

The fashion transition from the late 1950s into the early 1960s was almost seamless. For a while, women would continue wearing hats for most of their daytime and evening activities.

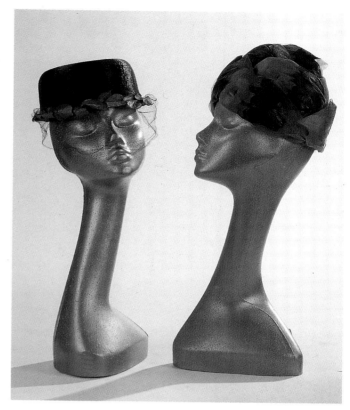

Forest green feathers are stripped and shellacked to form a sleek derby, from Mr. John. Variegated green feathers are swept into a netted turban, from Christian Dior. *Courtesy of (both): Maureen Reilly.* Value (each): $75-125.

For luncheon, they might pair a nubby wool suit with a feathery turban. For evening, a diminutive hat was popular, dubbed the "toy." This was not so much a revival of the 1940s doll hat, as a new breed of cocktail hat.

In typically breathy prose, *Vogue* described it in March 1960 as:

> *"Educational toy...one of the enchanting new toy hats that are converting even the hat-haters this season."*

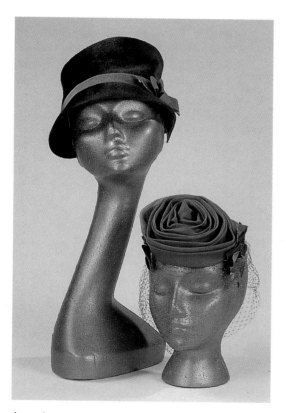

Avocado green was popular in the 1960s, for everything from fashion to kitchen appliances. Seen here in a fur felt toque by Leslie James, and a chiffon-rose toy by John-Frederics. *Courtesy of (both): Maureen Reilly.* Value (each): $55-75.

Women might choose a toque in the popular avocado green to go with a stadium coat and slacks, for sports or suburbia. Even those women who would otherwise favor classic attire, willingly donned the most ridiculous beach hats for fun in the sun!

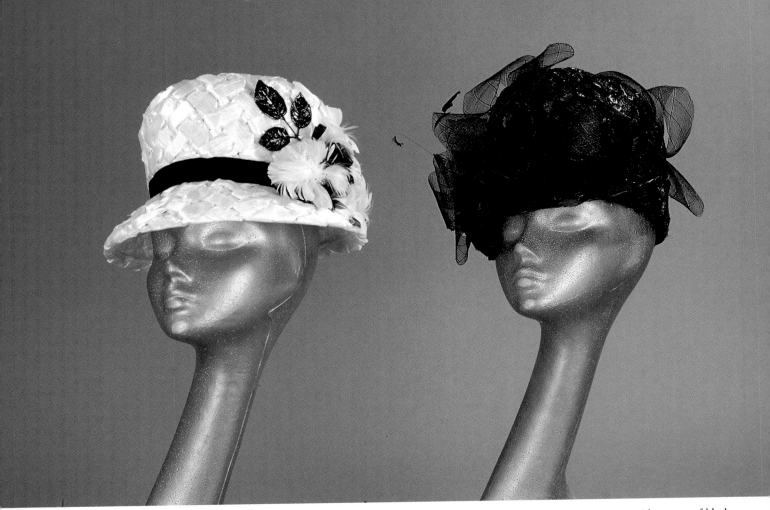

Two straw helmets. The black hat is bursting with braided ribbon and white feathers. The white cellophane straw calls attention with a spray of black velvet flowers. Label (left): Miss Eileen. *Courtesy of (both): Maureen Reilly*. Value (left): $45-65. Value (right): $25-45.

Mink was still in style, joined by such exotic skins as leopard and lynx. Fun fur was a big item—expressly designed for the budget of a young woman, but quickly adopted by those who wanted to look young. Cossacks and toques were often styled in fur to match a coat for an outdoor ensemble. Fur "chechias" were considered fine for dressy occasions, as with a brocaded cocktail dress or satin theater suit.

Flowered hats continued in popularity, styled in the pillbox and almost any other shape that could support a bouquet.

These hats were often graced by a veil, and were the ultimate in frothy femininity. On the other end of the fashionable scale, menswear was again copied by milliners in shako Homburgs and felt fedoras.

Unlike their counterparts of the 1940s, these hats featured blended colors, matched to the revival of Chanel's tweed suits (e.g., olive green and turquoise or magenta and burnt orange). They also differed from earlier menswear styles in their oversized crowns, and their characteristic of sitting squarely on the head rather than at a tilt.

This chilli-pepper beach hat is so hot, it's cool. *Courtesy of: Banbury Cross Antiques*. Value: $45-65.

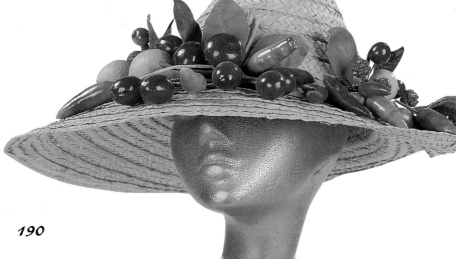

The nightcap, and its forerunner the fez, surely inspired the pillbox. This was a fashion icon of the 1960s, the hat that Jackie Kennedy wore to the Presidential Inauguration in 1961.

Halston designed the hat worn by Jackie that day, and for that reason he is often credited with its design. However, it was also a staple in the collections of Oleg Cassini, who designed most of Jackie's wardrobe while she was in the White House.

In any event, Jackie favored the pillbox, and brought this style into the fashion limelight. She was the embodiment of style for a generation of American women, and her clothes were slavishly copied nationwide.

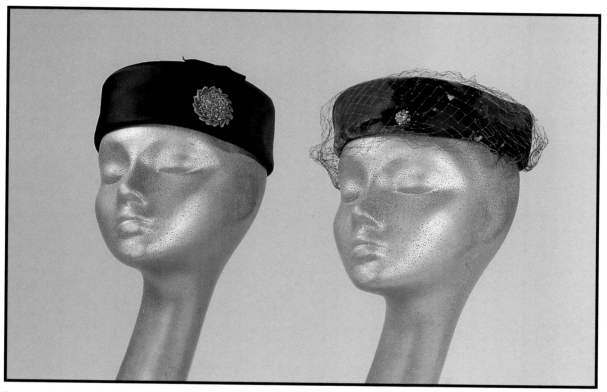

Two queenly pillboxes for evening. A braid medallion glows like a jewel against black satin, and a single pearl holds veiling in place on patterned velvet. Label (left): Mark III. Label (right): Mr. John. *Courtesy of (both): Banbury Cross Antiques.* Value (left): $25-45. Value (right): $35-55.

The beehive, the bubble, and other teased hairdos were popular in the early 1960s. Hats grew in size accordingly, until it seemed as if the sedate pillbox and toque of the previous few years had exploded.

Many hats were brimless, but with ballooning crowns too large to be mistaken for a cloche. This style was often trimmed with silk flowers and feathers. An alternative was the wide-brimmed hat, reminiscent of the Molyneux collection in 1940. This style was often severely styled, all in black and with only a hatband for trim.

In fashion magazines, even the new collections from France were frequently photographed on hatless models. It was the "sexy sixties" when starlets went bareheaded in the movies, and on television. The carefully-tousled hairstyles of Marilyn Monroe and Bridgette Bardot were widely copied, and women were reluctant to cover the results with a hat.

Cocktail parties were a favorite form of entertaining, and helped to keep hats in style for many years during this decade. What woman could resist the chance to flirt from behind the brim of a feathered Pamela, or showcase her curls with a darling tilted toy?

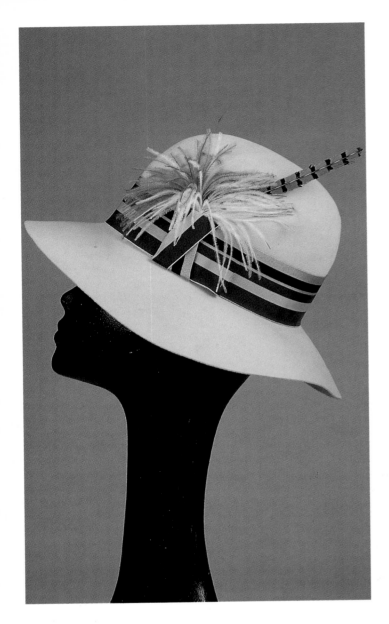

Play it Again, Sam. A classic felt fedora with multi-colored grosgrain hatband. Label: Frank's Girl. *Courtesy of: Lisa Carson.* Value: $55-75.

In London, the Carnaby look propelled street style to the height of fashion. In France, Andres Courregès created a runway furor with his vinyl mini skirts and "go go" boots. His neo-helmet was in wide circulation, part of the famous collection that inspired many milliners to trim hats with leather, white vinyl, and see-through plastic.

Glowing red satin and a black chiffon rose create a fabulous cocktail toque. *Courtesy of: Maureen Reilly.* Value: $75-125.

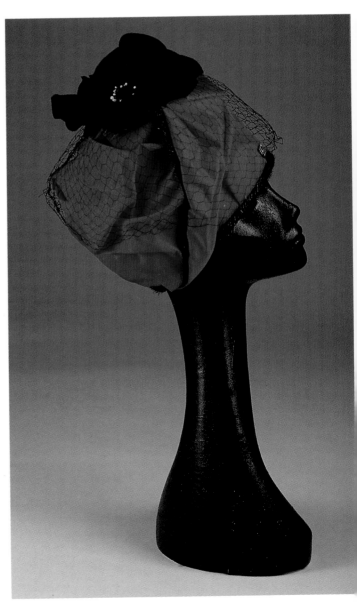

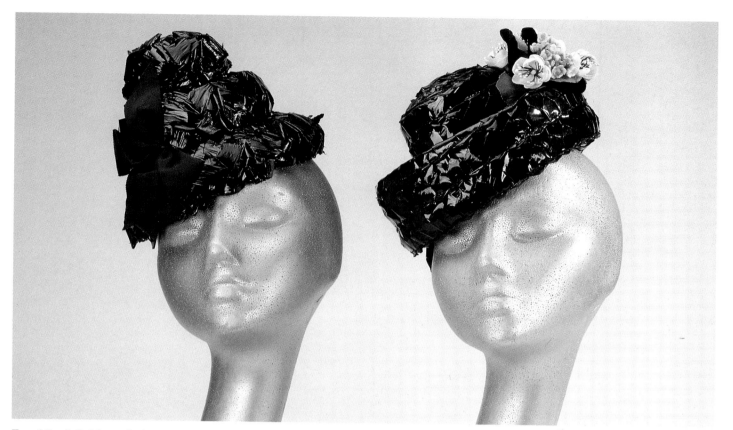

From Miss Sally Victor, the bridge line introduced in 1962, a three-stage cone is tilted for take-off. Shown with a Breton in the same black lacquered straw. *Courtesy of (both): Banbury Cross Antiques.* Value (left): $55-75. Value (right): $35-55.

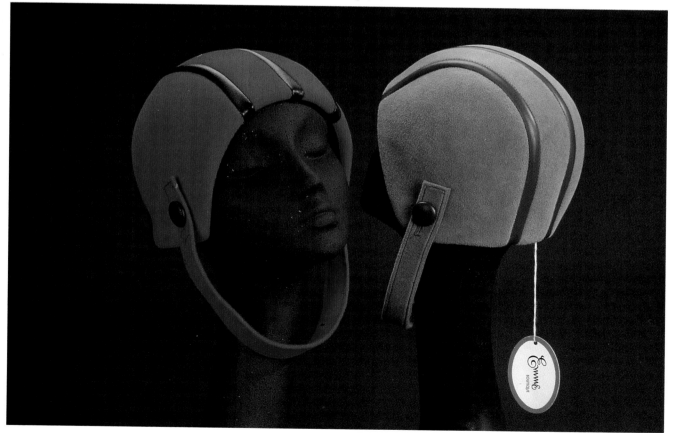

These two helmets in scarlet and fawn were never worn, and still bear the original nametags from Emme. Note the Courrèges-inspired black leather strips, and the chinbands. *Courtesy of: The Way We Wore.* Value (each): $125-175.

In Italy, fashion went psychedelic through the vision of Emilio Pucci. His wildly clashing prints in man-made fabrics are now treasured by museums and collectors. Pucci inspired wildly patterned knock-offs that were ultimately formed into fedoras, berets, and turbans.

In America, Halston experimented with pantsuits, doubleknits, and a streamlined form. He began his career in haute couture, and branched into custom-made millinery in the 1960s. In later years, he designed for the mainstream, with a bridge line in J. C. Penney's.

The decade of the 1960s was the beginning of "street style" and the end of hats. The flower children walked off the streetcorner of Haight and Ashbury in San Francisco and into the annals of fashion history. They were wearing macrame vests, tie-dyed skirts, and ethnic jewelry—but not hats.

It was a time for freedom of expression, and hats were viewed as restrictive. Indeed, some social historians have speculated that hats were spurned by the "flower power" generation as an emblem of class distinction. By the late 1960s, the cultural revolution was upon us. It shook haute couture to its foundation, and all but eliminated hats from fashion's lexicon.

Given the cyclical nature of fashion, hats may come into vogue again. We certainly hope they do! If not, the hat collector can still enjoy the beauty and charm of this unique accessory.

Haute Couture

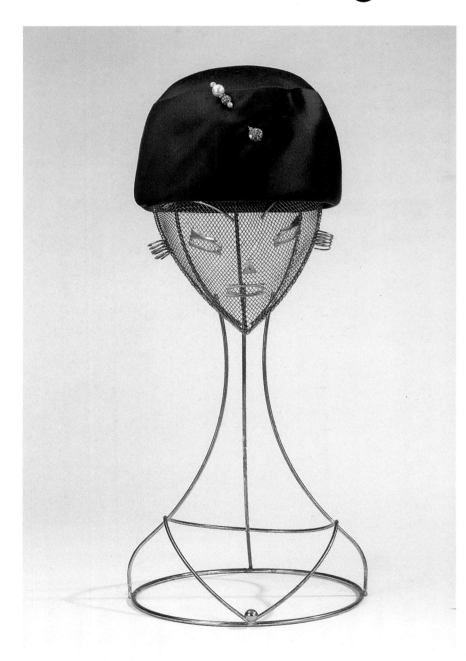

Sleek satin pillbox with rounded crown and pearl-tipped hatpin. Label: Galanos. *Courtesy of: The Way We Wore.* Value: $200-300.

Camelot

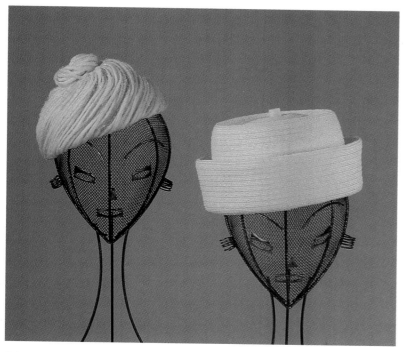

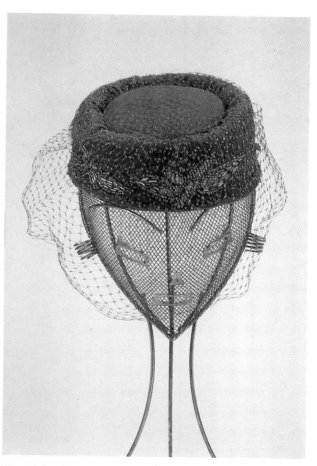

A beanie updated in swirling silk taffeta, and a button-tufted pillbox in white Milan, both from Hattie Carnegie. *Courtesy of (both): Maureen Reilly.* Value (each): $65-95.

Fine gilt beading sparkles on a field of grass-green felt. *Courtesy of: Banbury Cross Antiques.* Value: $35-55.

Whirling Around

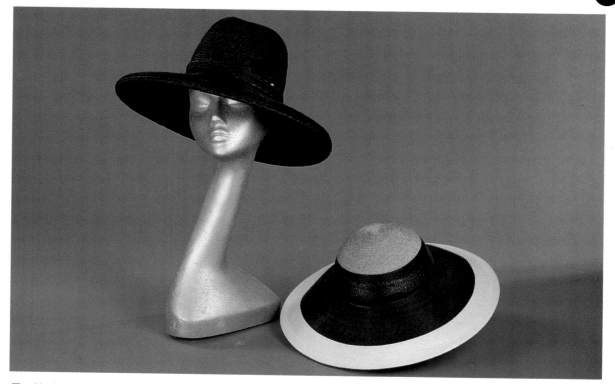

Two black straw cartwheels, one enlivened with a bullseye pattern in pink and white. *Courtesy of (both): Connie Beers.* Value (each): $55-75.

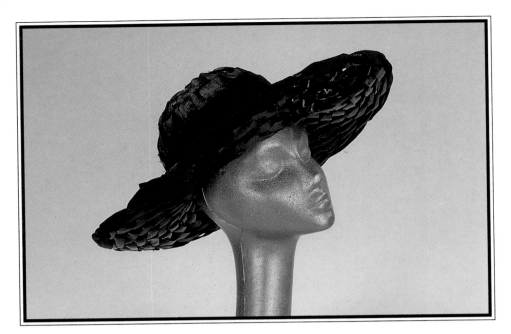

Designer Models

A coarsely-woven wood straw Pamela with great city style. It is a matte finish on top, and lacquered underneath—a subtle surprise from the salon of Lilly Daché. *Courtesy of: Sharon Hagerty.* Value: $75-125.

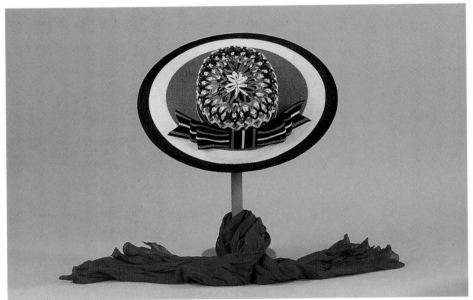

A beauty from Yves St. Laurent, in fresh watermelon, navy, and white. Note the fine detailing on the open-weave crown. *Courtesy of: Maureen Reilly.* Value: $75-125.

City Lights

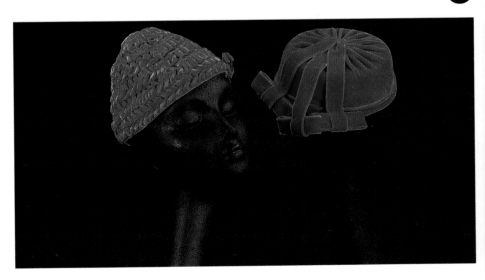

Two hats in magenta velvet. Bands form a cone on one; the other is bow-tied in back. These hats are known to have been purchased in 1966. Label (both): Fannye's. *Courtesy of (both): The Way We Wore.* Value (each): $45-75

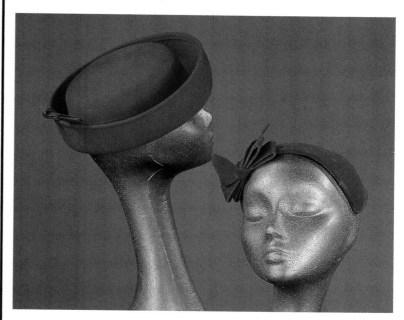

Black felt forms a sculpted toque for evening, topped for luck by a rhinestone die. Label: Coralee. *Courtesy of: Banbury Cross Antiques.* Value: $35-55.

A felt Breton and a velvet half-hat, both in the same vibrant shade of tangerine. Label (left): Patrice. *Courtesy of (both): Maureen Reilly.* Value (each): $35-55.

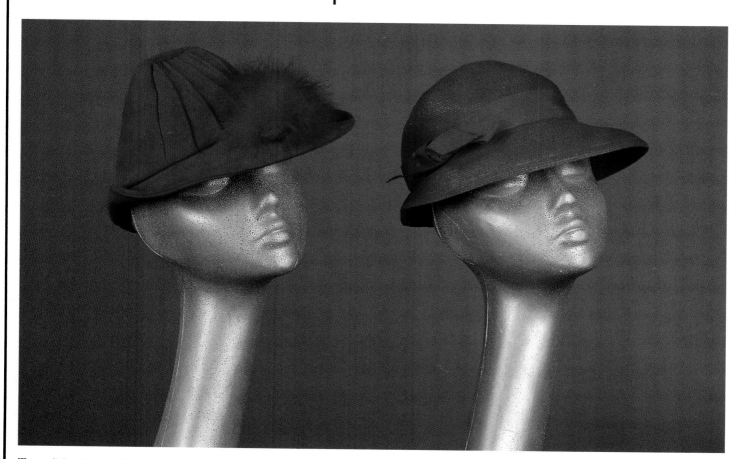

Two stylish red caps. To the left, a pleated red suede Tyrolean with a dashing plume. To the right, a similarly-shaped scarlet straw. Label (right): Knox 5th Ave. *Courtesy of (both): Banbury Cross Antiques.* Value (each): $35-55.

Tam O'Shanters

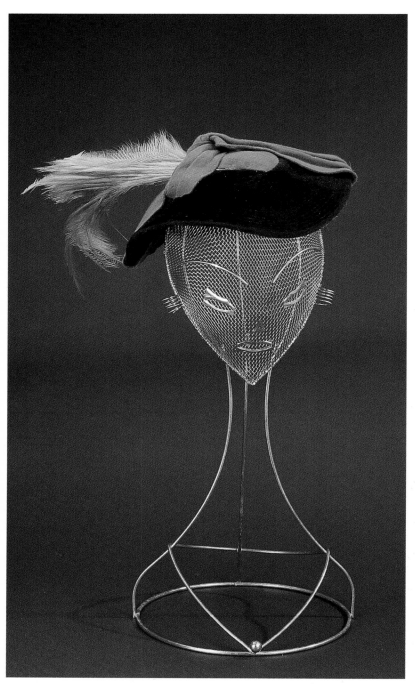

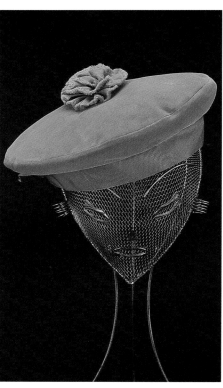

A delicious beret in pale butterscotch velvet. Label: Fannye's. *Courtesy of: The Way We Wore.* Value: $35-55.

Malachite green and black form a stylistic velvet beret. *Courtesy of: Banbury Cross Antiques.* Value: $35-55.

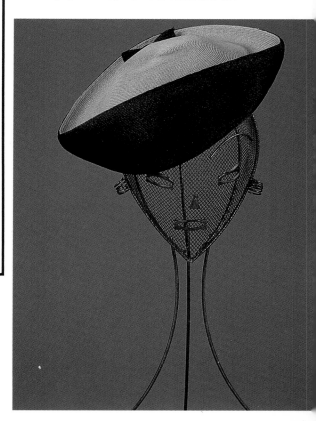

Snappy, highly-stylized straw, in a duotone of wheat and black. Label: Schiaparelli. *Courtesy of: Sharon Hagerty.* Value: $95-145.

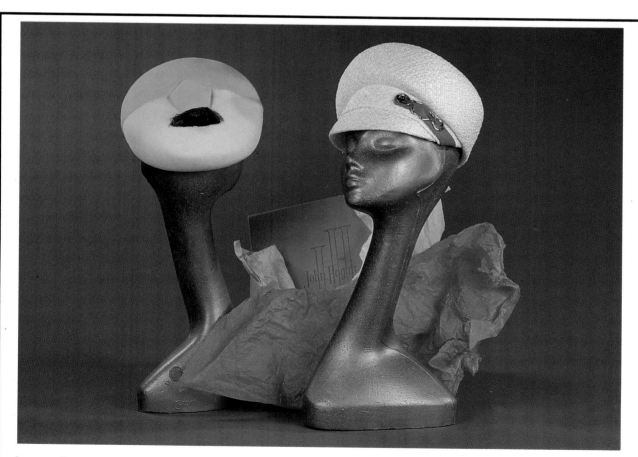

Striped silk taffetas, posed like big and little sisters, from the salon of Mr. John. *Courtesy of (both): Banbury Cross Antiques.* Value (each): $55-75.

Lemon yellow and citrus orange shine against white newsboy caps. Label (left): I. Magnin & Co. Label (right): John Hogan. *Courtesy of (both): Maureen Reilly.* Value (each): $35-55.

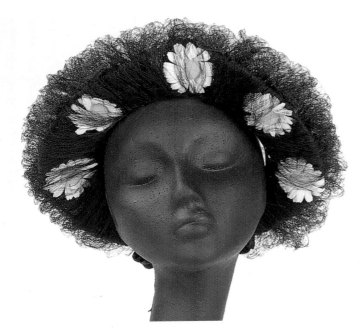

Angelic in stiffened tulle, sprigged with daisies. Label: Switzer's. *Courtesy of: Banbury Cross Antiques.* Value: $45-65.

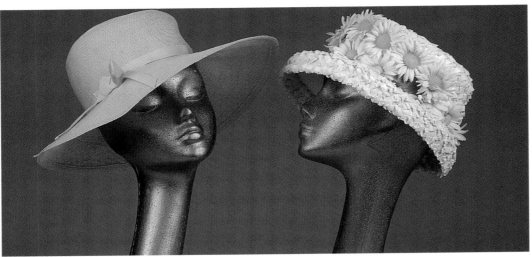

A picture hat in buttercup Milan, shown with a toque in white cellophane straw with daisy garland. Label (left): The Paris Boutique. Label (right): Joseph Magnin. *Courtesy of (left): La Cat & Co. Courtesy of (right): Maureen Reilly.* Value (each): $45-65.

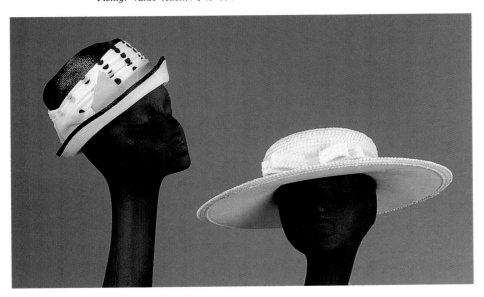

Q: What's black, white, and yellow all over? A: The straw derby from Dachettes. Shown with a cool white straw cartwheel from Schiaparalli, softened with a pat of butter yellow. *Courtesy of (both): Maureen Reilly.* Value (left): $75-125. Value (right); $95-145.

...and Winter Warmth

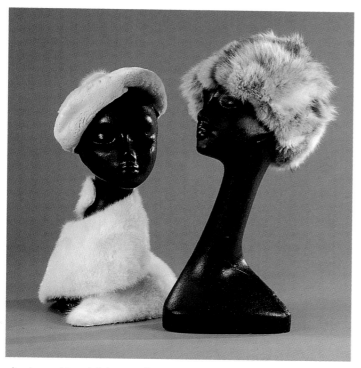

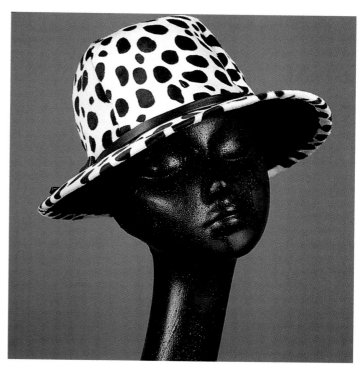

A winter white mink beret and matching scarf snuggles up next to a luxurious lynx Cossack. Label (left): *Custom Made by Reggy Wyatt.* Label (right): *Marshall Field & Co. Courtesy of (both): Barbara Griggs Vintage Fashion.* Value (left, set): $75-125. Value (right): $95-145.

Stenciled ponyskin shapes a safari style. Label: *Emme. Courtesy of: Barbara Griggs Vintage Fashion.* Value: $75-125.

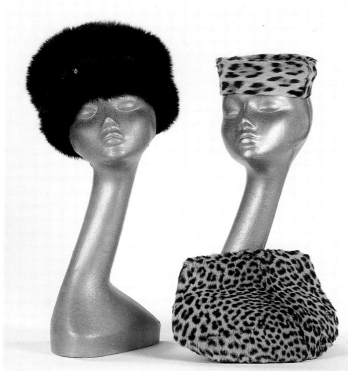

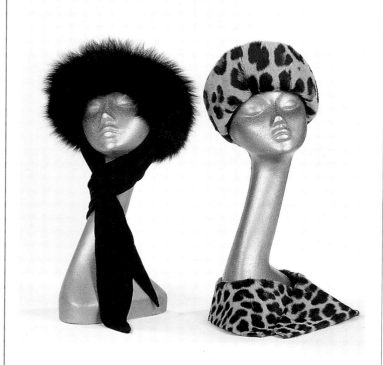

Black nutria makes a toasty toque. Shown with a pillbox and muff, ladylike in leopard. *Courtesy of (both): Barbara Griggs Vintage Fashion.* Value (left): $55-75. Value (right, set): $125-175.

A foxy fur shako and leopard toque with scarf, bred for the wilder side of city life. *Courtesy of: Banbury Cross Antiques.* Value (left): $75-125. Value (right, set): $125-175.

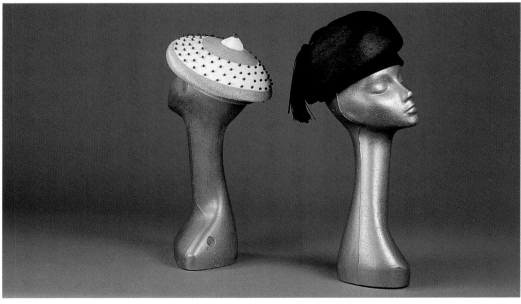

The enduring beret, in steel and white straw. The black Milan straw is puffed, to accommodate a bouffant hairdo. Label (left): Coralee. Label (right): Christian Dior. *Courtesy of (both): Banbury Cross Antiques.* Value (left): $35-55. Value (right): $65-95

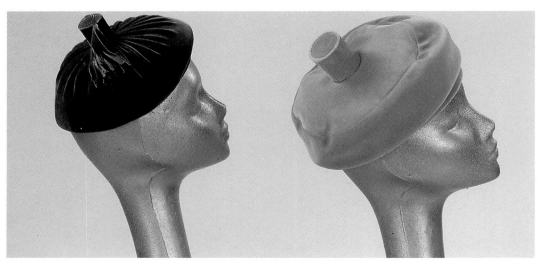

These berets in coffee and cream velvet would have accessorized many fall outfits. Label (left): Irene of New York; I. Magnin & Co. Label (right): Emme. *Courtesy of (both): Maureen Reilly.* Value (each): $55-75.

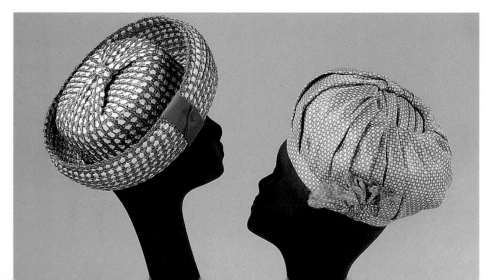

Biscuit and white cellophane straw in a Breton by Coralie. The same color scheme is shown in jersey, draped and shaped in a toque by Kirsten (who was a custom milliner in the Sacramento area). *Courtesy of (both): Maureen Reilly.* Value (left): $35-55. Value (right): $55-75.

Candy Store

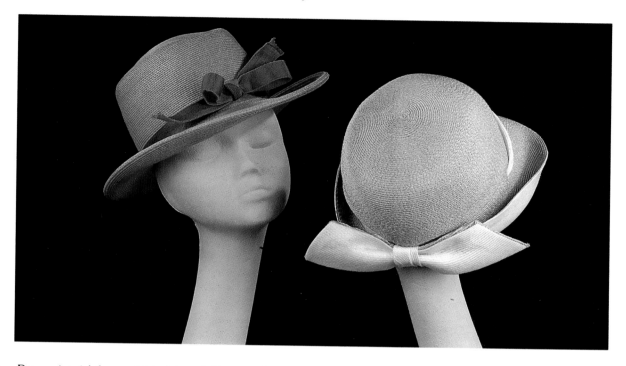

Peppermint pink for a sprightly fedora, tied in green. Its companion, a tart toque in lime, with a vanilla underbrim. Label (left): Lonette Original, L.A. Label (right): Frank Olive. *Courtesy of (both): Maureen Reilly.* Value (left): $35-55. Value (right): $55-75.

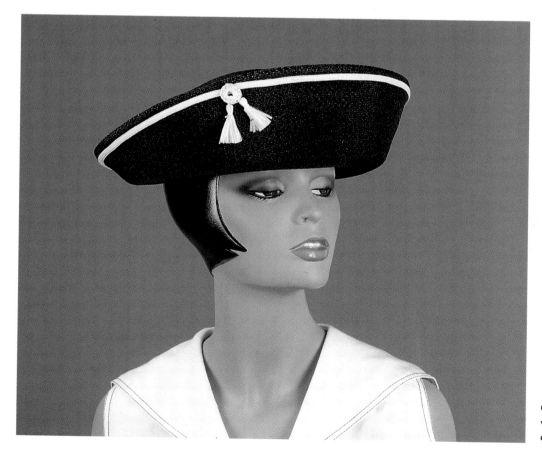

Crisp & Clean

Outsized nautical Breton in black and white Milan. Label: Patrice. *Courtesy of: Connie Beers.* Value: $45-65.

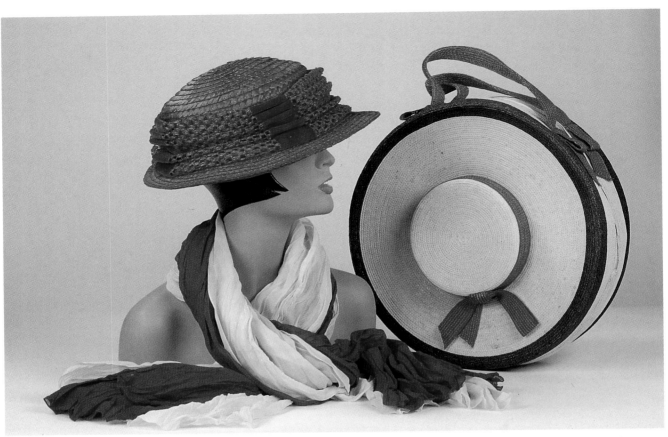

Summertime scarlet with scrunchy banding. Shown with a trompe l'oeil "hat box," a functional purse in patriotic colors. Label (hat): Chanté. *Courtesy of (both): Barbara Griggs Vintage Fashion.* Value (hat): $45-65. Value (purse): $125-175.

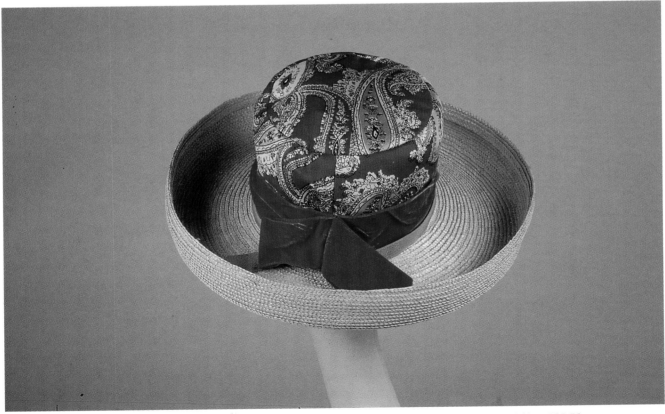

Paisley silk crowns this natural straw picture hat from Mr. John Jr. *Courtesy of: Barbara Griggs Vintage Fashion.* Value: $55-75.

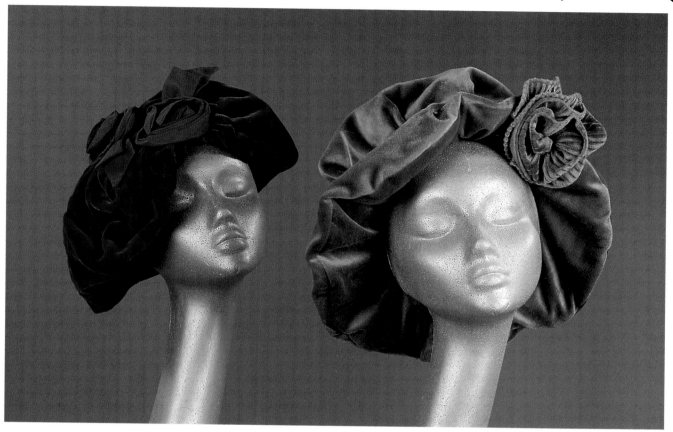

These floppy velvet tams reflect a recurring romantic theme. The burgundy is brightened with silk roses; a rosette accents the aquamarine. Label (left): Livingston Bros. *Courtesy of (both): Maureen Reilly.* Value (each): $55-75.

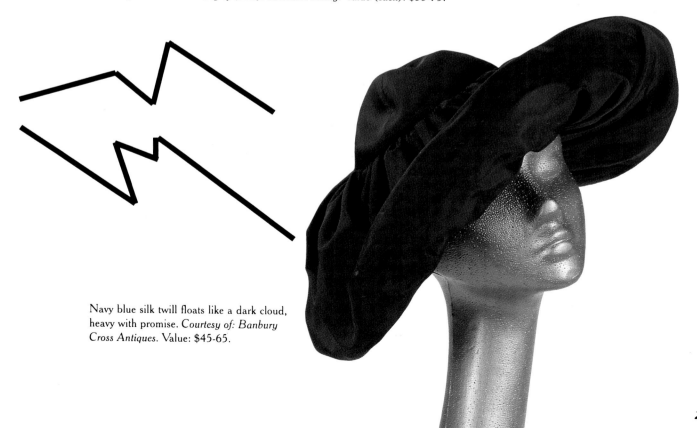

Navy blue silk twill floats like a dark cloud, heavy with promise. *Courtesy of: Banbury Cross Antiques.* Value: $45-65.

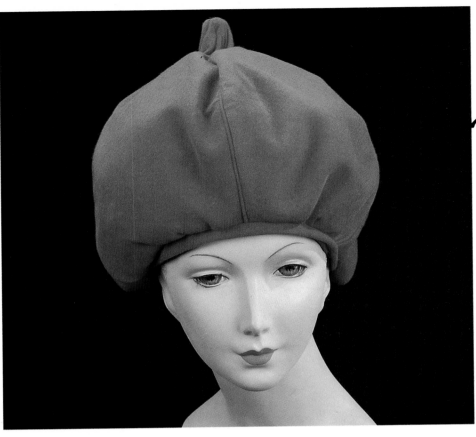

Pumpkin Patch

A beret, round and plump, in felt the color of
a ripe pumpkin. Label: Eleanora Barnett—
San Francisco. *Courtesy of: The Way We
Wore.* Value: $125-175.

Groovin'

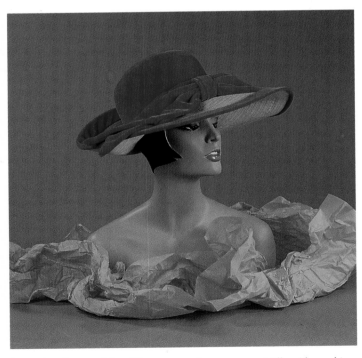

Hot colors for a cool hat. The orange velvet contrasts vividly with sunshiny
rayon. The brim holds its shape with trapunto stitching, over a buckram
form. Label: Hale's. *Courtesy of: Maureen Reilly.* Value: $75-125.

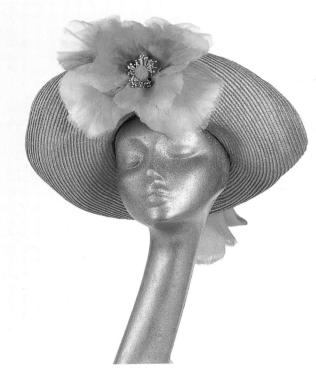

A large sunny poppy pins a spectacular brim in place. Label: Mr. John.
Courtesy of: Banbury Cross Antiques. Value: $75-125.

Persimmon felt and a single perfect
rose. Label: Dorée. *Courtesy of:*
Banbury Cross Antiques. Value: $35-55.

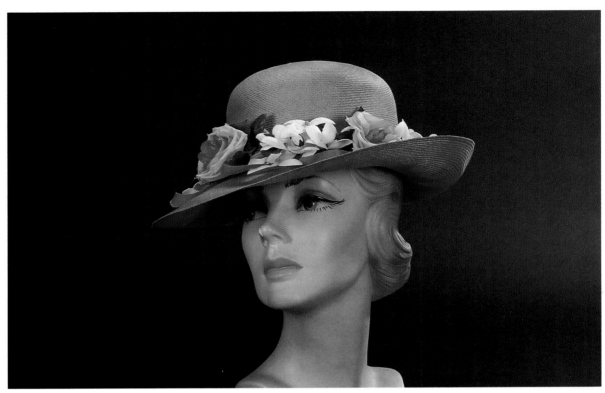

Candy pink straw with roses and gardenias. Label: Adolfo II.
Courtesy of: Banbury Cross Antiques. Value: $75-125.

Spring Fever

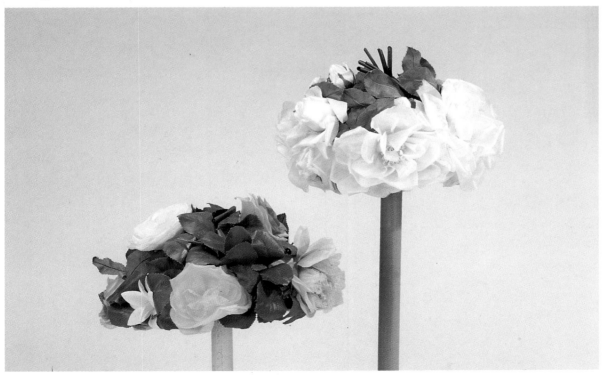

Two allover floral hats, one a riotous garden and the other a wreath of pure white. *Courtesy of (both): The Way We Wore.*
Value (each): $55-75.

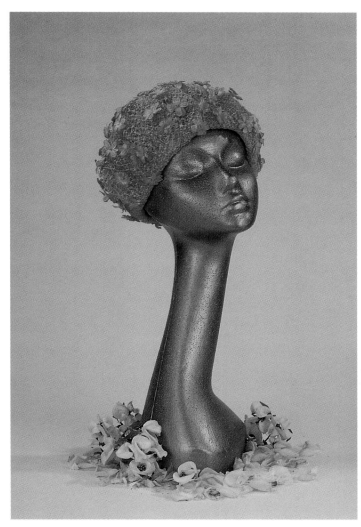

A stiff net "bubble hat" planted with pinks. Label: Christian Dior. *Courtesy of: Maureen Reilly.* Value: $75-125.

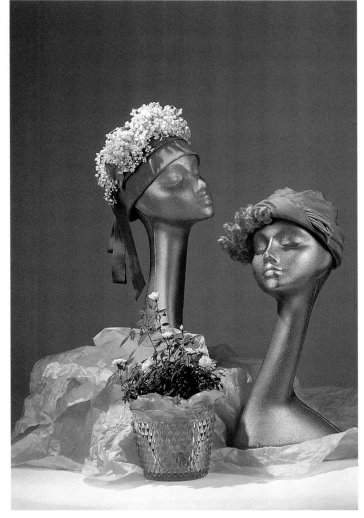

Lilies of the valley bloom on a green silk band, while hot pink roses fold into pleated linen. Label (left): Kirsten. Label (right): Noreen. *Courtesy of (both): La Cat & Co.* Value (left): $75-125. Value (right): $35-55.

Savoir Faire

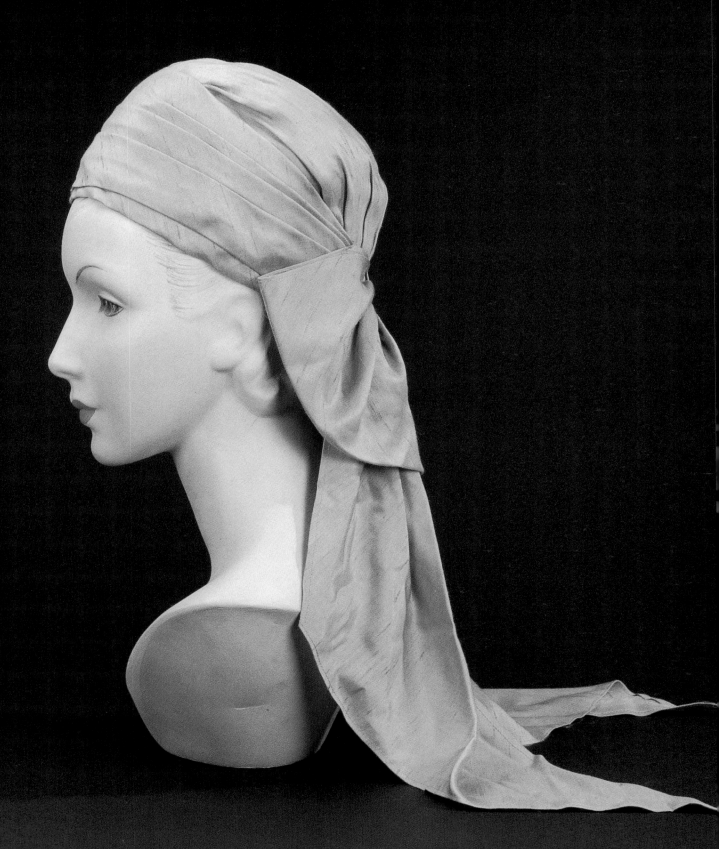

Turbans with a Twist

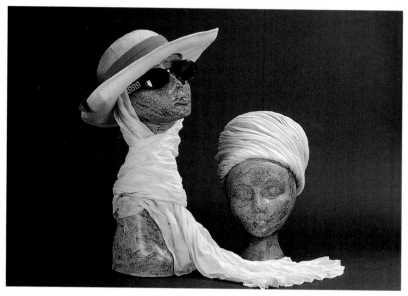

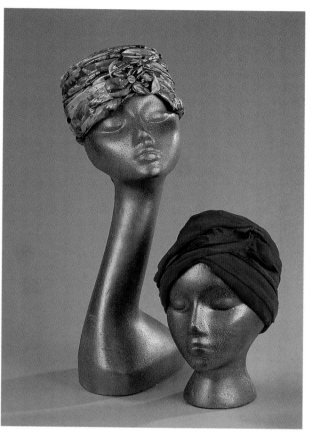

For town and country. A pleated ivory silk turban nestles in the shade of a sky-blue and white straw picture hat. Label (left): Mr. John Clasics. Label (right): Christian Dior. *Courtesy of (both): Maureen Reilly.* Value (both): $65-95.

Turbans in shades of rose and moss green. One is custom-made, in pleated silk. The other is from Dior, in twisted silk velvet. *Courtesy of (both): Banbury Cross Antiques.* Value (each): $75-125.

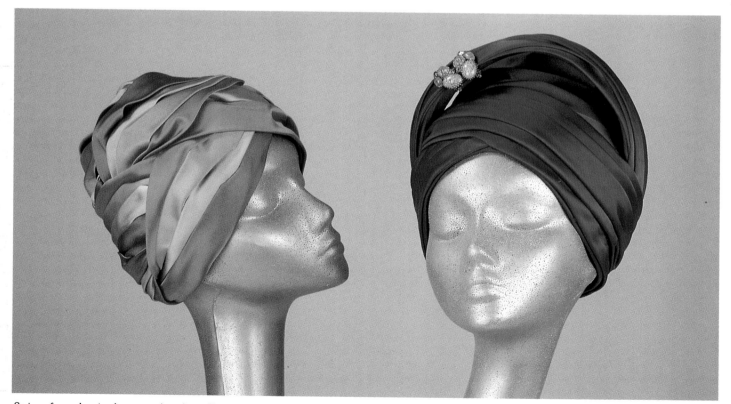

Strips of pastel satin shape a turban from Christian Dior. Straps of satin in sapphire blue form an arched turban from Jack McConnell (the pin is added). *Courtesy of (both): Barbara Griggs Vintage Fashion.* Value (left): $75-125. Value (right): $75-125.

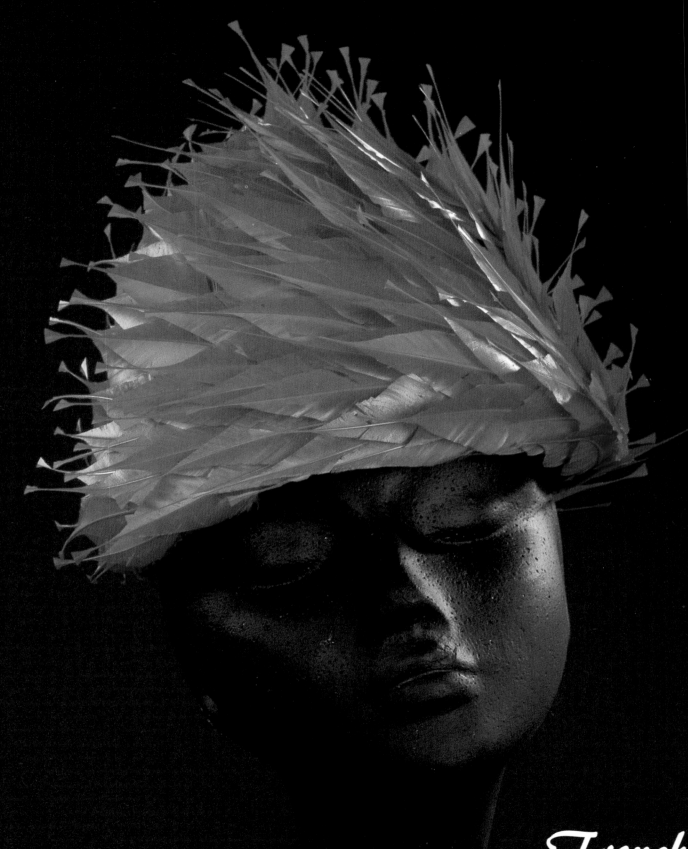

Deep scarlet feathers are scored at
the tips, and light up this hat like a
flame. Label: André Denis—Paris.
Courtesy of: Banbury Cross Antiques.
Value: $150-225.

*French
Flame*

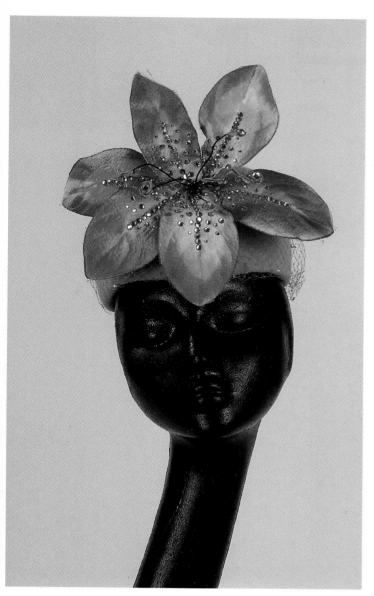

After-five glamour in silvery satin petals, sparkling with rhinestone dew. Label: Jack McConnell. *Courtesy of: Banbury Cross Antiques.* Value: $95-145.

Making Headlines

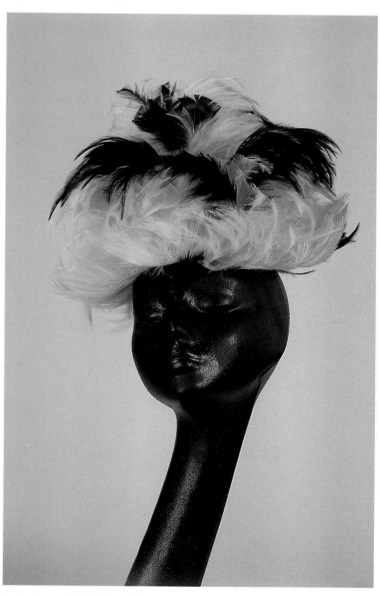

A glorious ostrich feather cocktail hat in striking pink and black. Label: John-Frederics. *Courtesy of: Barbara Griggs Vintage Fashion.* Value: $125-175.

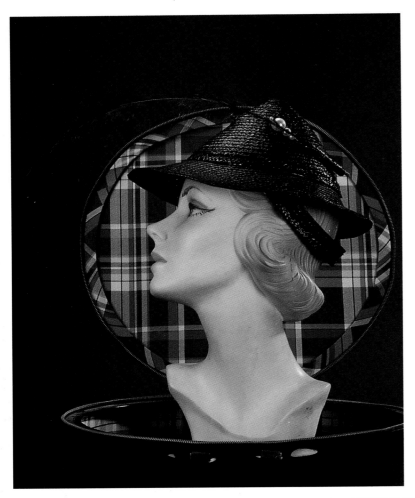

Enduring Chic

Black straw rises to a witch's peak, stabbed by a pearl hatpin. Shown in a jaunty, plaid-lined hatbox. Label (hat): *Adolfo II. Courtesy of (both): Banbury Cross Antiques.* Value (hat): $65-95. Value (box): $55-75.

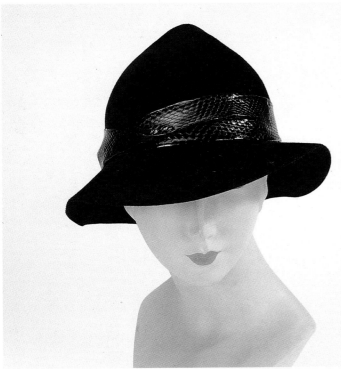

A simply elegant black felt fedora, banded in patent reptile skin. Label: Frank Olive; Neiman Marcus. *Courtesy of: Banbury Cross Antiques.* Value: $65-95.

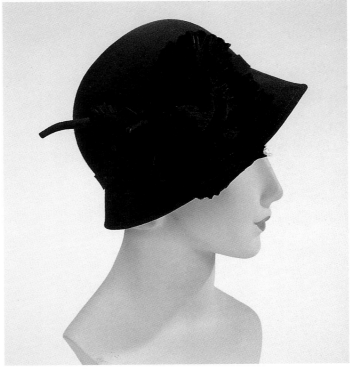

Deep purple felt and a sassy black flower make a classic cloche. Label: Mr. John Classics. *Courtesy of: Banbury Cross Antiques.* Value: $55-75.

A Starring Role

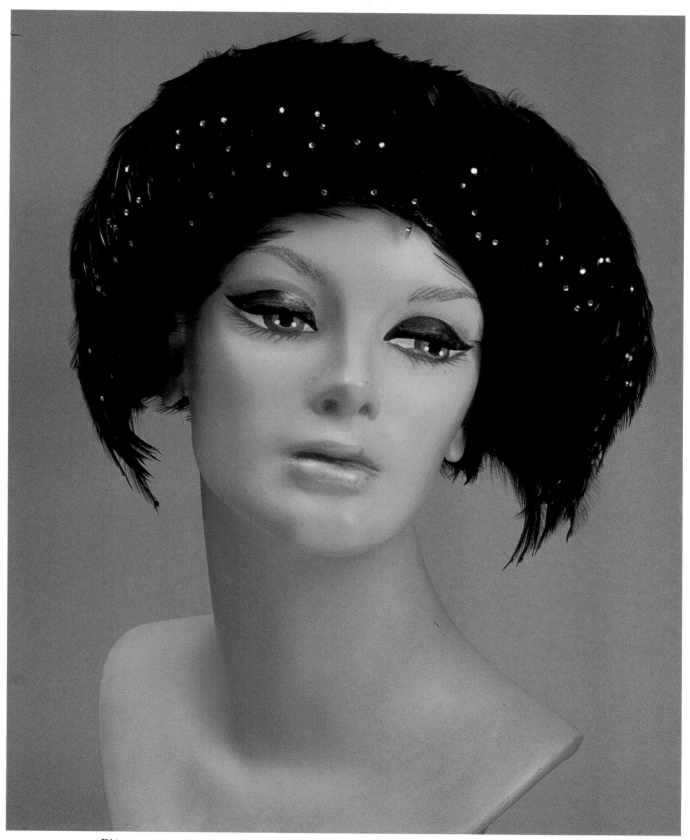

Rhinestone stars glow on a midnight-blue feathered cocktail hat. Label: Jack McConnell. *Courtesy of: Banbury Cross Antiques.* Value: $150-225.

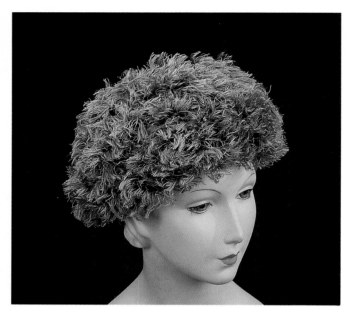

Dusty blue fabric is fringed into a "wig hat"—great for bad hair days! Label: I. Magnin. *Courtesy of: The Way We Wore.* Value: $45-65.

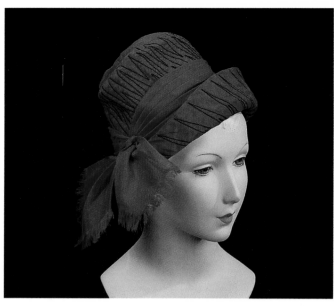

Red silk in an unstructured toque, with tiny beads for trim. Label: Mode Mirondor—Firenze—Lungarns. *Courtesy of: Banbury Cross Antiques.* Value: $95-145.

Grande Finale

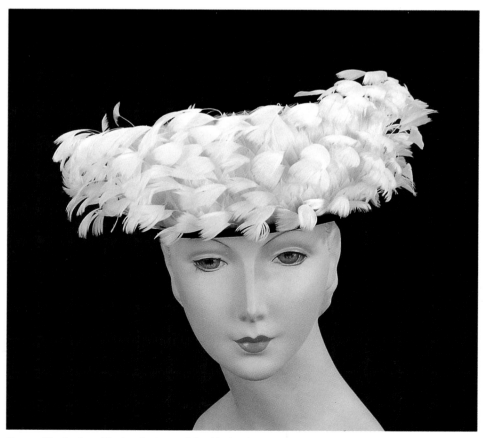

Snow white feathers blanket the brim of this black velvet hat from Jack McConnell. *Courtesy of: The Way We Wore.* Value: $150-225.

XI. The Art and Craft of Millinery

Early hatmaking techniques were complex and labor-intensive, especially in preparing the felt or weaving straw forms. The invention of a straw-sewing machine and other devices in the late 1900s greatly improved this process, but many steps in making a quality hat are still performed by hand.

Consider the fur felting process, one of the "lost arts" that was only re-discovered by Europeans circa 1200. As the story goes, St. Clement made the first fur felt from the skin of a rabbit, which he trod upon to ease his travel-sore feet. For many years, he was the patron saint of male milliners, the same role played by St. Catherine for midinettes of the fair sex.

Rabbit fur remains the most popular for felts, as it was in feudal times. This fur was rivaled only by beaver during the 1800s and early 1900s. But all furs require hours of meticulous work before the pelt can be blocked, and put to good use by a milliner.

In the first stage of processing, the fur must be sheared from the skin, then chemically treated to raise the fibers or barbs that will twist together into felt. It is then graded by hand into its various tensile strengths, and bagged for delivery to the hat manufacturer. There, it undergoes several mixing and refining processes before it can be shaped.

Shaping the felt is even more time-consuming. Each pelt, now loose without its skin, is placed into a forming machine with a three-foot high copper cone. There, it is rotated and steamed so as to shrink the barbs evenly. Further shrinking occurs in the next, critical stage of processing. Using hot water and rollers, the large and loose pelt is felted down successively until it takes its final size as a hat form.

In the finest hats, most felting work is still done by hand, little changed since feudal days—except that, back then, *wool* felt was pressed by hand after having been processed in mercury. The poisonous effect of the fumes led to delirium and hallucinations. It was an occupational hazard for milliners of the day—hence the term, "mad as a hatter."

In the early 1900s it was commonplace for women to make their own hats, or at least trim factory forms. It was a chance to express artistic talent, at a time when women had few creative outlets that could be appreciated outside the home.

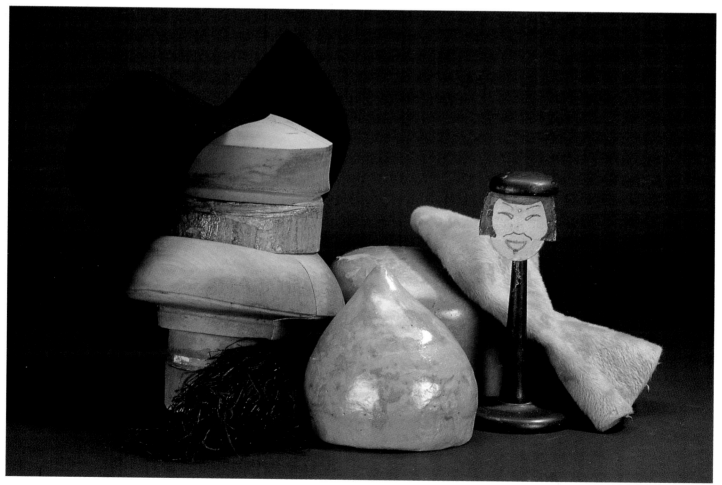

A fur felt, dyed the color of ripe wheat. Shown with hardwood hatforms that were used for shaping felts. Note the amusing Geisha hatstand. *Courtesy of (felt): Sharon Hagerty. Courtesy of (stand): Lottie Ballou.* Value (felt): $35-55. Value (stand): $75-125.

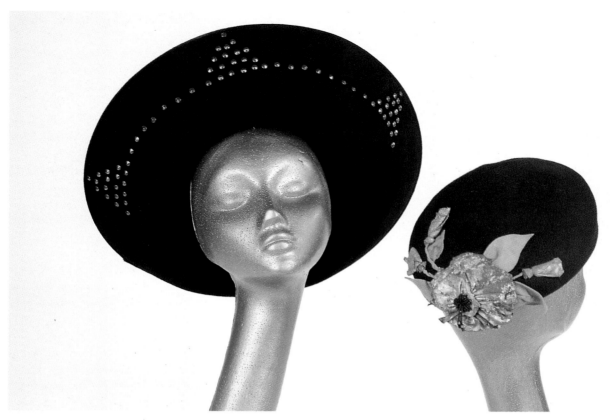

Two felts from the 1930s. The halo-brimmed Breton is trimmed with brass studs; the beret, with gilded suede flowers. *Courtesy of (both): Connie Beers.* Value (left): $55-75. Value (right): $25-45.

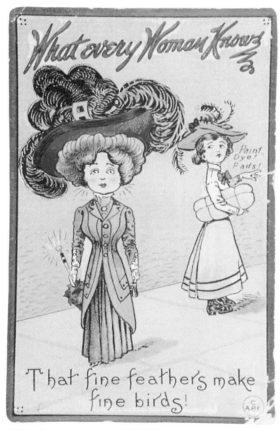

"Fine feathers make fine birds!"

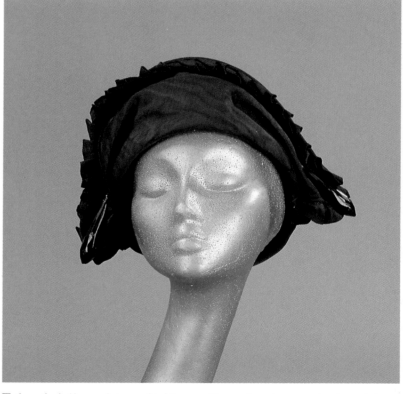

To form the half-moon brim on this bicorne, silk was shaped onto a wire rim and then carefully ruched for the trim. The addition of large jet hatpins highlights the delicacy of design, which was probably executed by the nimble fingers of a female milliner circa 1915. *Courtesy of: Sharon Hagerty.* Value: $150-225.

In 1879, *Ehlrich's Fashion Quarterly* urged its readers to try their hands at home millinery, with this advice on the use of feathers:

> *"Feathers should be selected of colors to match the materials used in trimming... A long feather should always be set in front of the crown, and drooped thence toward the back and side. Short feathers, on the contrary, should have a forward droop. The latter, when properly arranged, aid greatly in producing that coquettish effect in which so many young ladies delight."*

Fashion periodicals also offered instructions in how to trim specific styles. These appear disarmingly vague to the modern eye! A case in point, direct from a fashion plate circa 1900:

> *Exceedingly pretty is the hat with its full ruche of taffeta with pinked edges...Toward the back is a large bow with two forward loops and another backward, fastened with a long, loose knot."*

Of course, most women possessed basic seamstress skills. The editors of an Edwardian magazine would have rightly presumed that their readers knew the difference between pinking and scalloping, and the properties of silk vs. velvet.

For the truly talented home milliner, there was also the opportunity to launch a full-fledged career. In 1894, the *Delineator* ran articles on "Employments for Women." Number six in the series was on millinery, as shown in part here:

> *"There are several weighty reasons which recommend the milliner's trade...In the first place, it is essentially feminine. Because of that quality, there is comparatively little rivalry between men and women in this avocation.
> "The question of woman suffrage over which we have all been either sharpening our wits or losing them, has emphasized the fact that in whatever pursuit man's efforts are pitted against woman's, the man usually makes the more money. (W)e must conclude that any business in which we are able to engage with the least chance of opposition is likely to afford the best results."*

To the modern eye, the Victorians seemed overly concerned over the suitability of activities for women. But in this article, it was couched in startlingly modern terms: the perennial issue of parity in pay!

If you have a special interest in the techniques of millinery during this era, we are pleased to recommend a book for further reading: *Edwardian Hats: The Art of Millinery*, penned by Madame Anna Ben-Yusuf in 1909 and reprinted by R.L. Shep in 1992. It contains fascinating details on making wire rims, sewing silk flowers, ruching ribbon, and curling ostrich feathers.

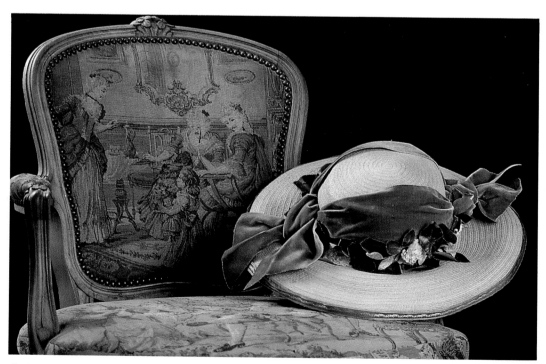

A "light reception chair" such as might have been used in a millinery establishment circa 1909. The straw hat with large velvet band is from the same era. *Courtesy of (all): Banbury Cross Antiques.* Value (hat): $150-225.

Madame Anna's details of construction are useful for the purpose of dating hats and appreciating their fine workmanship. But perhaps the most interesting chapter concerns the business of selling hats. We excerpt below her description of how to furnish a salon for a high-class clientele:

> *"The room should be simply but tastefully furnished; no bright colors or glaring contrasts, even if you must repaper and paint it yourself.*
> *"You cannot have too many mirrors, and certainly one or two long ones, where the entire figure can be seen. Near each mirror have a small table with a hand mirror, pin cushion, hat and short pins, and a tray with hairpins...*
> *"A couple of easy chairs and several light reception chairs; this, with soft green or gray walls, and a floor covering to match—makes an attractive room. [I]n a high-priced trade*

> *divisions formed by screens, each containing a long mirror, chair and little table, will be necessary, as many women insist on privacy in being fitted to hats, as much as if they were being fitted with gowns.*
> *"In elaborate establishments the screened partitions are developed into delightful little arbors, or boudoirs, of mirror, gilding and lace. Nowadays, when the evening or restaurant hat is made a special feature, a dark room with brilliant electric light is necessary to test colors and effects..."*

A scant generation or two ago, it was the dream of many women to turn their hatmaking hobby into a profession. The art and craft of millinery may never be revived, but it is still recorded in the hearts and memories of the "living historians" who were its practitioners.

Interview With a Milliner

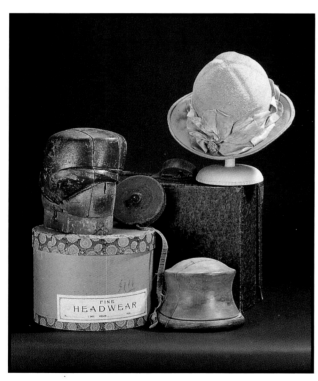

Hatforms with moveable parts allowed "blockers" to shape the felts, working over steam tables for hours on end. The trade was so physically demanding that it was practiced almost exclusively by men. *Courtesy of (all): Banbury Cross Antiques.* Value (hat): $65-95. Value (box): $25-45.

The authors were fortunate enough to speak with one of these women, who was born in 1906 and retired some decades ago in our home state. The story of Miss Lucy Pope echoes the fashion history reference books, but resonates with the freshness of her personal experience.

Mrs. Lucy Pope grew up in a large family of limited income in the midwest. Now aged 88 years, she delightfully recounts her early experiences in hat-making.

"I remember mother making hats for the family. Although millinery shops abounded, we did not have the means to buy what we wanted. Instead, we created our own. If you bought a crown block and had a tea kettle, you were in business!"

As a young girl, Mrs. Pope became fascinated with hat-making, and used "anything handy" as a hat form. Wooden mixing and salad bowls served her purpose, as well as her father's porch lamp shade (which she promptly broke). Even the toilet seat was put to fashionable use, making a wonderful block for a Breton hat!

Millinery schools and apprenticeships existed in the early 1900s, but finances were a problem. It was later, as a married woman and home economics major at Louisiana Tech, that she completed a course in millinery.

At the outbreak of World War II her husband was shipped to China. To "keep out of trouble" she took a job as a "maker" at a wholesale millinery house in Los Angeles. There, samples were created, or more often copied, from leading French fashion designers.

Mrs. Pope recalls, "the sample was made and the company's photogenic Russian lady modeled it" for photographers. The sales force then went to retailers with these pictures. Orders were placed specifying colors, trimmings and quantities.

Back at the wholesale workshop, a "floor lady" organized the work to be done. First the material used, often felt, went to the blocker. This job was usually held by men, as it required the stamina to work long hours over hot steam tables. The blocker shaped the felt, or other form, which then went to the maker (a job traditionally held by women as it was considered artistic). It was the maker who did the trimming, according to the retailer's order. The finished product was then sent to the store, which affixed its own label.

Mrs. Pope continued to create hats at home, including a celebratory hat that was meant to be worn on a special night—when her husband returned from the war. However, his war experiences had so depressed him that it was not until years later that the hat finally debuted.

In her youth, Mrs. Pope also worked in the millinery salons of some fine depart-

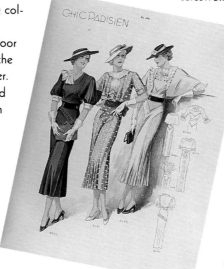

Coordinated ensembles from *Chic Parisien*, a fashion folio published in May 1936, showing how hats and dress trim were angled in the same manner.

ment stores. "We provided dressing tables with large mirrors. The customer was seated and select hats were brought to her by the saleswoman," she recalled. "It was nothing like the way women buy hats today, right off the shelf!" Standing behind her, the hat was carefully placed on the lady's head. Judging her expression in the mirror helped the saleswoman know which hat to promote!

The tilt of the hat was important. Hats that had been designed to be worn tipped were fashioned that way on the block. The millinery rule was "up on the left, down on the right," which seemed to enhance the balance of a woman's costume.

According to Mrs. Pope, the side on which a lady parts her hair is not the true criterion for the angle at which a hat should be worn. Instead, it is the millinery rule. In this same manner, corsages and jewelry were routinely worn on the left side of the dress. Tall hat trim, such as feathers were placed on the left; hanging trim, such as tassels, on the right.

Mrs. Pope went on to teach adult education classes in home economics and millinery for many years before her eventual retirement in Sacramento.

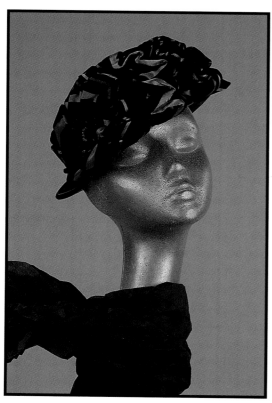

A lovely capote constructed from rich pinstripe silk, rippled into shape. Surely this is a "celebratory hat" such as Mrs. Pope might have created for her husband's homecoming. *Courtesy of: Past Perfect.* Value: $95-145.

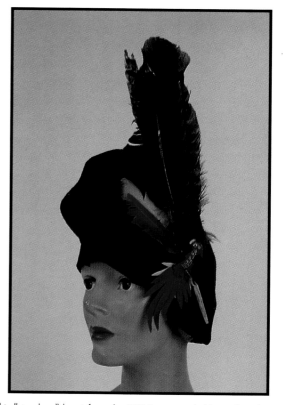

This "stand-up" beret from the 1930s was probably made at home from scraps of felt. The parrot's tailfeathers soar on the right side, according to the millinery rule. *Courtesy of: Banbury Cross Antiques.* Value: $25-45.

XII. *Storing, Restoring, and Displaying*

Hats are not as portable as many other fashion collectibles, such as handbags or jewelry. Thus, any serious collector must soon consider methods of storage. Hatboxes, vintage or otherwise, are a natural choice. In and of themselves, round and oval hatboxes lend a note of charm to home interiors. They are now being reproduced and sold through major retail outlets—fortunately for hat collectors!

Storage boxes should be lined with acid-free tissue paper, especially for hats from the Victorian or Edwardian periods. The inside crown of the hat or bonnet should be stuffed with this same paper and laid with the brim down. Be careful not to use plastic bags as they do not allow sufficient air flow for the fabric to "breathe." Also, try not to crowd several hats into one box—delicate flowers and feathers become damaged, often beyond repair.

Straw hats may be displayed in the open air, but most felt and fur hats should be stored in a covered box with moth repellant. If you must display the latter, consider rotating them into boxes for protection, during the warm months. Beware of storing or displaying any hat near extremes in temperature,

which can cause cracking or splitting. Also, avoid direct sunlight, as it can easily fade delicate trimmings and vintage fabrics.

If your hats do become crumpled, or if you are intent on rescuing a flea-market find, consider steaming. We have had fantastic results using steam to revive crushed silk flowers, felt, and straw.

If you care to invest in a hand-held steamer, this is certainly the most convenient method. However, even a blast of steam from an old-fashioned teakettle will do the trick! We do not recommend steaming for any hat that is already showing signs of mildew, however.

As for cleaning, we know of dealers who will dunk vintage lace into hot water—but we are not so brave. Certainly, any hat on a wire rim should not be submerged. The same is true for felts, which would shrink or otherwise lose their steamed-in shape. Water of any temperature will turn straw limp and straighten the careful curl of a feather. There is also the risk of creating mold or shrinkage, in the cloth lining of any hat.

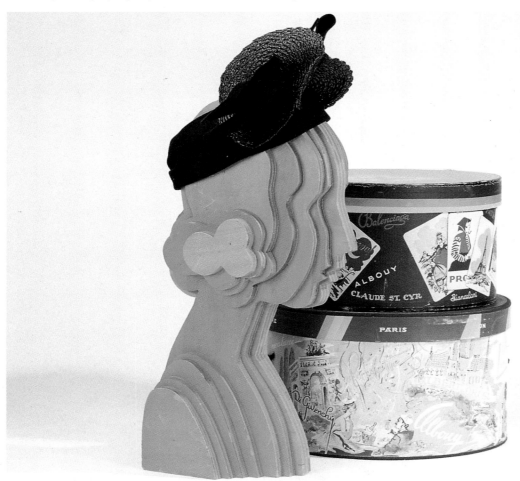

An unusual wooden hatstand, with an Art Deco flavor. Shown with a 1920s felt hat and vintage hatboxes, for a charming display that doubles as storage. *Courtesy of (stand): The Way We Wore. Courtesy of (rest): Banbury Cross Antiques.* Value (stand): $75-125. Value: (boxes, each): $45-65.

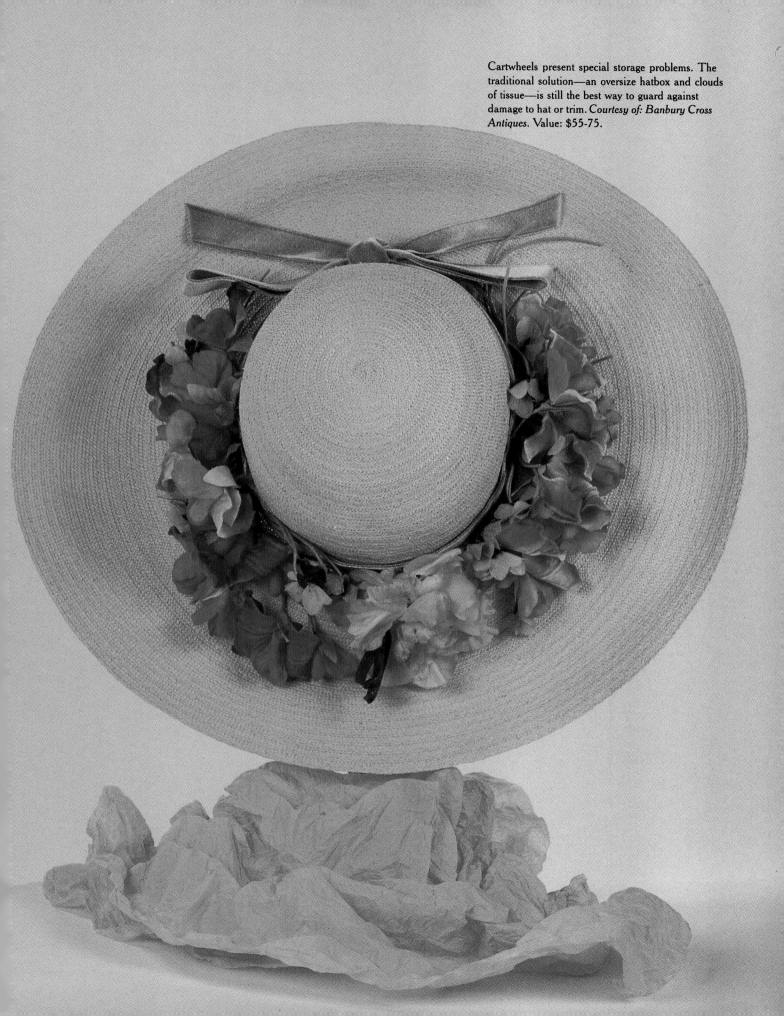

Cartwheels present special storage problems. The traditional solution—an oversize hatbox and clouds of tissue—is still the best way to guard against damage to hat or trim. *Courtesy of: Banbury Cross Antiques.* Value: $55-75.

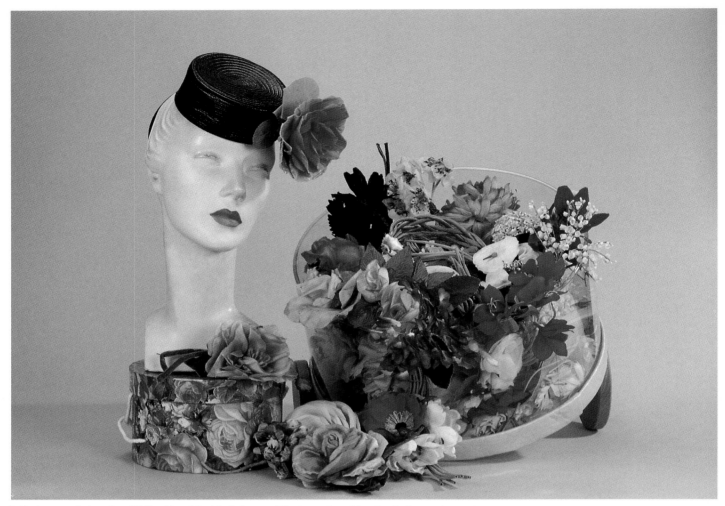

A black straw tilt hat circa 1945 with original fuchsia rose. The box is brimful with silk flowers that took years to accrue, but were well worth the effort! *Courtesy of (hat): Banbury Cross Antiques. Courtesy of (rest): Sandra Headley.* Value (hat): $45-65. Value (box): $25-45. Value (flowers, each): $25-55.

● ══════════════════════════════ ●

Suffice it to say, we do not recommend wet cleaning; nor ordinary cleaning solvents, as their chemicals are too harsh for vintage hats. Instead, try an organic dry agent such as cornstarch or salt. They are effective in removing grease and other stains, and can be used in sequence. Just take care not to overwork a felt nap or stretch a delicate lace by repeated cleaning efforts.

We have had particular success brightening beaver pelts with cornstarch, sprinkled liberally, then gently dusted off with a fine brush. Some collectors report good results with dried bread crumbs, similarly applied.

You can remove stray fur or feather tufts, and bits of dried felt or shredded lace, with the sticky side of a piece of tape. Special hat brushes are also sold for this purpose. Also, professional hat-blockers recommend brushing felts with a stiff wire brush, in the direction of the nap, on a regular basis.

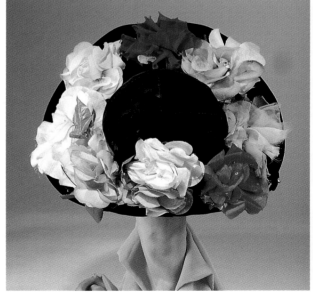

A cartwheel in deep blue velvet, carpeted with hand-made silk roses that the authors revived with steam. *Courtesy of: Cheap Thrills.* Value: $55-75.

From Mme. Anna Ben-Yusuf, a milliner who wrote authoritatively on the subject of renovation in 1909, came the following practical advice for cleaning straw:

> "To clean leghorns, panamas, milans and other fine straws, make a solution of oxalic acid and hot water, one teasponful to the pint, and brush [it on] thoroughly with a long-handled nail brush, taking care that the acid does not touch the hands. Rinse immediately in clear hot, then cold, water.
>
> "Wipe off as much moisture as possible, then pin a bit of rag to the brim and thereby pin it up to dry in the air or heat. When partly dry, press into shape with a hot (but not scorching) iron with muslin over the straw, on the wrong side.
>
> "Black straw hats may be freshened by brushing over with a mixture of good black ink and gum Arabic—after thoroughly brushing and cleaning—or if only a slight new gloss is wanted, brush over with white of egg."

Some collectors acquire volumes of silk flowers and other vintage trimming from the same sources as they find hats. These can be stored or displayed, then used to replace worn or damaged trim on later acquisitions.

Women have retrimmed hats throughout the centuries. This is so, even with hats that bear investment-grade price tags. There is just no assurance that the original owner did not experiment with trim to match a dress. The moral is—if you come across a ravishing cloche with feathers added on, don't hesitate to buy the hat and pluck the plumage!

With the exception of museum quality hats, or those with couture labels, you should certainly experiment with repairs if you prefer hats in mint condition. Veils are especially susceptible to harm, and it is all but impossible to find vintage hats without some damage in this area

If you choose to make repairs or replace trim entirely, take care to match the color and mood of the hat. With diligent searching, we have successfully located the proper replacement trim for many hats (as noted when they are shown in this book). Of course, vintage goods are always preferable, but they are becoming harder to find and are often high-priced.

Fortunately, many companies now offer a line of reproduction veils, flowers, and fruit clusters. These are sold to milliners or hobbyists who remake vintage hats, but are also ideal for renovations. You should be able to purchase these products at vintage clothing shows, or through nationally-advertised catalogs.

We realize that some purists would rather leave antique and vintage hats alone, whatever their state of disrepair. To them, the detritus that occurs naturally with age and use is a fascinating aspect of their collections. The choice, of course, is up to you!

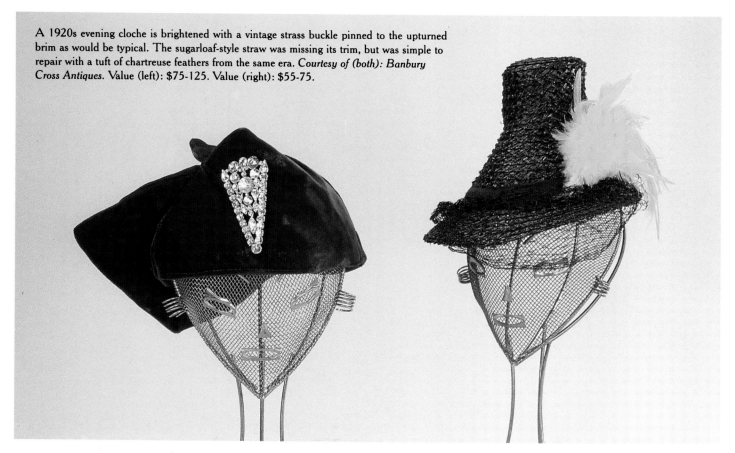

A 1920s evening cloche is brightened with a vintage strass buckle pinned to the upturned brim as would be typical. The sugarloaf-style straw was missing its trim, but was simple to repair with a tuft of chartreuse feathers from the same era. *Courtesy of (both): Banbury Cross Antiques.* Value (left): $75-125. Value (right): $55-75.

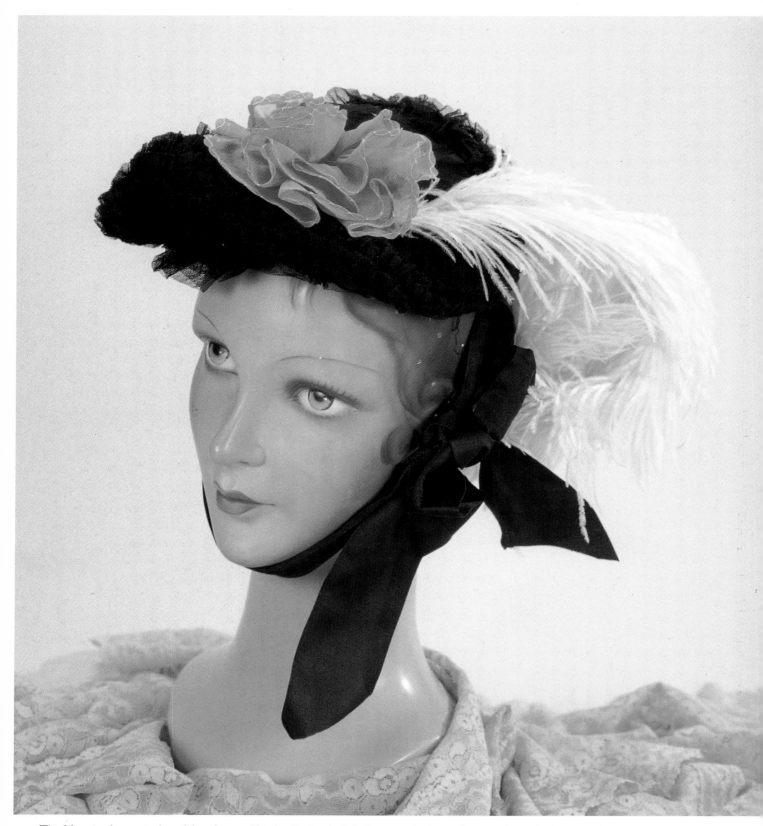

This Victorian bonnet is shaped from layers of black tulle, hand-stitched onto a wire frame. Its original ostrich plume was damaged, and replaced with a vintage hand-curled pink feather. *Courtesy of: Maureen Reilly.* Value: $75-125.

Part of the allure of hat collecting is purely aesthetic appeal. Some hats are the essence of romantic femininity, dripping with feathers, lace, and flowers. Others are almost sculptural in their simplicity, a pure sweep of felt or fabric.

All hats evoke a mood, and can be displayed to good effect in almost every room of your home. It has been the experience of many antique dealers that hats are also wonderful accents for a grouping of bedroom furniture or tabletop displays.

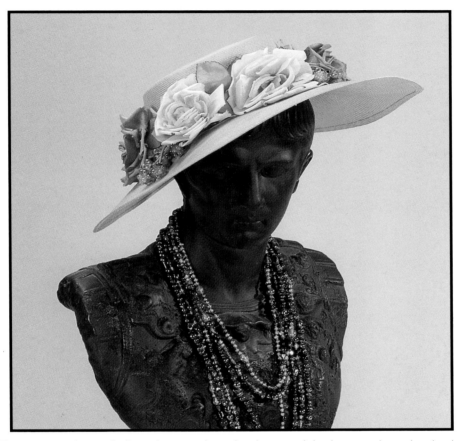

Great Caesar's Hat! This serious reproduction of a Roman bust gains charm when the emperor's head is crowned—not by a laurel wreath, but a floral-wreathed straw Pamela. *Courtesy of: Maureen Reilly.* Value (hat): $35-55.

❖ Use billowy chiffon curtains in a bedroom or dressing area; for tiebacks, substitute doll hats.

❖ As part of a display of vintage hats, you could display similar styles on antique or vintage dolls.

❖ Top a classical bust or other sculpture with a whimsical hat, for a casual note in an otherwise formal room.

❖ Cover an entire wall with straw hats; let their various shapes and colors form a pattern.

❖ Toss a beribboned Pamela at the foot of a guest bed; set a romantic straw picture hat on a pretty chair; top the poster of a bed with one or more deep-crowned boaters.

❖ Arrange favorite hats on a vanity or other tabletop in your bedroom, grouped next to dresser accessories or perfume bottles.

❖ Create a vignette with a flock of feathered hats, come to roost on or around a lovely vintage birdcage.

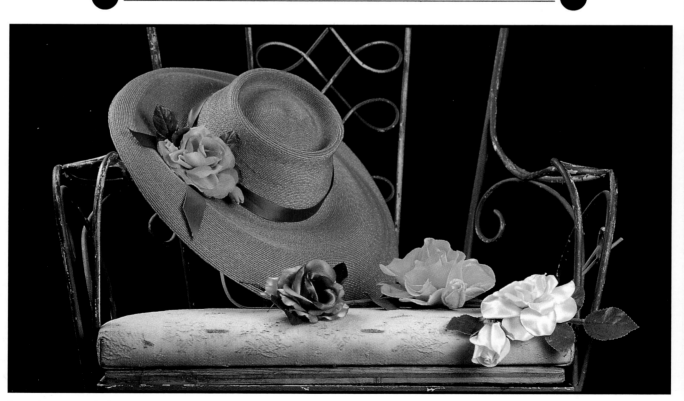

Languid as a summer's day, a vintage straw cartwheel on a wrought iron chair. *Courtesy of: Banbury Cross Antiques.* Value (hat): $95-145.

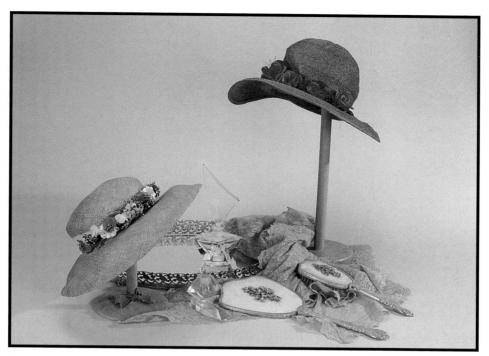

For a stylish dressing table, display two straw garden hats with floral trim in dreamy shades of apricot, blue, and white. *Courtesy of (both): Sandra Headley.* Value (each): $65-95.

❖   Welcome visitors to your home with a halltree in the entry, and cover several hooks with country bonnets or boaters.

❖ Instead of an arrangement of real flowers on your luncheon table, why not try a floral hat?

❖ Seek out interesting hatboxes and mannequin heads to line a shelving unit with your favorite styles; rotate those stored in boxes with those on display, from time-to-time.

❖ If you come across old prints or photographs of women in hats, frame these in chased silver or other vintage frames, and prop them next to hats from the same era on a shelf or table.

❖ Hang your hat on an interior doorknob. Or proclaim your hobby to the world by hooking a weathered straw—wreathed in roses—on your front door.

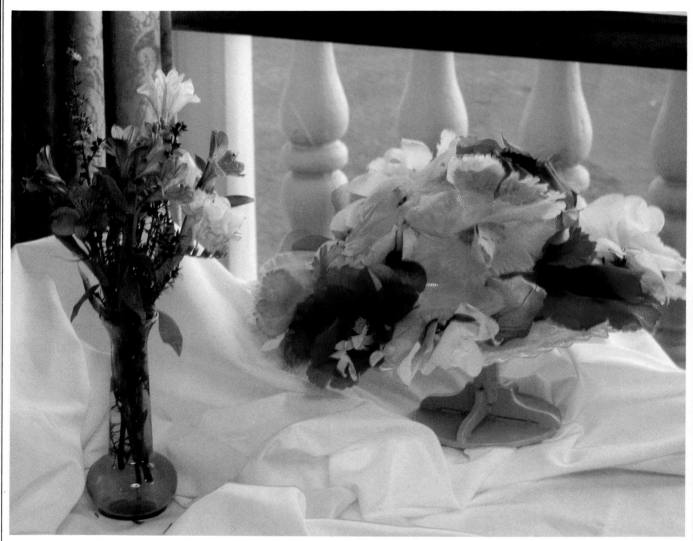

A tabletop centerpiece of real flowers can hardly be distinguished from its counterpart, a floral "bubble hat" circa 1960. Label: Mr. Almo. *Courtesy of: The Mad Hatter.* Value: $55-75.

XIII. *From Start to "Finishing Touch"*

It has been said, "There is not so variable a thing in nature as a lady's head-dress" (Joseph Addison). It is this variety that makes hats so much fun to collect! If you are not such a purist as to avoid trying on your vintage hats, it is like combining a history lesson with playing "dress up."

Whether you are just starting up, or adding the finishing touches to your collection, you share a common interest: Where can I find collectible hats? For the budget-minded, there are garage sales, flea markets, thrift stores, secondhand clothing shops, and even the local church bazaar. Don't forget, many women bought dozens of hats each year! They are often donated to charitable causes, when it comes time to clean out the closets.

Collectors who want to upgrade should become familiar with the antique shops in their vicinity. Let the dealers know what you are looking for. Often, they'll call you when something special comes in. Contrary to popular belief, the prices in shops may be no higher than other venues, since dealers may pass on a good price, or discount for multiple purchases.

The most desirable Victorian and Edwardian hats can be found at the vintage clothing shows, sponsored once or twice a year in most major metropolitan communities. Rarely, one of these older hats will come on the market through an individual estate sale, auction, or classified ad. If you are focusing on a particular type of hat, you might try advertising your needs in a newsletter geared to the antique trade.

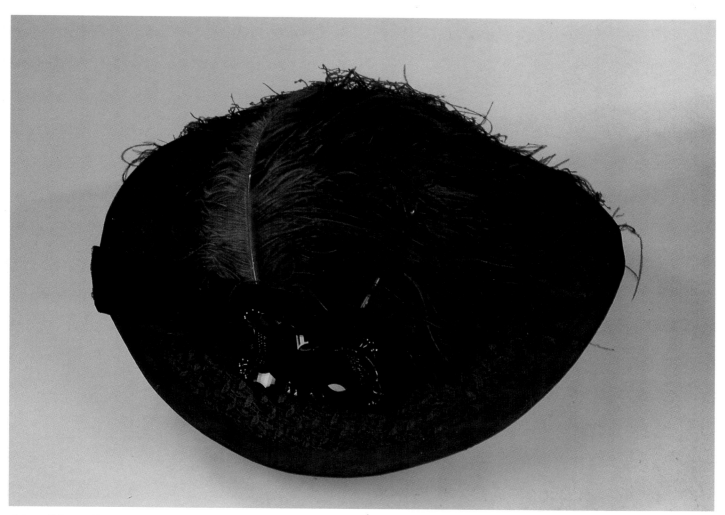

A beautiful straw Pamela from the late Belle Epoque, with curled and dyed ostrich plumes and a cut-steel buckle on the velvet hatband. This type of quality hat is much sought-after by collectors and museums alike. *Courtesy of: Mary Aaron Museum.* Value: Special.

If you can bear to part with any of your treasures—which we realize is a rare quality—then you are ready to upgrade or otherwise "finish" your collection. Consider which hats best satisfy your personal standards of beauty, quality, and rarity.

You may fall in love with the hats of a particular era, perhaps one to which you relate personally or that you feel has the greatest expression of artistic design. Or, you may be drawn to a certain style and mood, such as the boater with its air of gamine grace.

If you have seamstress skills, or can otherwise recognize the beauty of fine workmanship, you might build a collection around the method of construction. You can readily find wonderful and witty hats that made entirely from felt, fur, flowers, or feathers.

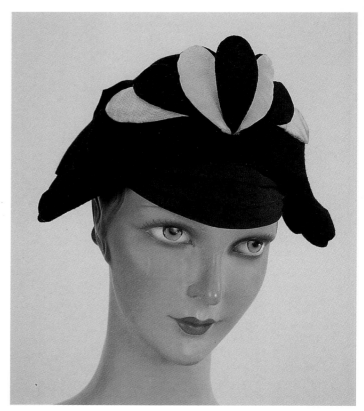

Many women favor the flair of Art Deco, exemplified by this stylized cloche in pink and black felt. Label: Poppy Hats of New York. *Courtesy of: Lottie Ballou.* Value: $75-100.

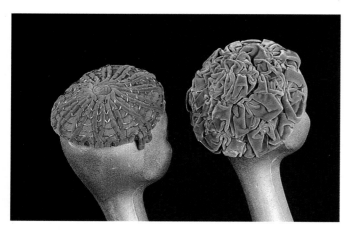

Bugle beads and smocked pink velvet make a cute cap. With it, a scrunch of turquoise velvet forms a beret. These two softies would have capped late-day ensembles, circa 1955. *Courtesy of (both): Banbury Cross Antiques.* Value (each): $35-55.

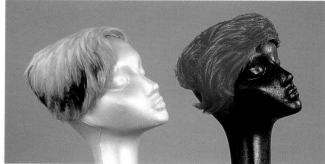

The same colors in a froth of feathers form close-fitting caps, circa 1965. *Courtesy of (both): Maureen Reilly.* Value (each): $35-55.

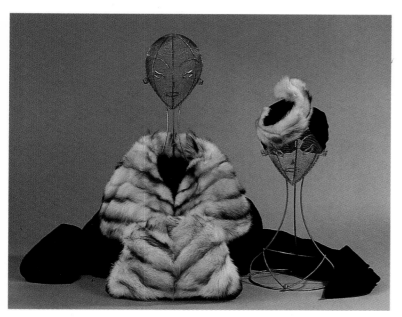

Fur is in disfavor, given the worthwhile goal of protecting wild animals. But when it comes to vintage skins, the point of discussion is dead! Shown here, a fabulous custom-made ensemble trimmed in chinchilla, from the late 1930s. *Courtesy of (all): Maureen Reilly.* Value (ensemble): $200-300.

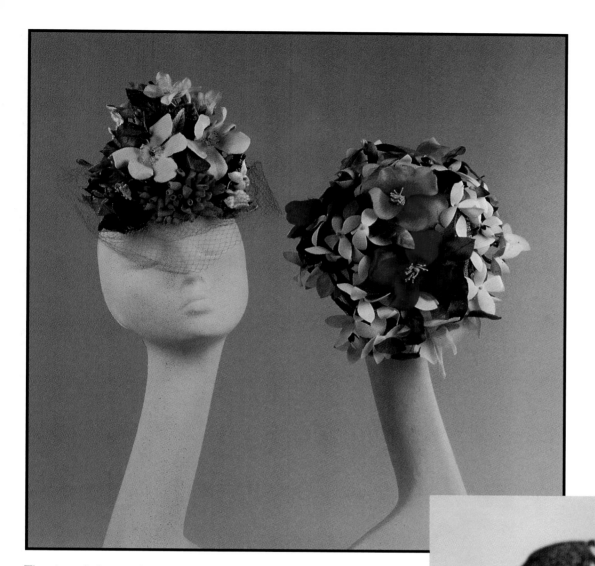

There is much charm in the allover floral hat. A 1950s toy hat is shown, with a "bubble hat" inspired by the popular hairstyle of the same name. Label (left): Lilly Daché. Label (right): Bullock's Victorian Room. *Courtesy of (left): David Mejia. Courtesy of (right): Banbury Cross Antiques.* Value (left): $65-95. Value (right): $45-65.

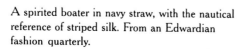

A spirited boater in navy straw, with the nautical reference of striped silk. From an Edwardian fashion quarterly.

Unusual veiling is yet another point of interest. Veils add allure and mystery to any hat, and can be found in a myriad of shapes, sizes, and trim. Concentrate on unique veils, be they oversize or studded with velvet beauty marks.

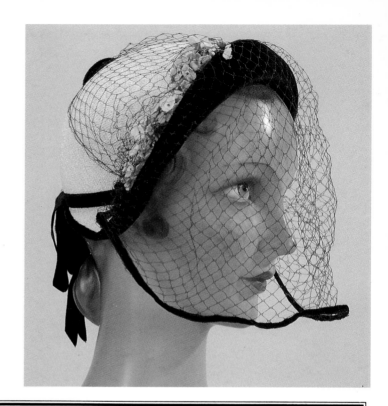

A full-face veil, banded in the same navy blue velvet as on the button on the "beanie" crown. This sweet straw, circa 1935, relays a mixed message of ingenue allure. *Courtesy of: It's About Time.* Value: $45-65.

Theme Hats

In every era, milliners created truly unique styles for special purposes. Some hats are anomalies, interesting to the collector by reason of their curious usage more than intrinsic style. This genre might include military headgear, ethnic headdress, and bridalwear.

Huge headdresses were in demand for masquerades and other themed balls at the French court. These Follies are chiefly known to us from journal accounts and paintings of that era. But similarly fantastic theatre hats have survived intact from the mid-1800s, affording a glimpse of atypical but skillful millinery.

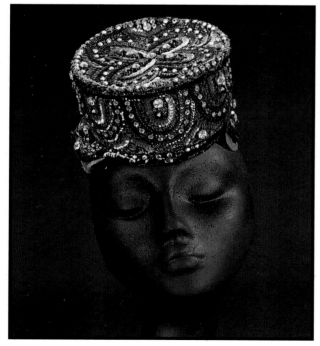

This rare "cigarette girl" cap is encrusted with sequins and rhinestones. A true work of art! *Courtesy of: The Way We Wore.* Value: $300-500.

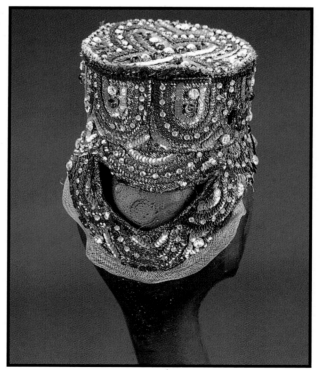

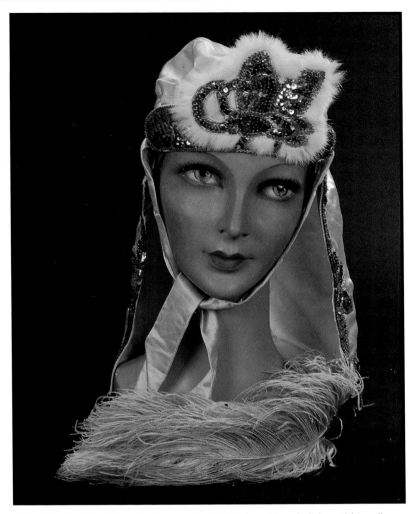

A "goddess headdress" from the theatre, circa 1920. It is delicately fashioned from silk, embellished with a whoosh of silver sequins and tufts of white fur. *Courtesy of: Banbury Cross Antiques.* Value: $150-200.

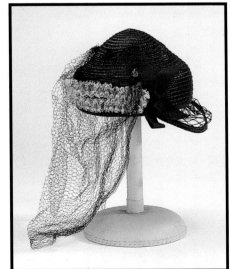

This diminutive straw capote is unremarkable, except that it is reputed to be a "salesman's sample." *Courtesy of: Rich Man, Poor Man.* Value: $65-95.

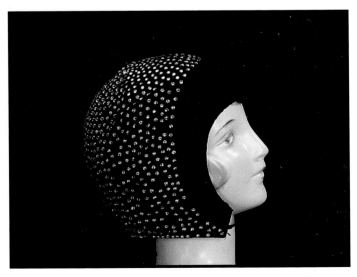

A chorine's cloche, outlined in rhinestones, circa 1925. The overall effect is one of barbaric splendor in the manner of Erté's stylized sketches. *Courtesy of: The Way We Wore.* Value: $200-250.

Dior styled many turbans during the 1950s and 1960s. He often used jewel-like colors, that match the mood of his bijoux. Shown, his cocktail turban twisted from strips of glowing satin. *Courtesy of: Banbury Cross Antiques.* Value: $75-125.

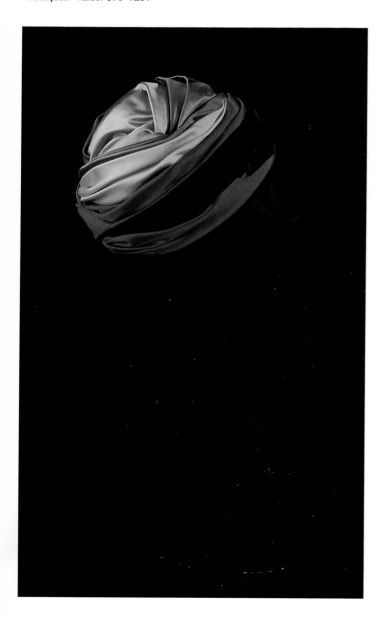

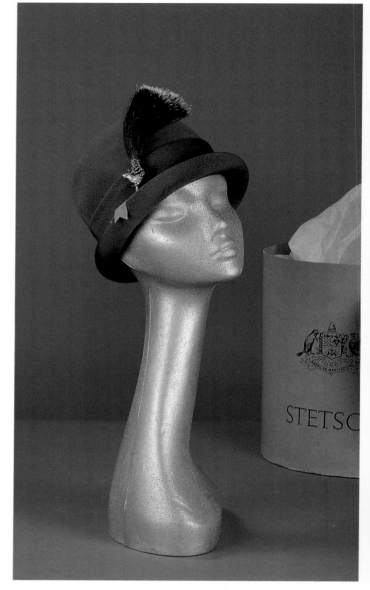

The Stetson label is usually associated with a man's ten-gallon, but the company also produced a Lady Stetson line. Shown, one of its sportier models circa 1945. A pewter stags-head pins a brush of feathers to the hatband. *Courtesy of (both): Sheryl Birkner.* Value (hat): $75-125. Value (box): $35-55.

If you enjoy searching for the finest quality, and have the purse to support such a habit, you might enjoy a collection of hats from the haute couture. However, scarcity is a problem with this genre. Values are going up, and for this reason designer hats from the 1960s are a good investment for the serious collector.

Many hats were custom-made to suit a select clientele, and may bear no label at all. Instead, the inside crown may have the milliner's signature in silk skein, or the inner hatband may be finished with a small flower or feather. Some designers emulated this look, with special touches on their salon labels. Jack McConnell affixed a small red feather; Bernard Workman and Mr. Arnold used rhinestones.

Now comes the inevitable link between collecting hats along with other items from the same designer. If you quest for jewelry by Schiaperelli or dresses by Dior—what could be more natural than to expand your collecting horizons, with hats?

For vintage clothing fans, hats are obviously one of the accessories that make the look. Carefully matched ensembles were *de rigueur*, particularly in the 1930s through the 1950s. It's a rewarding challenge to complete each outfit with matching gloves, shoes, and jewelry. The final touch is the perfect hat!

Any collection would be upgraded by pairing hats with their original hatboxes, or those of the same label and era. Your search must be diligent, however, as these have become collectible in their own right. Some dealers cannot bear to part with them, so useful are vintage hatboxes for storage and display.

Hats have rightly been considered the personal stamp of an individual, and a revealing clue to the spirit and culture of an era. One thing we know—given the truly wonderful hats that are still available—whatever your particular collecting interest, you will find the hat to satisfy it.

A rhinestone-studded dandy prancing for the Bernard Newman label. Shown inside the crown of a black silk toque, circa 1950. *Courtesy of: Maureen Reilly.* Value: $35-55.

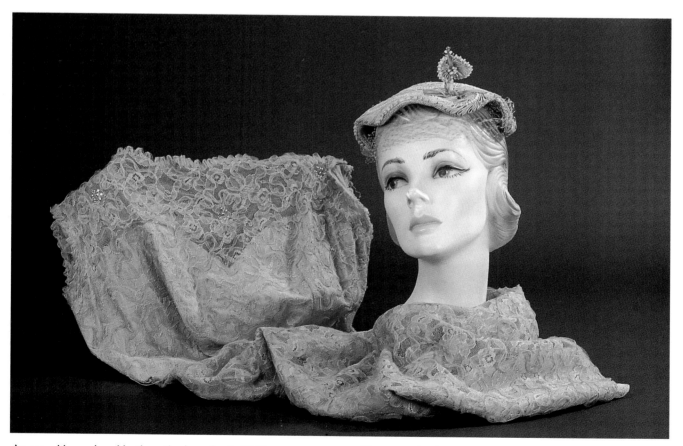

An ensemble purchased by the author's mother in 1947, to wear as matron of honor at a family wedding. The cap's beading and rhinestones are perfectly matched to the sheath. *Courtesy of: Maureen Reilly.* Value: Special.

"When dolly is to be taken out for an airing, she needs have something to put on her head in order to prevent her taking cold, as well as for adornment."

The Doll's Dressmaker, 1892.

Home millinery was promoted as a suitable and productive pastime for little girls of the 19th century. "Essentially feminine" girls were thought to have the delicacy of touch required to handle frail materials used in hat making.

Periodicals such as the *Delineator, Harper's Weekly,* and *Godey's* offered cut-out patterns for doll hats as well as very detailed instructions on fitting, shaping, sewing, and trimming. Girls were advised to check mother's old sewing basket or the attic for unused materials. A scrap of lace, a single feather, perhaps a bit of blue china silk—all could be used in making a fine Paris creation!

Straw hat forms are still a staple of doll wardrobes, as they have been for many years. The forms, typically sold through yardage shops, are easy for little fingers to trim with flowers and ribbon. They may also be used by collectors to enhance a display of vintage summertime straws.

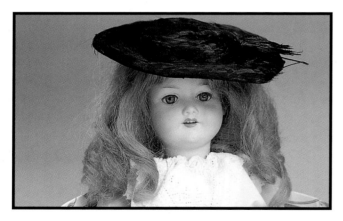

This circa 1890 doll's hat may have been made by an older child. It is crafted from sleek black feathers, layered on a stiffened fabric form. A rogue feather adds the only accent. *Courtesy of: Banbury Cross Antiques.* Value: $95-145.

For dolly's summer outing: a choice of two straw boaters, circa 1930. Shown with an old trunk, of a type that may have held doll clothes. *Courtesy of: Banbury Cross Antiques.* Value (each): $45-75.

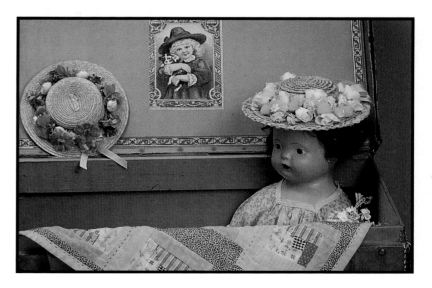

XIV. Valuation Guide

For most collectors, one question is paramount: Where can I find the best for the least? The corollary for dealers is: How do I make a profit without outpacing the market? Of course, there are no sure answers.

It's not just a matter of supply and demand, but also regional interests and national fads. Prices may fluctuate widely, even on a street of clustered antique stores, for no apparent reason. That much said, we can offer overall advice.

Generally speaking, the older a hat, the more valuable it is. The link between age and cost of a hat is especially strong on the East Coast and in the South, where the concept of

heritage is deeply rooted. But the value of a hat cannot be measured by its age alone! The collector or dealer must also weigh such intrinsic factors as condition, quality, and style.

In the popular perception, hat styles changed clearly from one decade to another. In actuality, when changes occurred they were gradual, and blurred by the frequency of revivals and alterations.

Variations in age, size, values, and personal taste have resulted in stylistic inconsistencies in every era. We have found that the only way to date hats with any accuracy is to search for clues that appear in the body of the hat itself.

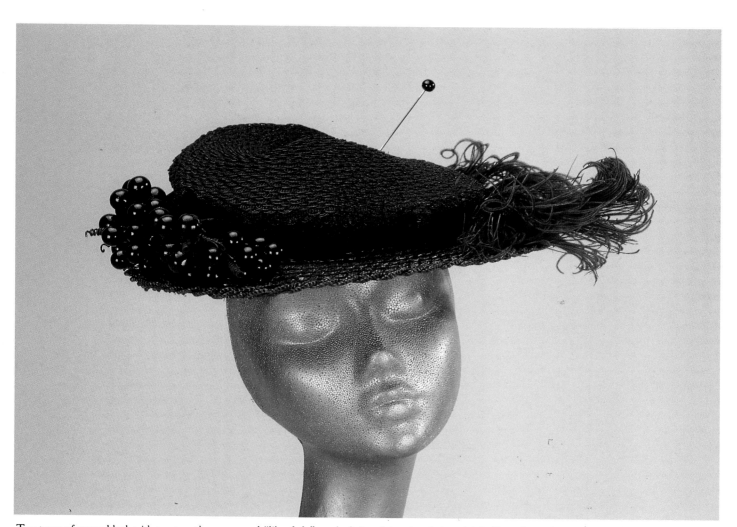

Two tones of straw, black with toast on the crown and "lilac fade" on the brim. A hand-curled ostrich feather, vintage but not original to the hat, was sewn at the site of a broken feather shaft. The grape clusters were also added, to disguise a frayed brim. Repairs diminish value, but this hat still has great style. *Courtesy of: Maureen Reilly.* Value: $75-125.

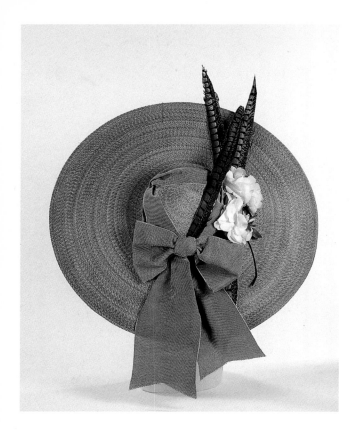

The dramatic cartwheel at the left is Edwardian in mood, although it was made in the late 1930s. It could have been inspired by the cartwheel to its right, which dates from 1915. Label (left): Fleur de Paris, New Orleans. *Courtesy of (left): Barbara Griggs Vintage Fashion. Courtesy of (right): The Mad Hatter.* Value (left): $125-175. Value (right): $175-250.

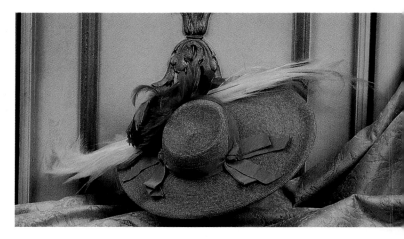

Tips on Dating

An Edwardian Pamela, fashioned from a spiral of horsehair. It was hand-stitched, as shown by the irregular swirl on the crown. *Courtesy of: The Mad Hatter.* Value: $150-225.

Victorian and Edwardian hats were usually constructed on a wire rim. They typically incorporate a drawstring bag in the inner lining of the crown, meant to be stuffed with tissue to ensure a custom fit.

The machinery necessary to pre-shape wire rims and spiral-sew straw forms was not available until the late 1900s. Thus, the irregularity of a hand-shaped form may indicate an earlier date of construction.

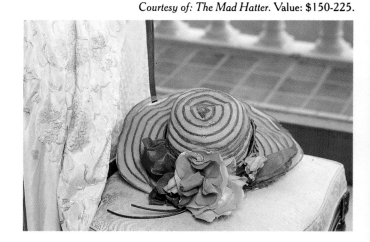

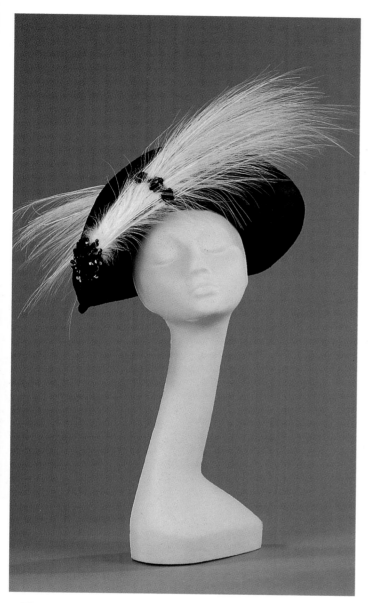

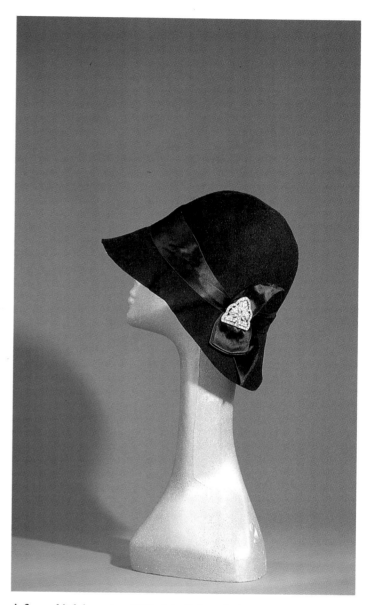

This sheared beaver Bicorne was formed on a wire frame, circa 1918. It is trimmed with snow-white malines swooping to the right and left, then clasped with black sequins on the upturned brim. *Courtesy of: Maureen Reilly.* Value: $95-145.

A floppy felt fedora, circa 1925. It is distinguished only by a rhinestone Bakelite pin on the right side. *Courtesy of: Lisa Carson.* Value: $75-125.

Bobbin-weave raffia, distinguished by a loopy pattern like crochet, helps date a hat as Edwardian. Another construction detail from this era was the use of a silk blouson to cover the crown of a straw Pamela. Horsehair was popular as a hatform, and was also used as a flouncy "skirt" on a straw brim. In later decades horsehair was usually relegated to the hatband, bow, or other form of trim.

Ribbons and bows were often wired on vintage hats , so as to swoop boldly to the side or poke dramatically into the air. The latter effect was a hallmark of the teens, adding drama to small-scaled hats. Milliners also used feather "antennae" to achieve a vertical line during this era.

Beaver felt was extremely stylish in the early 1900s. It may have been dyed a snowy white, or left a natural dark brown or black. It may have been sheared, or shaggy in the manner of angora. It was not unusual to pair furs with sprightly trim, such as plumage and silk flowers.

Wool felt was chic in the 1920s, especially a soft variety that could be artfully draped into a clingy cloche. Look for spare ornamentation, such as a brooch of Bakelite or strass. Given the influence of Art Deco, milliners favored asymmetrical lines.

Rubberized fabrics were discovered in the mid-1920s, when they were used for bathing attire. Be careful not to dismiss any hat made from rubber-backed fabrics as a novelty of the 1960s!

Silk was emblematic of the 1930s, and was used extensively by milliners in a variety of new weaves and textures. Silk velvet, renowned for its near-transparency, was ideal for the slinky and bias-cut styles in clothing and hats.

Most hats of the 1930s sat at a rakish angle. The crown kept a low profile, and the brim was often soft. Early in this decade, the brim was scant; it later flared up in an halo effect.

Given the depressed economy of the decade, few 1930s hats could boast expensive fabrication. Instead, chenille "pipecleaners" might be woven through a horsehair form, or cellophane straw might be twisted into an improbable but witty shape.

Cellophane was also woven raffia-style, often in a deep mahogany with russet highlights. This is a glowing color that catches the light, given the transparent property of the material. We have also seen cellophane hats advertised in a "steel" color, circa 1935.

Almost every method of construction was employed by milliners during the heyday of the hat, from the late 1930s through the 1940s. The hat most associated with this period is the doll. Boldly tilted forward, this hat was secured in back by a ribbon cage or wire hoop.

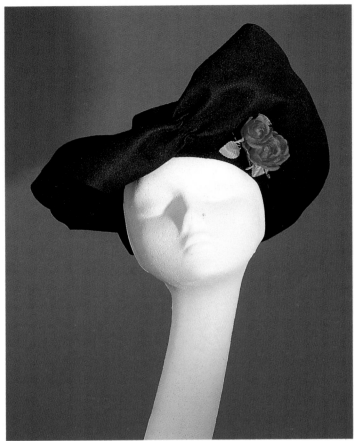

A halo-brimmed beret in black felt, typical of the late 1930s. *Courtesy of: Sheila Parks.* Value: $75-125.

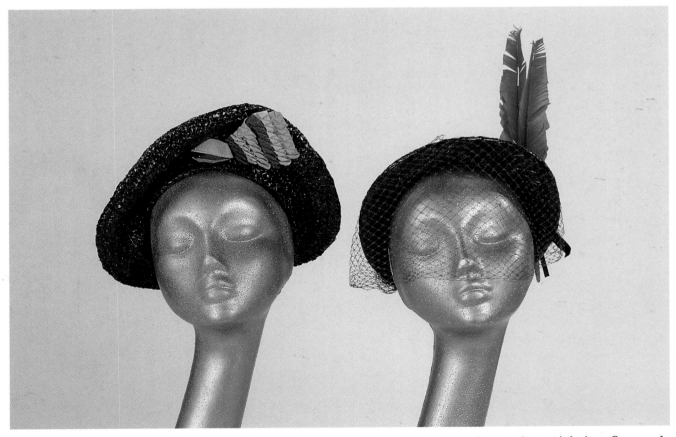

Two cellophane straws, in the popular mahogany shade. The beret sports a ribbon cockade, while the bonnet salutes with feathers. *Courtesy of (both): Banbury Cross Antiques.* Value (each): $45-65.

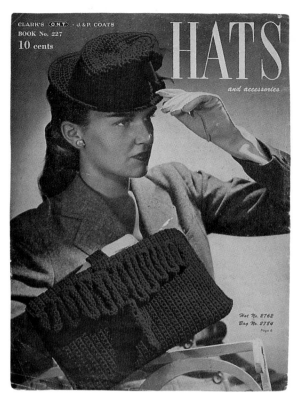

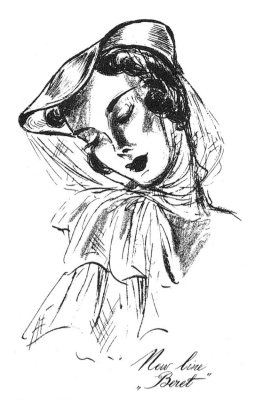

In 1945, Coats & Clark Co. sold patterns for "a collection of eyecatchers" in hand-knit or crocheted hats, complete with matching scarves and bags.

From a 1949 pattern book for home seamstresses, titled the *Originator*, sketches of straw and cloth hats that could be trimmed to coordinate with the featured ensembles.

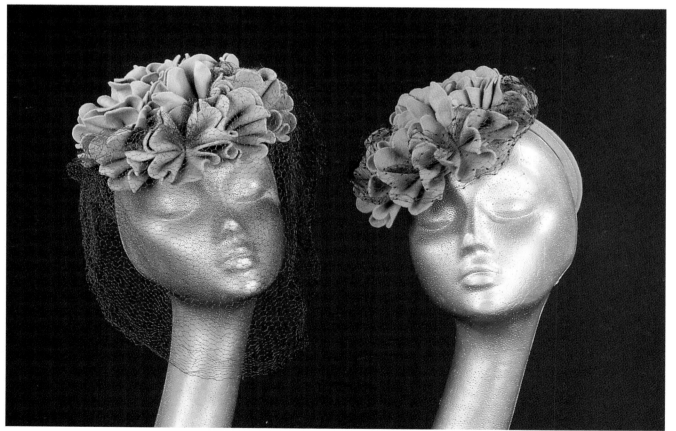

A froth of felt forms the crown, which tilts at a rakish angle thanks to the rear hoop on these nearly identical hats. *Courtesy of (both): Maureen Reilly.* Value (each): $35-55.

Allover floral hats were in vogue during the 1950s; as were crownless picture hats, half-hats, and bandeaux (little more than headbands).

The Space Race brought helmet shapes and metallic shine to millinery, as the decade drew to a close. Cellophane straw was popular again, especially in a rough weave and often in white. Faux fur was a fad in the 1960s, along with vinyl and leather. Given the influence of Op Art, wild prints and psychedelic colors were in wide use, even for staid styles.

Labels offer another important clue to dating in their typeface, which should generally correspond with the artistic style of a given era (e.g., thin and elongated for the 1920s).

If a label indicates an unusual head size, it is probably from the 1920s or 1930s, when hats were still offered in a wide range of sizes. If it boasts of Parisian origins, it may well pre-date the 1940s, which is when American designers began to gain name recognition.

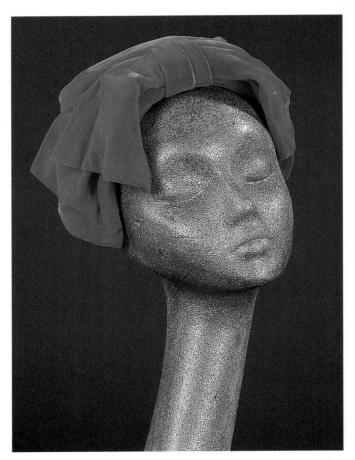

Perfect for cocktails circa 1955, a candy-box bow on a pert candy pink pillbox. This hat is held on with a headband, covered in the same rich velvet. Label: Sonni. *Courtesy of: Maureen Reilly.* Value: $35-55.

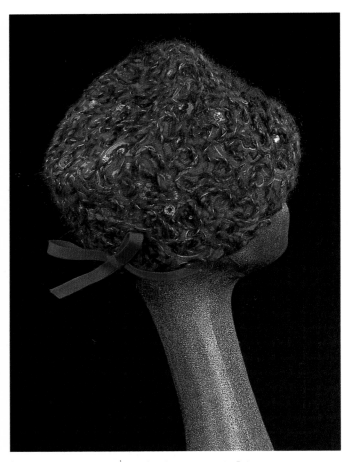

Imagine wearing this toque to lunch, circa 1965. Otherwise conservative, it goes psychedelic with a paisley swirl of vibrant color outlined in pink yarn and sprinkled with rhinestones. Label: Patrice. *Courtesy of: Maureen Reilly.* Value: $35-55.

These tips were gleaned from fashion history books, vintage fashion magazines, and hands-on experience. You will, no doubt, develop your own ideas as your collection grows.

If we had to choose a single tip, it would be: Try the hat on! How the brim sits on your own head, and how the crown tilts over your own hairdo, is an invaluable clue to the era in which it was made. The boater that was pinned to a pompadour in 1900 is far different from the revival that would have tilted over a French twist circa 1950. If unsure of how to wear a hat, remember that the label or inside seaming will always go in back. If combs are sewn into the inner hatband, these indicate how the hat should be situated.

You can learn to gauge value by comparing the wares offered at large vintage clothing shows, and by frequenting antique and vintage clothing stores. Also, try to attend vintage fashion shows that may be offered by museums and other organizations in your area.

From these sources, you can develop a sense of the details that denote quality. But style is another matter. It is a chimera born of wit and charm, and its valuation is more art than science.

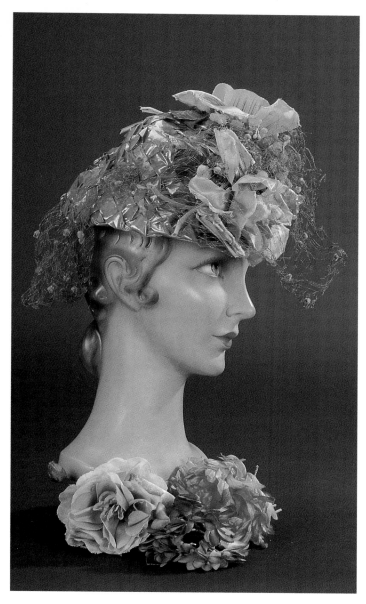

In every era, hats with style capture a certain mood, one that is born of gaiety and charm. They may be starkly simple, or trimmed to the nines. Either way, they will shine with the clarity of beautiful lines.

The crown and brim of a stylish hat will be in proper scale, each to the other. The fabric and trim will also balance, as a harmony of texture and color. A beautiful hat may indeed have exaggeration in scale or off-kilter balance, but it will be clear that this is by design.

The quality of construction is also an important element of style. Does the ornamentation advance a look, or does it appear to be an afterthought? If the crown is flat, will it situate well on the head or slide about in disarray? If the brim is wide and floppy, will it wilt or does it properly frame the face?

If there is veiling, is it proportionate to the "heft" of the hat? Does it reach a proper level—eyebrow, nose, chin, or waist? If backswept, does the veil conform in shape to the crown and brim?

This hat is a revival, as revealed by several clues. It is fashioned from cellophane straw; the color combination is atypical, and the crown is designed to tilt forward, circa 1939. *Courtesy of: Banbury Cross Antiques.* Value: $95-145.

Two Edwardian toques, piquant in scale. Both have oversize hatbands—ecru lace for the black bombazine, watered silk for the claret velvet. *Courtesy of (both): Lisa Carson.* Value (each): $125-175.

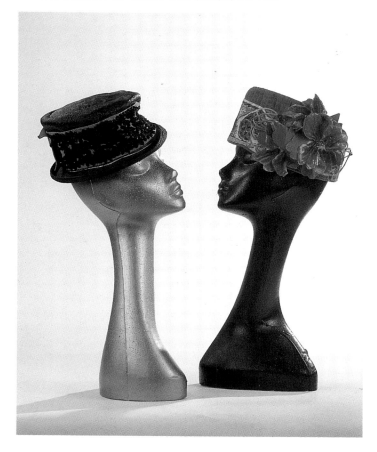

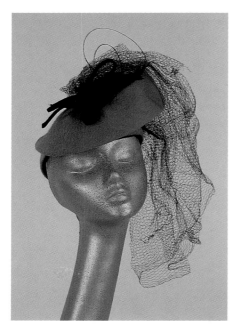

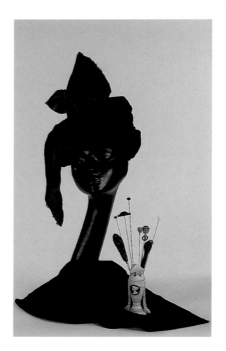

From Lilly Daché, a fabulous periwinkle felt with forward brim, circa 1945. Her signature asymmetry appears in the bold swoop of veiling. *Courtesy of: Barbara Griggs Vintage Fashion.* Value: $95-145.

Victorian and Edwardian hatpins were typically displayed on a dressing table in special holders. This one, in hand-painted porcelain, is marked Shafer and Vater. *Courtesy of: Banbury Cross Antiques.* Value (hatpins, each): $45-125. Value (holder): $250-300.

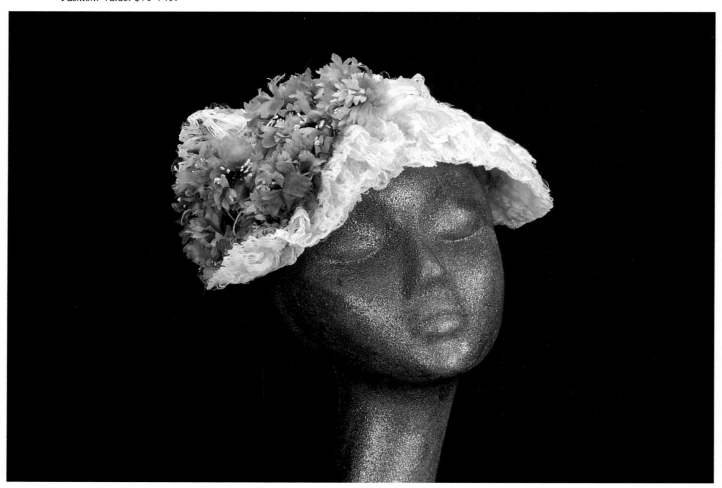

This hat is collectible by reason of its sweet shape and simple chic. It is hand-made in silk and horsehair, a classic rendering of violets in snow. Label: Juanita—Altman Bldg. *Courtesy of: Banbury Cross Antiques.* Value: $75-125.

Our discussion of valuation would be incomplete without reference to hatboxes and hatstands, and you will see that these are valued whenever they appear in photos. Other accoutrements are hatpins, plumes, and silk flowers. We recommend pricing hatpins in the books by experts, such as Lillian Baker.

Expect to pay $10 to $25 for a medium-size ostrich plume, more if it is beautifully curled or dyed. The largest plumes may be priced $25 to $50, as they are hard to find in good condition. Hand-made silk and velvet flowers will sell for $10-$25 apiece.

It should come as no surprise that exact pricing is next-to-impossible in this genre. In assigning values, we have deliberately used a range, or guideline. You should assume that all prices are based on hats in mint condition, unless otherwise indicated in the photo caption. Likewise, assume that the original trimming and veiling is intact.

Our primary source for valuation was vintage clothing stores and shows on the West Coast, especially Northern California. We believe there may be a greater emphasis on designer labels in this part of the country—perhaps a harbinger of the trend in this genre.

The High Cost of Hats

"The fashionable female hat is nothing, after all, but a caprice. Let those who pay for it—fifty dollars, more or less—grumble about the cost. We, as spectators, shall be satisfied if it prove an ornament."

Harper's Weekly, *1857.*

In their day, hats were one of the most costly of fashion accessories. It is well-documented that Josephine caused a minor scandal when she ordered thirty-eight new bonnets in one month. The feathers alone cost 1800 francs—a princely sum, even for Napoleon.

But no remarks are so charming, or informative, as a full-page article that appeared in *The Ladies Home Journal* of April 1917. In it, Marguerite Jacobs chronicles her visit to a millinery wholesaler. Her mission was to learn "Why Women Pay From $20 to $50 for Hats." Considering inflation, this would be the equivalent of $200 to $500 in today's dollars, all the

more remarkable since the article ran in a magazine marketed to the average American homemaker.

As an author, Ms. Jacobs displays a fine wit and keen powers of observation. The article offers insight into the construction, jargon, marketing and mark-up of the elegant hats worn during the teens. Particularly noteworthy is her commentary on the trade's efforts to revive the fashion for ostrich feathers, which dovetails with the origin of Fifth Avenue's Easter Parade.

Altogether, it is a captivating text, of interest to both fashion buff and historian. For that reason, we reprint the article virtually intact.

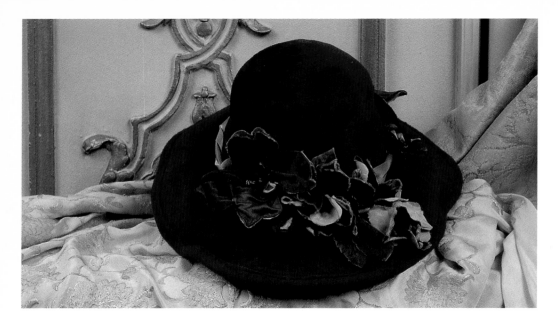

Oh, you yard of velvet and (in this case) a few pansies! A hat straight from Marguerite Jacobs' fashionable world of 1917. *Courtesy of: The Mad Hatter.* Value: $200-300.

Why Women Pay $20 to $50 For a Hat

"I sat at the dressing table in the French room at Madame Dunstan's. I had what almost any woman would acknowledge to be a "dream of a hat" poised on my head as only a dreamer of hats would poise it. The "dreamer"—Madame herself—looked over my shoulder into the mirror at my face. In her eyes was an expression of rapture for my beauty, or style, or piquancy—or something.

I looked more closely to find just what it was she did see—and then, in answer to my question, she lightly mentioned the price. My dream of a hat dissolved. I might put the milkman off for a week, but I couldn't murder him.

"But why should it cost so much?" I protested. "There is nothing on it but this rose—no, aster—with blue leaves."

"Both the flower and the velvet are imported," informed Madame. "Then the style—observe this high side effect."

I observed—all round. Oh, my sisters, you all know the feeling! It was my hat, perfect in line and color for me! "Is that the best you can do on it?" I asked.

"It is very closely marked," said Madame. "I could not afford to let it go for less."

Couldn't afford! Stuff and nonsense! The idea of charging a fairly prosperous man's weekly salary for a piece of velvet and a rose—I mean, aster. I left, and determined to turn my planned pleasure trip to New York into a quest. I would learn just how much too much, our milliners charge us!

I am sometimes very lucky. Several years before I had met a college friend's aunt who had opened a millinery shop in a basement. This aunt, a charming widow, was on my train, eastward bound to do her season's buying. I learned that she now had the leading shop of her city, a son in college, and expected to retire in another year. Oh, you yard of velvet and single aster!

Before many hours, I told her of my mission. She laughed, but gave me some startling information. In all legitimate milli-

nery firms, she said, practically the same method of pricing hats was followed: Twenty per cent of the cost would be added to cover the buyer's expense while in the market, and then that total would be doubled. She confessed it!

That was the general system; but often expensive hats had to be marked more closely, and cheap hats a little higher to strike a balance; therefore the real profit lay in the latter.

"But why charge us double what you pay?" I asked. She explained the cost of overhead, and slow seasons. Even with doubling, it required all a milliner's cleverness and care to meet competition and come out a little ahead.

"Meet me at ten o'clock Thursday morning and go buying with me," she suggested. That was splendid of her and would help me get at the heart of my hat problem.

"I have been buying for three days," said my friend when we met, "and am going to select some patterns this morning." Now, I knew that a pattern was a trimmed hat or "model." Although it was in advance of the season, my friend was already wearing one, with a smart silk dress and comfortable shoes.

The entrance to the big establishment we first went to was a long room, paneled in Circassian walnut, with settees of the same wood along the wall. It looked like the hall of a country manor, and the young man who came to greet my friend might have been our host. He chatted about everything except hats.

Upstairs, the country house vanished, however, and I could see through the glass doors of the elevator one vast floor devoted to bare hats—"flats" my friend called them Another floor to feathers, another to ribbons, and when we finally stepped off at our floor it was into an octagonal enclosure, paneled in gray, with an Oriental rug and gray settees.

Immediately a gray door popped open and a young man appeared. Without apology he asked my friend's name, place of residence, firm name and whether she had a choice as to saleswomen. I fully expected him to follow with "Age?" and "Married or single?"

But he was not the census man. He merely wanted to know that we were bona-fide buying milliners. Otherwise we should have been gently urged to take the elevator down. That was the purpose of this room. I stepped into its duplicate in all the uptown shops we afterward visited, where "models" were displayed. From its quiet, one never would have dreamed of the seething "show rooms" beyond. They burst upon me all unexpectedly as my friend opened another door.

Milliners from all over the country were gathered about hat-covered tables that seemed mile-long. Clerks and messengers rushed about. Above the giant hum of voices now and then there called from a graphophone arrangement in the wall a name, the owner of which straightway hurried to the telephone booth. And dominating the scene, distinctive in the crowd and turmoil, moving as if in a world apart, were the hat models or saleswoman.

Softly clad in satins and Georgette crepe, freshly powdered and tinted, hair coaxed into fluffy, wonderful effects, they glided through the throng, tried on hats, posing with that slow, luring turn of head and eyes we have seen in the "movies." Some of them, I was sure I had seen before; but no, it was their pictures in the fashion magazines, advertising the company's hats.

Now one of the fluffiest approached us, and her voice made me bubble with secret delight—it so matched her. Her a's were very broad indeed, her r's had long since been dispensed with, and her inflections were cooing velvet.

Again my friend was greeted as a guest and taken to the busy tables. And here I learned another name for hats. Here they were not hats or patterns or models, they were numbers— or, as the models have it, "numbahs."

"You must not miss this little numbah, Madame," she says, poising a foot-and-a-half circumferenced hat on her curls. They are so called because the milliner does not buy the pattern before, but an exact reproduction of it, ordered by its number.

There were dozens of stunning "numbahs" from four to ten dollars each in this room. We looked, tried on, bought, and changed our minds about them for hours, until they all began to look exactly alike to me. That, I learned, was one of the difficulties of buying—"buyer's fag," it is called. For while the buyer orders her untrimmed hats by the dozen, her models she selects always with an individual or type of individual in mind, and only as she can keep to this plan does she suit her trade.

Now my friend suggested that for a "rest" we go downtown and find a certain new, purple untrimmed hat, that sold for eighteen dollars a dozen and would be trimmed to sell for five dollars each. The uptown houses were sold out of them.

We took the Subway and went to Bond Street. The delight of contrasts! If a life history was necessary to get into the uptown houses, here the head of the firm stood in the doorway, decided you were a milliner, and beamed. If you looked uncertain he came out and asked if he could be of service. He would do anything to "get you for a customer, Madame."

He had no "poiple" hats, but he would have a shipment in the morning. He would lay some aside for your inspection, he would bring them to your hotel, he would give his watch or kill his child—I'm sure he would—anything to "get you for a customer, Madame." We went to one after another of these shops, but our "poiple" hat was not to be had.

Disappointed but dauntless, we stopped on our way uptown at a house which handled feathers exclusively. Again I exclaimed at the prices of the little feather hats and novelties for trimming, which were higher than I had expected.

While my friend was selecting some, the proprietor took me back where, at tables, hundreds of girls were gathered— sorting, bunching, cutting, evolving them. So many fingers, so many brains! I began to see the reason for their cost.

He showed me the dye rooms with the huge copper cal drons and the men in their color-stained aprons. He pointed to a jar of peroxide, tripled in price since the war. He explained the risk of a business of changing fashions, how the passing of the ostrich plume had nearly ruined many feather firms. One of these had spent fifty thousand dollars this season trying to revive them into favor; had paraded models all over fashionable New York, with ostrich parasols, hats, boas and purses.

It was now three o'clock, and we had not lunched. We did so hastily and returned to the scene of our model buying of the morning. Again our saleswoman, immaculate as we had left her, came to us. My friend said she wanted to be shown the higher-priced models. I, who had asked if any hat cost more than ten dollars wholesale, followed eagerly to the French rooms.

Here the lights were softened and the mirrors more cunningly placed—and the hats! Ten dollars up, they were, and the "up" seemed limitless. I learned that even higher prices prevailed in the world-famous pattern shops on Fifth Avenue.

At one of these a milliner had to contract to buy two hats before she was permitted to see any, the lowest priced one being thirty-five dollars. Once a milliner had protested that she couldn't tell if she'd like their designs until she had seen them.

"Our designs are correct, Madame; there can be no question as to your liking them," had come the calm response.

That shop, of course, was not for the small city milliner, even though she claimed a high-priced trade.

Just then our saleswoman brought us a model which consisted of a high drape of velvet in rich amethyst shades. I exclaimed over the severe beauty of it. It was twenty-three dollars and a half, wholesale.

"But why should it cost so much?" I asked, echoing a former moment.

"It is one of our newest and best designs, Madame."

"But is it not imported?"

The model gave me a hurt look, but saw my ignorance. The materials were imported, but big houses imported very few of their models now. New York claimed as fine designers as Paris, and each house took pride in having its own designs. There never had been as many hats imported as was supposed anyway.

Formerly milliners had sewed tags with French names in their hats. Probably owners of those names never existed, but it was part of the humbugging that Barnum said Americans loved. But now most firms used their own tags, and so advertised their own names.

As for this "numbah," it was by Veron, their own artist, and so highly paid that his models were necessarily high priced. Our saleswoman returned to her selling: "I want to see you have this numbah, Madame. What difference if you don't get your money out of it? It will give tone to your opening and be a hat for your trimmahs to copy again and again."

I sank on a chair. As my friend had said, it was complex, but I thought I had traced the price of the hat to its source. We paid our milliner for choosing hats for us to select from; she paid the wholesaler for manufacturing them.

And in back of the manufacturer stood the artist; he who watched the sky for new colors, the world's workshops for his materials, and with his finger on the pulse of the moment bent the creative gift within him for the winning of feminine fancy. He it was who chose the shapes, colors, textures, weaves, trimmings used all up and down the world; copied in the French rooms, the twenty-five-cent stores and the country kitchens.

And then the wheel turned back to us. So long as we women bought our hats as artistic expressions of ourselves rather than as utilitarian protections, we would have to be content to have their material value figure as a by-product of their price. We were responsible for the vast, complicated industry built up to the artist in back of it.

If ever a time came when women adopted a comparatively uniform headgear, we would be able to order by size, wholesale, and save the milliner's profits. But my friends and I would much prefer to continue supplying the Easter magazines with their comedy. At least, now we know why we spend from twenty to fifty dollars, according to our several purses—for a tiny satin head covering or a flat of felt or straw. We continue to buy, but perhaps with truer judgment!

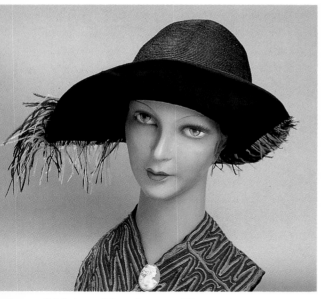

Celebrity models in the teens? This mannequin seems about to ask if Madame would like to see a special "numbah." *Courtesy of: Banbury Cross Antiques.* Value: $75-125.

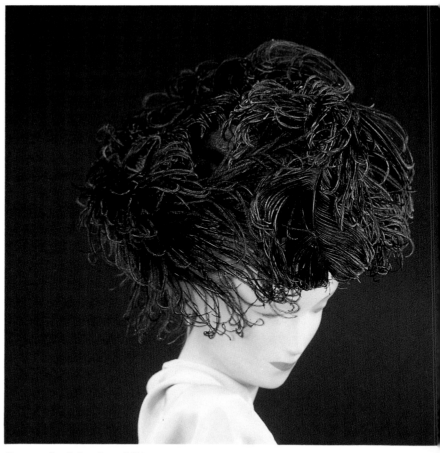

Smart and stylish, a "poiple" hat trimmed with costly ostrich plumes that had been curled and dyed-to-match. Ms. Jacobs recounts that this type of trim was outmoded by 1917, much to the chagrin of the feather merchants! *Courtesy of: Mary Aaron Museum.* Value: Special.

Aigrette A stiff tuft of rather tall feathers, originally those of the egret, used as an ornament.
Aureole French for halo; a hat with large, half-moon brim swept up from the back crown, so as to halo the face; a.k.a. halo hat.

Ballon French for balloon; used to describe a hat of that shape.
Balibuntl A very fine weave of straw used in hats, and to describe a hat of that material.
Bandeau A band worn around the forehead à la the dancer Irene Castle (1920s); a type of half-hat (1950s).
Batting Densely-packed wool cotton or straw, used to interline large, stiff hats (e.g., helmet).
Bavolet A drape of material attached to the back of a bonnet to shade the neck.
Beret A round, soft brimless hat; associated with artists.

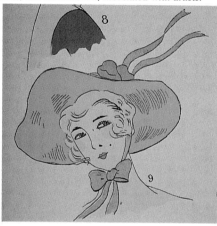

Bergere French for Shepherdess; used to describe a flat straw hat trimmed simply with ribbons and flowers.

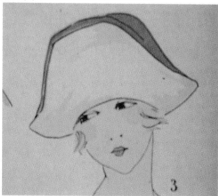

Bicorne A hat with brim turned up in back and front, sometimes secured by a cockade (à la Napoleon).
Block To shape a felt or straw hat with steam (verb); the wooden form on which the hat is shaped (noun).
Boater A hat with flattened crown and small brim, usually in straw with ribbon hatband; a.k.a. "sailor."
Bobbin Lace Lace formed in loopy patterns on a bobbin, from thread or raffia; may be machine-made or hand-made.
Bonnet A close-fitting crown that covers the back of the head, and a peaked crown; secured by streamers tied under the chin.
Bowler A domed crown and narrow rolled brim, usually in stiffened felt; a style of riding hat; a.k.a. derby.
Breton Like the boater, but with a larger upturned brim (both styles were originally worn by French sailors).

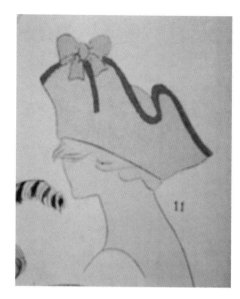

Brim Part of a hat, below the crown.
Brocade A patterned textile; usually a rich, figured silk; often the pattern is emphasized in two tones.
Bucket A hat with stiff, sloping brim and no crown; like an upside-down bucket; a.k.a. lampshade.
Buckram A stiff, woven fabric used to interline the brim or to shape an entire hat.

Calash French for hood; a bonnet with oversize brim that is stretched over a series of hoops so it may collapse, accordian-style.
Cap A close-fitting brimless hat; it may have a visor.
Capote A little hat with shallow brim, usually oval in shape.
Cartwheel A type of picture hat, with exaggerated brim and low crown.

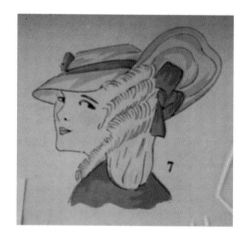

Cavalier A broad-brimmed hat, one side of which is upturned and pinned by a cockade; usually plumed.
Cellophane A man-made, transparent straw (acetate base).
Chechia An allover fur toque, little cousin of the Cossack.
Chiffon A lightweight, diaphanous, plain-weave fabric.
Chou French for cabbage; used to describe any round and puffy ornament, or style of hat.
Cloche French for bell; a close-fitting, brimless hat in that shape, very popular in the 1920s.
Cockade A round ornament, like a button with fluted ribbon edging.

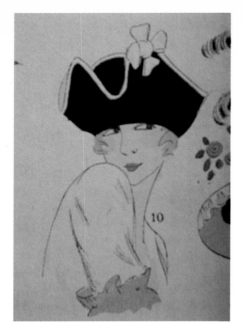

Cocked At an angle (tilted down, or turned up).

Cocktail Hat The dressy and dramatic type of hat worn to cocktail parties.

Comb Used as a hair ornament, or sewn into the hatband to hold a hat in place.

Coolie Like the Chinese field hat, a shallow cone-shaped brim with no crown; usually in straw; a.k.a. pagoda.

Coptain A type of Cavalier, with exaggerated plumes.

Cording A cord of any diameter, covered with bias-cut fabric, used to tie a bonnet, finish a brim, or as a general sort of trim.

Cossack A tall, brimless fur hat worn by the Russian cavalry.

Crown The top part of a hat, covering the crown of the head.

Doll Hat A diminutive hat, usually tilted forward.

Dormeuse An oversized soft cap, with ruffled crown; see mobcap.

Derby A style named for the Earl of Derby; see bowler.

Esparta An early type of interlining; see buckram.

Eyelet Lightweight cotton with small, thread-bound holes forming a lacy design.

Fedora An oval-shaped hat with medium brim; the crown is creased front-to-back and pinched at the sides; usually in felt.

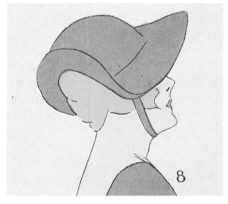

Felt A material formed from interlocking the fibers of wool or fur; may be smooth or napped, and is often dyed.

Fez A tall, brimless hat with small flat crown; usually in felt and often tasseled; associated with Arabia.

Gainsborough A low-crowned hat with broad brim, worn slightly raised off the head; trimmed with plumes.

Grosgrain A matte-finish, ribbed ribbon.

Halo Hat A halo-brimmed hat popular in the 1930s; see aureole.

Hatband A band or ribbon used to trim the juncture of crown and brim; often merely decorative.

Hatpin A long pin used to secure a hat as stabbed into a bun, pompadour or other "ratted" hairdo; usually with ornamental tip.

Headband A cloth band worn at the crown of the head over a hairdo; a horseshoe-shaped clip used to secure a half-hat.

Helmet A military style similar to the bicorne or bucket; popular in the Directoire and Edwardian eras .

Hennin A towering, cone-shaped headdress affected by ladies in the Middle Ages.

Homburg A man's stiff felt hat with narrow rolled brim and creased crown; similar to the fedora.

Hood A fabric headdress, draped over the head and about the shoulders; may be worn under a hat.

Horsehair Hair from the mane and tail of a horse, in an openwork weave, used for hats and stiff ribbons; a.k.a. "crin."

Jacquard A cutwork pattern used to finish textiles.

Jersey A type of plain, knit fabric with a soft drape; often made from wool.

Juliet Cap A petite skullcap, often edged with pearls.

Kerchief From the french "couvre chef," a fabric scarf or shawl used to cover the head.

Knife-Edge Denotes the edge of crisply-pleated fabric.

Lace A method of forming thread, raffia, horsehair, or other material into an open-weave design; a net fabric or ribbon.

Lampshade A style of hat made popular by Dior in the 1950s, shaped like a lampshade; see bucket.

Leghorn A finely-ridged straw from Livorno, Italy; a wide-brimmed hat with high crown, made from the straw.

Linen A type of fabric with a tight weave and flat finish.

Liripipe One of the earliest hats, a cloth cap that ends in a flattened cone draped to the side.

Mantilla Spanish for mantle; a long shawl in lace, draped from a high comb over the head and shoulders.

Matador A Spanish bullfighter's cap; like a small bicorne.

Mobcap A large, puffy fabric cap popular in the late 1700s; see dormeuse.

Nap The finish of a fabric or felt (i.e., high or low).

Net Silk or other thread, woven to form a veil.

Nightcap Small, close-fitting cap worn at home by men and women to keep the head warm at night.

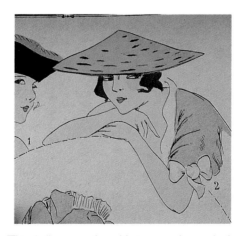

Pagoda This shallow cone-shaped hat was made popular by Dior in the 1950s; if small, a pagodine; see coolie hat.

Paillettes French for sequins; flat, rather large spangles used to trim a veil.

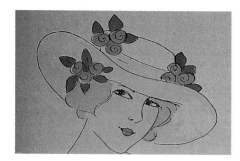

Pamela A shallow-crowned hat with a slightly-curved brim that slopes down in front and back; often in straw.

Panama A type of very fine straw, woven from the fiber of an South American plant; a straw fedora.

Pancake A wide-brimmed hat with almost no crown, shaped like a pancake; see platter.

Phrygian Bonnet One of the earliest hats, in soft fabric with a self-flap draped to one side like the liripipe; a symbol of freedom.

Picture Hat A hat with shallow crown and a large brim that frames the face, like a picture.

Pile The depth of a fabric or felt nap (i.e., deep pile).

Pillbox A type of hat, shaped like a pill and worn low on the crown of the head; very popular in the 1950s

Platter A version of the picture hat with a stiff brim and low crown; see pancake.

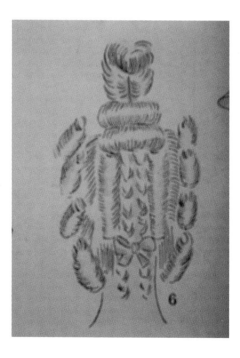

Plume A long, arching feather used to trim a hat.

Pom-Pom Ball of chenille or yarn used as trim—if small, may decorate a veil.

Porkpie A man's soft hat with snap brim, creased around a flat crown; a brimless cap popular for women in the 1860s.

Poke Bonnet A bonnet with very deep brim, projecting like a visor for sunshade.

Raffia A fibrous straw, woven from the raffia palm of Madagascar.

Rhinestone A glass jewel, often simulating a diamond.

Rosette Ribbon that is formed into a rose, as an ornament.

Ruching Ribbon or other fabric that is pleated and tucked into a ruffle.

Satin A finish that is smooth and lustrous; any fabric with that finish.

Sequins Small, lustrous acetate disks of any color, used as trim; may be sewn together in a motif, or sprinkled on a veil.

Silk A type of fabric, lightweight and supple, formed from the cocoon of a Chinese silkworm.

Shako A fur hat, shaped like a Cossack.

Snood A woven or crocheted net, worn to cover or contain the hair.

Smoking Cap A type of pillbox worn by men to protect their hair from the odor of cigar smoke; often highly embellished.

Strass Lead glass used to make an artificial jewel.

Straw The non-edible and fibrous part of a grain plant; any material woven from straw; any woven or plaited fibrous material.

Top Hat A man's tall-crowned hat in silk or brushed beaver cloth, with a slightly rolled and narrow brim.

Toque Any small, close-fitting brimless hat with a stiff crown.

Tricorne A hat with brim turned up, to form three corners.

Turban A hat formed by strips of fabric wrapped around the head, of Turkish origin; any hat with beehive-shaped crown and no brim, usually with the appearance of wrapped fabric.

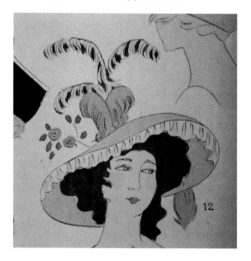

Tyrolean A type of fedora, but with slightly peaked crown; styled after an Alpine hunting hat; often in felt, with a tuft for trim.

Tulle A fine, machine-made net with a hexagonal mesh.

Veil Netting used to cover all or part of the head or face, as draped from a hat; the weave may be fine or coarse, intricate or plain.

Velour French for velvet; any extra-plush velvet.

Velvet A type of fabric with a thick pile that may be sheared, plush, or cut (a.k.a. jacquard); usually of wool, cotton, or silk.

Wimple A scarf, usually linen, coifed over the head and folded under the chin; worn by women in the Middle Ages.

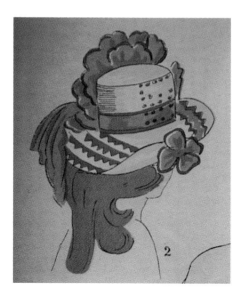

Selected Bibliography

Baker, Lillian. *Hatpins & Hatpin Holders*. Collector Books, 1992.

Ball, Joanna Dubbs, and Dorothy Hehl Torem. *The Art of Fashion Accessories*. Schiffer Publishing, Ltd., 1993.

Battersby, Martin. *The Decorative Twenties*. Walker & Co., 1969.

Bawden, Juliet. *The Hat Book: Creating Hats for Every Occasion*. Lark Books, 1992.

Bell, Jeannene. *Old Jewelry*. Books Americana, Inc., 1992.

Blum, Stella. *Everyday Fashions of the Twenties*. Dover Publications, Inc., 1986.

_____. *Everyday Fashions of the Thirties*. Dover Publications, Inc., 1986.

Campione, Adele. *Women's Hats*. Chronicle Books, S.F., 1994.

Clark, Fiona. *Hats*. London, B.T. Batsford, Ltd., 1982.

Dolan, Maryanne. *Vintage Clothing*. Books Americana, 1995.

Ettinger, Roseann. *50s Popular Fashions for Men, Women, Boys & Girls*. Schiffer Publishing Ltd., 1995.

Ginsburg, Madeleine. *The Hat: Trends & Traditions*. London, Studio Editions, 1990.

_____. *Paris Fashions—Art Deco Style*. London, Bracken Books, 1989.

Harris, Kristina. *Victorian & Edwardian Fashions for Women*. Schiffer Publishing Ltd., 1995.

Horsley, Edith. *The 1950s*. The Mallard Press, 1990.

Howell, Georgina. *In Vogue*. Penguin Books, 1978.

Madsen, Axel. *Chanel*. New York, Henry Holt & Co., Inc., 1990.

McCormick, Terry. *The Consumer's Guide to Vintage Clothing*. New York, Dembner Books, 1987.

McDowell, Colin. *Hats*. New York, Rizzoli Publishing, Inc., 1992.

_____. *McDowell's Directory of 20th Century Fashion*. New York, Rizzoli Publishing, Inc., 1994.

Millbank, Caroline Rennolds. *New York Fashion*. 1995.

de Pietri, Stephen, and Melissa Leventon. *New Look to Now: French Haute Couture, 1947-1987*. Rizzoli Publishing, Inc., revised 1996.

Probert, Christina. *Hats In Vogue*. Abbeyville Press, 1981.

Shep, R.L. *Edwardian Hats: The Art of Millinery by Mme. Anna Ben-Yusuf (1909)*. Medocino, 1992.

Smith, Desire. *Hats: with Values*. Schiffer Publishing, Ltd., 1996.

Smith, Pamela. *Vintage Fashion & Fabrics*. Alliance Publishers, 1995.

Southern, Anne. *Millinery*. Arco, 1962.

Victoria editors. *The Romance of Hats*. Hearst Books, N.Y., 1994.

Wilcox, R. Turner. *The Mode in Costume*. Charles Scribners' Sons, 1958.

_____. *The Mode in Hats and Headdress*. Charles Scribners' Sons, 1959.

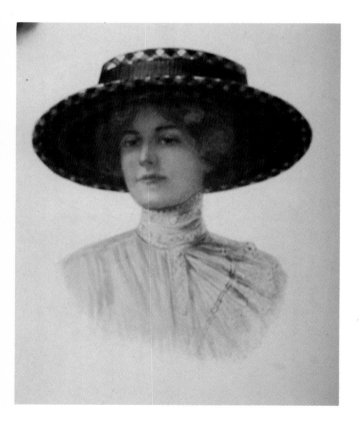

* Please note that we have listed at least a few hat styles for each of the major designers, and many of the hat styles, although this index does not exhaust every style\label pictured in the book.

It is said, if a milliner
leaves a pin in her hat, then
it will return to her.

And so, we end this book.

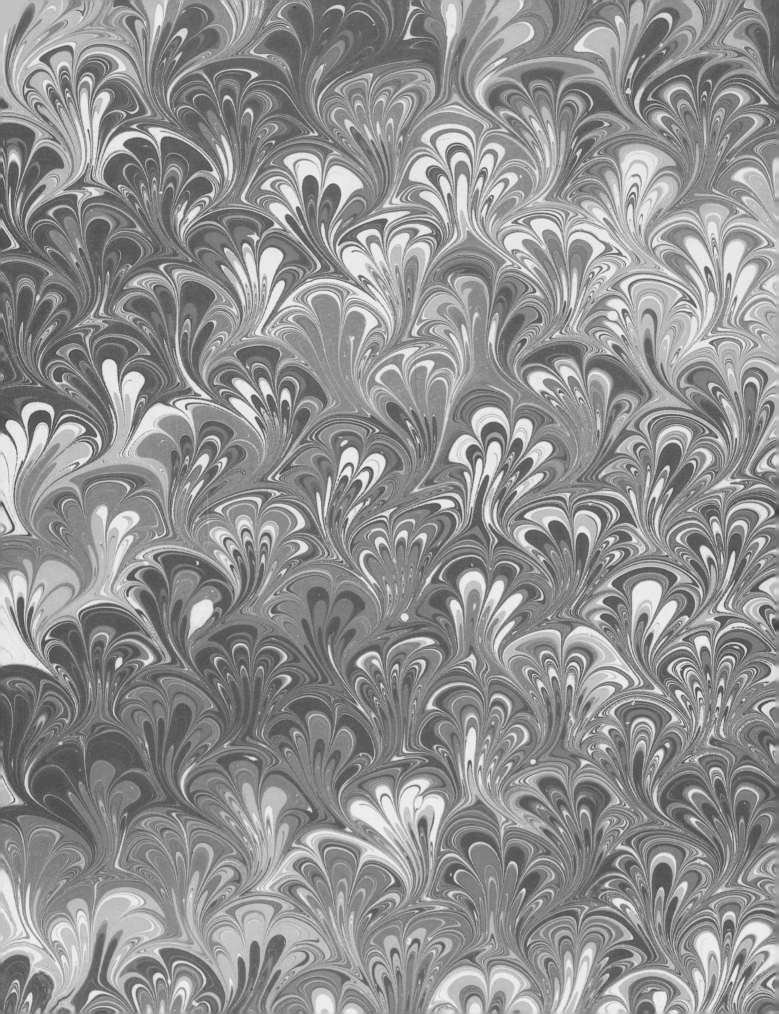